Improving Prognosis for Kidney Disorders

Improving Prognosis for Kidney Disorders

Edited by

Morrell Michael Avram
Long Island College Hospital, Brooklyn, New York, U.S.A.

SPRINGER-SCIENCE+BUSINESS MEDIA, B.V.

A C.I.P. Catalogue record for this book is available from the Library of Congress.

ISBN 978-90-481-6164-5 ISBN 978-94-017-1848-6 (eBook)
DOI 10.1007/978-94-017-1848-6

Printed on acid-free paper

Table of Contents

List of Principal Authors

Morrell Michael Avram
Long Island College Hospital
Brooklyn, New York
U.S.A.

Alessandra Boletta
Johns Hopkins University School of Medicine
Baltimore, Maryland
U.S.A.

Barry M. Brenner
Renal Division
Department of Medicine
Brigham and Women's Hospital
Harvard Medical School
Boston, Massachusetts
U.S.A.

Clinton D. Brown
State University of New York
Brooklyn, New York
U.S.A.

Ognjenka Djurdjev
University of British Columbia
British Columbia
Canada

Eli A. Friedman
State University of New York
Brooklyn, New York
U.S.A.

Gregory G. Germino
Johns Hopkins University School of Medicine
Baltimore, Maryland
U.S.A.

Esther A. González
Saint Louis University School of Medicine
St. Louis, Missouri
U.S.A.

Peter Hovind
Steno Diabetes Center
Gentofte
Denmark

George A. Kaysen
University of California Davis
Davis, California
U.S.A.

William F. Keane
University of Minnesota
Minneapolis, Minnesota
U.S.A.

Joel D. Kopple
Harbor-UCLA Medical Center
Torrance, California
U.S.A.

Gozewijn D. Laverman
University of Groningen
Groningen
The Netherlands

Adeera Levin
University of British Columbia
British Columbia
Canada

Nathan W Levin.
Renal Research Institute
and Beth Israel Medical Center
New York, New York
U.S.A.

Kevin J. Martin
Saint Louis University School of Medicine
St. Louis, Missouri
U.S.A.

William E. Mitch
Emory University School of Medicine
Atlanta, Georgia
U.S.A.

Neal Mittman
Long Island College Hospital
Brooklyn, New York
U.S.A.

Allen R Nissenson
School of Medicine
University of California at Los Angeles
Los Angeles, California
U.S.A.

Hans-Henrik Parving
Steno Diabetes Center
Gentofte
Denmark

S. Russ Price
Emory University School of Medicine
Atlanta, Georgia
U.S.A.

Margaret Spittle
Renal Research Institute
and Beth Israel Medical Center
New York, New York
U.S.A.

Maarten W. Taal
Renal Unit
Nottingham City Hospital
Nottingham
U.K.

Eric M Tong
School of Medicine
University of California at Los Angeles
Los Angeles, California
U.S.A.

Dick de Zeeuw
University of Groningen
Groningen
The Netherlands

Dedication

This volume derives from a career-long interest in understanding why patients with renal diseases develop clinical illness and how to treat it. As a teacher and clinical researcher, I have had the opportunity of learning from fellows, junior faculty and medical students. Few fields of medicine have evolved so rapidly as nephrology in which uremia changed from a universally fatal disease to a manageable and treatable morbid condition. It is this treatment necessity which now attracts my full-time energies. Because I believe that hypertension, anemia, nutrition and lipids contribute to sickness in my patients, both an investigative interest and the current book resulted.

My own career parallels, since 1960, the expansion and, indeed, explosion of informative generation and exchange in nephrology. I anticipate that the twenty first century, which we have entered, will witness a further experimental growth of our knowledge to detect and treat renal disorders by altering the immune response, better understanding of nutrition, diabetes, use of bionic devices and by prevention of genetic and acquired renal diseases, cytokine and biotechnology application.

It is toward this purpose that this conference, held at the Avram Conference Center, Long Island College Hospital, in which I spend the majority of my waking hours, was poised to inaugurate the third millennium.

I want to profoundly thank the authors who have contributed to this book, all longstanding, admired friends and colleagues. Loving thanks to my wife, Maria, and my children, Rella, Marc, Eric, Mathew and David, and their families for putting up with the rigors and excrescences of a medical practice, academia, and clinical research and for carrying the torch. I want to reaffirm my love for Brooklyn Heights and the City of New York for providing an exciting and productive lifetime medical home.

We all want to thank the National Kidney Foundation for releasing the copyright to this data in order for us to make this publication possible.

Morrell Michael Avram, MD, FACP
Brooklyn, New York
May, 2002

Introduction
Resumative Synthesis of Contents: It Is Time for Renoprotection

Over the final forty years of the twentieth century, irreversible kidney failure was gradually transformed from a hopeless, inexorably fatal disorder to a readily manageable entity for which treatment afforded life extension reaching, thirty-five years or longer, such as my patient, Mrs. Essie Rinehart. Several other Brooklyn dialysis patients are now well into their fourth decade after suffering total loss of renal function. Lessons learned that favor such enhanced survival include the critical importance of attenuating hypertension, metabolic bone disease, anemia, and, in diabetic patients, striving for euglycemia. Once life prolongation in end-stage renal failure (ESRD) became routine, study of comorbid extrarenal disorders in patients sustained by dialysis in the mid-1980s recognized the risk of coronary and other vascular disease imparted by dyslipidemia, stimulating a quest for strategies to normalize plasma lipids while maximizing nutrition despite persistent, partially corrected uremia. Next (current) in the evolution of odern nephrology was a concern over providing comprehensive renal care, identifying factors that promote renal injury and opening the potential for preventing their action thereby reducing kidney damage, a process termed renoprotection. This was extensively addressed at the Avram Center for Kidney Diseases, and manuscripts emanating from our world conference are presented herein. A resume of this work follows.

A growing and impressive body of evidence supports the thesis that proteinuria, irrespective of etiology, induces progression of kidney disease. It follows that reduction of the quantity of proteinuria will slow loss of kidney function. Toward that objective, inhibition of angiotensin-converting enzyme to preempt release of injurious kinins with reduction in proteinuria is a widely practiced treatment strategy made possible by a score of newly introduced drugs.

Having participated in uremia therapy since its inception, I marvel at the extent of changes in optimized treatment protocols that distinguishes productivity at the opening of the 21st Century from our relatively dark-aged past. With death in uremia reduced by dialysis and kidney transplantation, renal researchers seek means to retard progressive kidney damage. Comprehensive guidelines prepared by expert committees initially focused on malnutrition and hypertension as significant variables linked to reduced survival in dialyzed patients and is reviewed in several manuscripts that follow.

To collect and disseminate consensus thinking on renoprotection in general and perturbed nutrition and lipid metabolism in specific, international experts convened for the latest of a series of conferences devoted to enhancing renal care, periodically conducted at the Avram Center for Kidney Diseases at the Long Island College Hospital. This volume, a product of such a workshop conference and meetings, contains original investigations, reviews, and perspectives that, in total, comprise a manual for maximizing survival in kidney failure as well as delaying and /or preventing renal injury caused by several mechanisms.

Barry M. Brenner, a pioneer in the new field of renoprotective intervention in progressive renal disease, with Maarten W. Taal, brings rationality to a diverse literature by devising an action plan for utilizing interventions available today including: angiotensin-converting enzyme therapy, control of systemic hypertension, dietary protein restriction, reduction of proteinuria, treatment of hyperlipidemia and smoking cessation. Extending their perspective to probable future therapies, Taal and Brenner describe the potential of vasopeptidase inhibitors, a new class of drugs that simultaneously inhibit both angiotensin-converting enzyme and neutral endopeptidase. Endopeptidase, an ecto-enzyme in the brush border membrane of renal tubule cells, catabolizes natriuretic peptides, adrenomedullin and bradykinin. Vasopeptidase inhibition reduces hypertension in both low and high renin states. Omapatrilat, a vasopeptidase blocker, reduced blood pressure and delayed progression of renal disease in rodents to a greater extent than an angiotensin-converting enzyme inhibitor, affording the hope of its clinical application. Taal and Brenner also speculate that drugs like mycophenolate mofetil that blunt upregulation of cytokines, cell adhesion molecules and profibrotic growth factors may afford complementary renoprotection.

To Taal and Brenner's list, Allen R Nissenson and Eric M Tong would add the adverse consequences of the anemia of uremia. Noting that few studies have assessed the relationship between the level of anemia and hospitalizations in erythropoietin-treated patients, a case-controlled study found fewer hospitalizations and decreased length of stay compared with a matched group of patients who did not receive erythropoietin. Patients with hematocrit levels less than 30% had a 14-30% increased risk of hospitalization while those with hematocrit levels in the 33-36% range had the lowest risk of hospitalization. Evaluating darbepoetin alfa, termed by Nissenson and Tong: "a milestone in nephrology in the past 20 years," administered once-weekly in treating the anemia associated with chronic azotemia as effective as recombinant erythropoietin, simplifying anemia management.

The terrible toll of cardiovascular disease as the endpoint of unchecked hyperlipidemia becomes clear in Adeera Levin's careful analysis of 313 individuals of mean age of 56 years with a mean creatinine clearance of 36 ml/min in whom cardiovascular disease was present in 46%. In this cohort followed for a median of 23 months, either worsening of recognized cardiovascular disease or new cardiac events were noted in 20%. Predictors of new cardiovascular events were diabetes, advancing age, and high triglycerides. By documenting the high prevalence of cardiovascular disease in those with reduced renal function, Dr. Levin sets the stage for clinical trials of hypolipidemic drugs as a means of lowering the risk of cardiac complications. In a similar theme, William F. Keane agrees that even a modest decrease in estimated creatinine clearance to approximately 60 ml/min is associated with increased cardiovascular risk. Inhibiting angiotensin-converting enzyme will not delay or stabilize progression of renal disease but will reduce the incidence of stroke and myocardial infarction in these high-risk individuals. Keane believes that along with dietary modification and control of serum lipids, angiotensin-converting enzyme inhibition should be components of renal care regimens. Oxidative stress has emerged as an important cofactor for the development of endothelial dysfunction and atherogenesis. Nathan Levin et al. explores the relationship between oxidative stress and inflammation and examines their role in dialysis-related pathology. They demonstrated higher levels of oxidant stress markers, such as F 2 isoprostanes and ethane, in dialysis patients compared with control subjects. Their studies show that hemodialysis patients are exposed to both oxidative stress and inflammation, which add significantly to their morbidity and mortality risk. Levin et al demonstrate elevated levels of C-reactive protein (CRP) in dialysis patients, as well as a negative correlation of CRP quartiles with albumin, hematocrit, and creatinine levels, and a positive correlation with age, ferritin, hospitalization, rehospitalization, and death. High CRP levels have an additive effect with other known factors for mortality risk.

Morrell M. Avram et al., reexamining their finding that parathyroid hormone (PTH) levels can serve as uremic toxins, determined the correlation between enrollment serum intact PTH with mortality in 345 hemodialysis and 277 peritoneal dialysis patients monitored up to 14 years. An enrollment PTH was an independent predictor of survival for both dialysis modalities. Surprisingly, lower than expected levels of PTH in dialysis patients predict decreased survival. To explain this finding, Avram et al. hypothesize that inadequate protein and/or phosphorus intake impairs development of secondary hyperparathyroidism adding to the recognized excess mortality of malnutrition.

Neal Mittman et al., continuing the Avram group's incisive inquiry at elucidation of the significance of prealbumin as a marker of renal functional loss, prospectively assessed the relationship of enrolment prealbumin levels, as well as demographic characteristics and other biochemical markers, to all cause mortality in 130 hemodialysis and 128 peritoneal dialysis patients observed up to 10 years. Once again, enrollment prealbumin emerged as a strong independent predictor of long-term survival after adjusting for age, race, gender, and months on dialysis, diabetic status, and other nutritional markers in hemodialysis patients. Greater survival correlated with a prealbumin greater than 30 mg/dL and was the best single biochemical predictor of mortality irrespective of dialysis modality.

With the antiproteinuric response to antihypertensive treatment as the main predictor of renoprotective efficacy in long-term renal disease, establishing the optimal drug dose of angiotensin-converting enzyme inhibitors has not been judged as a correlate of maximal antiproteinuric effect. G. D. Laverman and Dick De Zeeuw et al. report an open-label, dose-response study using losartan in ten non-diabetic patients with proteinuria (5.8 ± 0.8 g/day) and a mean arterial pressure of 103 ± 3.7 mmHg. Consecutive doses of 50, 100 and 150 mg of losartan had a similar antihypertensive response, but optimal antiproteinuric response was reached at 100 mg losartan. That reduction of proteinuria peaked at 100 mg/day affords cost saving advice in dosage of an expensive drug.

For over a decade, it has been known that serum albumin level is a correlate of survival during maintenance hemodialysis and peritoneal dialysis. Exploring the basis of hypoalbuminemia, George A. Kaysen stresses that the first step in understanding is identification of pathogenesis of a reduced albumin concentration thus permitting directing therapy to correct the discovered cause. Inflammation, infection, and /or sources of albumin loss must be identified and, where possible, reversed. Manipulation of the angiotensin II system is an effective means of reducing urinary albumin leakage. Dietary protein supplementation may correct hypoalbuminemia providing that the protein catabolic rate is below 1g/kg/day. By contrast, intravenous albumin infusions are expensive and unlikely to improve outcome. Simply put, Kaysen advises: "Treat the cause of hypoalbuminemia not the albumin level."

William E. Mitch and S. Russ Price underscore metabolic acidosis as an important factor causing degradation of essential amino acids and protein in muscles in multiple steps mediated by enzymes that conjugate ubiquitin to a substrate protein. Ubiquitin, a small protein present in all cells, is a heat shock protein. Ubiquitin conjugation is initiated by an E1 enzyme that activates ubiquitin by an ATP-requiring reaction. Activated ubiquitin is then transferred to an E2 enzyme forming an ubiquitin-E2 intermediate complex with substrate specificity, because an E3 enzyme recognizes substitute as defective or abnormal proteins that should be degraded. The result of these reactions is conjugation of ubiquitin to the substrate protein. Protein degradation in the ubiquitin-proteasome system contributes to loss of muscle mass in kidney disease. Metabolic acidosis activates the system in muscle by a process that requires glucocorticoids. Inflammatory cytokines suppress the system, but glucocorticoids block the effect of cytokines to slow protein breakdown in the system. Thus how muscle mass is maintained is poorly understood but a critical factor is the stimulation of muscle protein degradation by the ubiquitin-proteasome system. Until much more is learned about this system, therapeutic methods to slow loss of muscle protein should avoid interfering with ubiquitin-proteasome or must be specific in blocking degradation of selected proteins.

Searching for a predictor of progression in diabetic nephropathy, Peter Hovind and Hans-Henrik Parving et al. call attention to increases in plasma total homocysteine with both rises in urinary albumin excretion in diabetes and plasminogen activator inhibitor-1 in increased matrix accumulation in glomerulopathies. There was a borderline significant relation between decline in GFR and total homocysteine as well as plasminogen activator inhibitor-1, though after adjustment for other established progression promoters, these markers were not independent predictors of progression.

Seemingly tangential to the main theme of renoprotection, Clinton D. Brown and Eli A. Friedman et al. explored the impact of excess advanced glycosylated endproducts (AGEs) in diabetic pre-endstage and hemodialysis patients by preventing AGE synthesis with aminoguanidine. Employing erythrocyte deformability, measured as surrogate for AGE damage, Brown et al. found that both erythropoietin and aminoguanidine corrected erythrocyte stiffness to normal after 12 months. The authors hypothesize that while erythropoietin may have reduced erythrocyte stiffness and influx of new and younger red cells, aminoguanidine protected erythrocyte integrity by blocking AGE formation.

Ultimately, renal disease may be prevented completely by identification and modification or elimination of an enabling gene. Autosomal polycystic kidney disease accounts for about 8% of kidney failure in the United States, afflicting all races and both genders equally. Alessandra Boletta and Gregory G. Germino et al. studied the most common form of autosomal dominant polycystic kidney disease resulting from mutation of the PKD1 gene on chromosome 16p13.3 resulting in the gene product, polycystin-1, that has a large extracellular portion postulated to be a plasma membrane receptor involved in cell-cell/matrix interaction. Biochemical characterization of recombinant polycystin-1 showed the protein is a 520kDa glycosylated polypeptide with an unglycosylated core of 460kDa. This initial characterization of polycystin-1 is an exciting first step and may ultimately lead to a genetic probe and corrective gene insertion before this decade ends.

After reflection on the extensive information imparted by conference participants, what is the clinician, eager to initiate renoprotection, to take home as "marching orders"? Joel D. Kopple emphasizes that the first concern is the prevention or treatment of hypertension. In those patients with advanced hypertension, dietary management alone will be insufficient; and drug therapy will be required. Nevertheless, appropriate dietary management may prevent onset of hypertension, may correct mild hypertension, and can be a useful adjunct to pharmacological therapy for the treatment of established hypertension. In obese individuals or those with a high NaCl intake, a reasonable approach is to start pharmacological anti-hypertensive therapy concomitantly with dietary management. Exercise training, after a careful medical evaluation, should be encouraged. To Kopple's prescription, I would add that incorporation of euglycemic strategies in diabetics, administration of vitamin D and erythropoietin, and avoidance of nephrotoxic drugs are reasonable measures to retard formerly inevitable but now sometimes preventable uremia. Bone disease is highly prevalent in patients with chronic renal failure resulting in high morbidity. Kevin Martin et al., in their article "How to Minimize Bone Disease in Renal Failure," discuss recent developments in the understanding of the pathogenesis of bone disease in renal failure patients, appropriate therapies, and the importance of controlling hyperparathyroidism. There is reason for optimism and a sense that nephrology is about to enter a wonderful era in which the formerly unavoidable path to uremia is commandeered by practitioners of effective intervention - renoprotection - delaying or bypassing the specter of chronic kidney failure.

Morrell Michael Avram, MD, FACP
Professor of Medicine
Long Island College Hospital, Brooklyn, New York

1 How to Achieve Maximal Renoprotection in Non-Diabetic Chronic Renal Disease

MAARTEN W. TAAL, MB.CHB. AND BARRY M. BRENNER, M.D.

Abstract

A rapid, global increase in the number of patients requiring renal replacement therapy necessitates that effective strategies for renoprotection are developed and widely applied. In this paper we review the experimental and clinical evidence in support of individual renoprotective interventions, including angiotensin-converting enzyme therapy, control of systemic hypertension, dietary protein restriction, reduction of proteinuria, treatment of hyperlipidemia and smoking cessation. We also consider potential future renoprotective therapies. Finally we suggest that, in order to achieve maximal renoprotection, a comprehensive strategy employing all of these elements is required and should be directed at normalizing clinical markers of renal disease in order to induce a state of "remission".

Introduction

Despite the dramatic progress in medical science over the past 50 years, there remain few effective treatments for specific renal diseases; and consequently, the population of patients requiring renal replacement therapy continues to grow rapidly worldwide. In an attempt to address this problem, attention has focused on the mechanisms whereby chronic renal disease (CRD) progresses to end-stage renal failure (ESRF). It has been appreciated for several decades that renal diseases of diverse etiology that result in substantial loss of functioning nephrons provoke a common syndrome characterized by systemic hypertension, proteinuria and a progressive decline in glomerular filtration rate (GFR), the rate of which depends more upon individual patient characteristics than specific disease etiology.[1,2] These observations suggested that CRD progresses via a common pathway of mechanisms and that therapeutic interventions inhibiting this common pathway may be successful in slowing the rate of progression of CRD irrespective of the initiating cause. In this article, we review experimental and clinical evidence in support of this hypothesis and discuss a comprehensive strategy for achieving maximal renoprotection with currently available interventions.

Experimental Studies

When rats are subjected to surgical ablation of 5/6 of their renal mass, they develop hypertension, proteinuria and a progressive loss of GFR, features very similar to those of human CRD; and this model has been extensively utilized in the study of mechanisms of CRD progression.[3] Brenner and colleagues, using micropuncture techniques that made possible the measurement of glomerular capillary hydraulic pressure (P_{GC}) and GFR in single nephrons (single nephron GFR – SNGFR), showed experimentally that when nephrons were lost, remaining nephrons underwent hemodynamic adaptations in order to partially compensate for the loss of glomerular filtration. Thus remnant kidney glomeruli evidenced substantial increases in SNGFR (glomerular hyperfiltration) and P_{GC} (glomerular capillary hypertension).[4] Furthermore, it was proposed that these hemodynamic changes, although initially adaptive, eventuate in damage to remaining glomeruli that results in a further loss of nephrons thereby establishing a vicious cycle of progressive nephron injury.[5]

Support for this hypothesis was provided by experimental studies showing that interventions that resulted in protection of remnant kidneys from progressive injury were associated with attenuation of the glomerular hemodynamic changes. Low protein diet feeding was associated with normalization of SNGFR and P_{GC} as well as substantial protection from progressive glomerular injury.[4,6] Treatment with an angiotensin-converting enzyme inhibitor had little effect on SNGFR but did normalize P_{GC} and afforded effective renoprotection, suggesting that P_{GC} rather than SNGFR was the critical determinant of glomerular injury in the remnant kidney.[7] Moreover, treatment with a combination of hydralazine, hydrochlorothiazide and reserpine was associated with similar lowering of systemic

M.M. Avram.(ed.), Improving Prognosis for Kidney Disorders, 1-8.

blood pressure to ACEI but did not lower P_{GC} or afford any renoprotection.[8]

Although angiotensin II (AngII) has emerged as a central mediator of the glomerular hemodynamic changes associated with progressive renal injury, experimental studies have revealed several nonhemodynamic effects of AngII that may also be important in CRD progression. These include mesangial cell proliferation and induction of TGF-β expression,[9] stimulation of plasminogen activator inhibitor-1 production by endothelial cells and vascular smooth muscle cells,[10,11] macrophage activation and increased phagocytosis,[12,13] as well as adrenal production of aldosterone.[14]

Angiotensin – Converting Enzyme Inhibitors

The publication of the first large randomized study to show the substantial renoprotective effects of ACEI among type 1 diabetics with established nephropathy[15] indicated that the above experimental findings were also clinically relevant. Several studies subsequently investigated the potential of ACEI to afford renoprotection in non-diabetic forms of CRD. Maschio et al. randomized 583 patients with CRD of diverse etiologies to treatment with benazepril or placebo. After 3 years of follow-up, the study found a 53% reduction in the risk of reaching the combined end point of doubling of base-line serum creatinine or the need for dialysis associated with ACEI treatment. However, a significantly lower blood pressure among patients receiving ACEI vs. placebo made it impossible to separate the beneficial effects of lowering blood pressure from any unique effects of ACEI treatment.[16] By contrast, in the Ramipril Efficacy In Nephropathy (REIN) Study, 352 patients with non-diabetic CRD, randomized to either ACEI or placebo, achieved similar control of blood pressure. Among patients with ≥3g/day of proteinuria at base-line, the study was stopped early due to a significantly lower rate of decline in GFR in patients receiving the ACEI (0.53 vs. 0.88ml/min/month).[17] In the next phase of this study, patients who had received placebo were switched to ACEI and those already on ACEI continued treatment. Consistent with the findings of the first phase of the study, there was a significant reduction in the rate of decline in GFR of patients switched to ACEI. In addition, patients continuing on ACEI treatment showed a further reduction in the rate of GFR decline, to levels similar to those associated with normal aging. Patients who received ACEI from the start of the REIN study had a significantly lower risk of reaching end-stage renal failure (ESRF) than those switched to ACEI after the initial phase of the study (relative risk = 1.86). Indeed from 36 to 54 months of follow up, no further patients in the former group reached ESRF.[18] Interestingly, a small number of patients continued on ACEI actually showed an increase in GFR after prolonged treatment.[19] REIN Study patients with <3g/day of proteinuria (n=186) were followed for a median of 31 months after randomization. Similar to the findings among those with more severe proteinuria, ACEI treatment significantly reduced the incidence of ESRF (relative risk = 2.72), particularly among those with a GFR of <45ml/min at baseline.[20] In addition to the renoprotective benefits of ACEI treatment, the recent Heart Outcomes Prevention Evaluation (HOPE) Study reported a substantial reduction in overall and cardiovascular mortality among patients receiving an ACEI vs. placebo among 9297 patients who were at increased risk of cardiovascular disease.[21] Since cardiovascular disease is the single largest cause of morbidity and mortality among patients with CRD, the HOPE Study data provide a further rationale for the use of ACEI therapy as the single most important intervention in CRD patients.

Antihypertensive Therapy

Even before the introduction of ACEI, marked reductions in the rates of decline of GFR were observed following initiation of antihypertensive therapy in insulin-dependent diabetic patients with diabetic nephropathy[22,23] implying that hypertension, an almost universal consequence of impaired renal function, also contributed to the progression of CRD. Data from the MRFIT study, which identified elevated blood pressure as a strong, independent risk factor for ESRD in 332,544 prospectively evaluated men, confirmed that systemic hypertension is also important in the pathogenesis of non-diabetic CRD progression.[24] The Modification of Diet in Renal disease (MDRD) Study directly evaluated whether lower than previously recommended blood pressure targets afforded greater renoprotection than "usual" blood pressure control. In addition to the dietary interventions described below, patients were randomized to a target mean arterial pressure (MAP) of 107mmHg or 92mmHg. Whereas the primary analysis did not show any overall difference in rate of GFR decline between these groups, patients randomized to the low blood pressure group evidenced an early rapid decrease in GFR, likely due to associated renal hemodynamic effects, that obscured a later significantly slower rate of GFR decline than that observed in the "usual" blood pressure target group. Furthermore, a higher level of baseline proteinuria was associated with a greater difference in GFR decline between "usual" and low blood pressure groups.[25] Secondary analysis revealed significant correlations between the rate of GFR decline and achieved blood pressure, an effect that was also more marked among those with greater baseline proteinuria. In study 1, rates of GFR decline increased above a MAP of 98mmHg among patients with baseline proteinuria of 0.25-3.0g/day, and above 92mmHg among those with baseline proteinuria >3.0g/day. In study 2, among patients with baseline proteinuria >1g/day, higher achieved blood pressure was associated with greater rates of GFR decline at all levels. The authors concluded by recommending a blood pressure goal of <125/75 (MAP=92mmHg) for CRD patients with >1g/day of proteinuria and <130/80 (MAP=98mmHg) for those with proteinuria of 0.25-1.0g/d.[26] Since not all the patients in the MDRD Study received ACEI, it remains unknown to what extent the level of blood pressure attained remains important in CRD patients receiving ACEI. Experimental studies have found systolic blood pressure to be a major determinant of glomerular injury in rats receiving either ACEI or angiotensin receptor blocker (ARB) treatment.[27] Moreover among patients with type 1 diabetes and established nephropathy receiving ACEI, randomization to a low (MAP=92mmHg) vs. "usual" (MAP=100-107mmHg) target blood pressure was associated with significantly lower levels of proteinuria after 2 years; although there was no significant difference in GFR.[28]

Dietary Protein Restriction

Based on the notion that reducing the excretory burden on the kidneys would slow the rate of progressive injury, dietary protein restriction was among the first interventions proposed to slow CRD progression. Experimental studies showed that low protein diet normalized glomerular hemodynamics in the remnant kidney model[4] and resulted in effective long-term renoprotection.[6] Unfortunately, clinical studies to date have failed to provide similar unambiguous evidence to support the use of protein restriction in human CRD. Following the publication of several smaller studies that generally suggested a beneficial effect from protein restriction, the MDRD Study was conducted to finally resolve the issue. 585 patients with moderate chronic renal failure (GFR=25-55ml/min/1.73m^2) were randomized to "usual" (1.3g/kg/day) or "low" (0.58g/kg/day) protein diet (study 1) and 255 patients with severe CRF (GFR=13-24ml/min/1.73m^2) to "low" (0.58g/kg/day) or "very low" (0.28g/kg/day) protein diet and followed for a mean of 2.2 years. All causes of CRD were included, but patients with diabetes mellitus requiring insulin therapy were excluded. Whereas the primary analysis revealed no difference in the mean rate of GFR decline in study 1 or 2,[25] secondary analyses revealed that dietary protein restriction probably did achieve beneficial effects. In study 1, an initial reduction in GFR, likely due to the functional effects of decreased protein intake, obscured a later reduction in the rate of GFR decline that was evident after 4 months in the "low"protein.[25] Further analysis of data from study 1 also showed that dietary protein restriction achieved the greatest renoprotective effect in those with the highest initial rates of decline in GFR.[29] In study 2, when data from both diet groups were combined and analyzed according to *achieved* dietary protein intake, a reduction in protein intake of 0.2g/kg/day correlated with a 1.15ml/min/year reduction in the rate of GFR decline, a 29% reduction in mean rate of GFR decline that implied a 41% prolongation in renal survival.[30] Further evidence supporting a renoprotective effect of low protein diet was provided by a meta-analysis of 5 randomized studies that included a total of 1413 patients with non-diabetic CRD (including those from study 1 of the MDRD) and showed a relative risk of 0.67 for renal failure of death in patients randomized to low vs. usual protein diet.[31] Thus, whereas no single study has yet provided conclusive evidence of the renoprotective effect of dietary protein restriction in humans, we believe that sufficient evidence exists to recommend moderate protein restriction of 0.6g/kg/day in patients with non-diabetic forms of CRD.

Proteinuria

Proteinuria reflects a loss of glomerular filtration barrier integrity, and the extent of proteinuria has long been used as an indicator of glomerular disease severity. Recently, however, it has been proposed that proteinuria *per se* also contributes to progressive renal injury.[32] In the REIN Study, higher baseline proteinuria was associated with more rapid rates of GFR decline and among patients with initial proteinuria of >3g/day, ACEI treatment reduced proteinuria to an extent that correlated inversely with the subsequent rate of GFR decline.[17] Furthermore, in the MDRD Study, a reduction in proteinuria, independent of blood pressure, was associated with slower progression of CRD and the degree of benefit achieved through blood pressure lowering was dependent on the extent of baseline proteinuria.[26] Experimental observations suggest mechanisms whereby an excess of filtered proteins may contribute to renal damage. Culture of tubular epithelial cells in the presence of a variety of plasma proteins has been shown to induce production of proinflammatory cytokines and extracellular matrix proteins[33-6], responses that may contribute to tubulo-interstitial fibrosis. *In vivo*, proteinuria induced by protein-overload was associated with renal expression of cell adhesion molecules and chemoattractants resulting in interstitial inflammation and fibrosis.[37] Together, these clinical and experimental data provide considerable support for the hypothesis that excessive filtration of serum proteins by injured glomeruli directly contributes to progressive renal damage. The strong association between the achievement of proteinuria reduction and renoprotection in clinical studies implies that minimization of proteinuria should be regarded as an important independent therapeutic goal in renoprotective strategies.

Treatment of Hyperlipidemia

CRD is commonly associated with abnormalities of plasma lipids characterized by elevated levels of the triglyceride-rich lipoproteins VLDL and LDL and reduced levels of HDL.[38] In addition to placing CRD patients at increased risk of cardiovascular disease, these lipid abnormalities may also accelerate the progression of CRD. In the MDRD Study, low serum HDL cholesterol was an independent predictor of more rapid decline in GFR;[39] and in another study, elevated apo-B containing lipoprotein levels were associated with more rapid deterioration of renal function.[40] Hypercholesterolemia has been associated with more rapid progression of renal disease among patients with diabetic[41-3] and non-diabetic forms of CRD.[44] The mechanisms whereby hyperlipidemia may contribute to renal injury are the subject of ongoing research; but studies to date have identified several different mechansisms, including stimulation of mesangial cell proliferation, cytokine expression and extracellular matrix synthesis,[45-6] oxidation of LDL to form reactive oxygen species[47] and elevations in P_{GC}.[48] In experimental studies, treatment of hyperlipidemia has resulted in attenuation of renal injury in a variety of models of CRD.[49-52] Whereas some clinical studies have found that lowering of plasma lipids was associated with reduction of proteinuria in patients with nephrotic syndrome,[53] this has not been a universal finding.[54-6] Large randomized clinical studies are, therefore, required to investigate the role of lipid-lowering therapy in renoprotection. Nevertheless, the fact that patients with CRD are at increased risk for cardiovascular disease alone justifies a policy of active dietary and drug intervention to correct hyperlipidemia.

Smoking Cessation

Smoking has been identified as a risk factor for the development of microalbuminuria, overt proteinuria and renal disease progression in type 1 and 2 diabetics.[57-9] Similarly, among patients with other forms of CRD, smoking has been identified as a risk factor for progression. Among patients with adult polycystic kidney disease or IgA nephropathy, smokers had a 10-fold increased risk of progression to ESRD vs. non-smokers;[60] the median time to ESRD was almost halved in smokers vs. non-smokers in patients with lupus nephritis;[61] patients with a primary glomerulonephritis and serum creatinine >1.7mg/dl were significantly more likely to be smokers than those with normal creatinine.[62] Though prospective studies showing re-nal benefit from smoking cessation are lacking, the above evidence suggests that the kidney may be adversely affected by smoking. The well-established benefits of smoking cessation for prevention of lung and cardiovascular disease as well as malignancy mandate that all patients with CRD should be counseled to stop smoking and assisted in achieving this goal.

Future Therapies

In the ongoing endeavor to achieve more effective renoprotection, many novel treatments are being investigated in experimental and clinical studies. Below we discuss some of the more promising of these potential future renoprotective therapies.

Angiotensin Receptor Blockers

Angiotensin receptor blockers (ARB) inhibit the renin-angiotensin system (RAS) by blocking angiotensin II subtype 1 (AT_1) receptors. Thus, ACEI and ARB differ in their effects on the RAS in ways that may be therapeutically relevant. First, ACEI are able to inhibit only angiotensin-converting enzyme (ACE)-dependent AngII production, whereas ARB block the effect of AngII from any source at the receptor level. In the presence of ACE inhibition, studies have shown that AngII may be produced by other proteases, including chymase and other serine proteases.[63] Second, there are at least two subtypes of the AngII receptor. Thus, blockade of AT_1 receptors in the presence of elevated AngII levels can be expected to result in stimulation of subtype 2 (AT_2) receptors. Whereas AT_1 receptors mediate most of the known effects of AngII, including vasoconstriction, stimulation of aldosterone synthesis and release, and renal tubule sodium and water reabsorption, the role of AT_2 receptors is not as clearly defined and may include fetal kidney development, modulation of pressure-natriuresis, mediation of AngII-induced renal production of nitric oxide, and renal conversion of prostaglandin E_2 to prostaglandin $F_{2\alpha}$.[64]

Despite the above theoretical differences, experimental studies have found that ACEI and ARB produce similar changes in glomerular hemodynamics and afford equivalent renoprotection in a variety of CRD models (reviewed in detail in [64]). Large randomized clinical studies of the renoprotective effects of ARB are still awaited, but preliminary data suggest that ARB will be as effective as ACEI. In small studies, ARB and ACEI produced similar antihypertensive and antiproteinuric effects among patients with essential hypertension[65] and among those with CRD.[66] In the study with the longest follow-up to date, ACEI or ARB treatment in type 2 diabetics with early nephropathy was found to afford similar reductions in blood pressure and albuminuria. GFR was not different between the groups after 1 year.[67] One important advantage of ARB over ACEI is their more favourable side effect profile. In clinical trials, ARB have been reported to have side effect profiles similar to placebo.[68-9] Importantly, ARB are not associated with the cough that may occur in up to 20% of patients receiving ACEI. Among patients converted from ACEI to ARB therapy, recurrence of a cough was significantly lower than patients rechallenged with an ACEI.[70-1] Thus, even in the absence of clinical trial evidence of the renoprotective effects of ARB, available evidence supports the use of ARB as an alternative in patients who are unable to tolerate ACEI due to side effects. Furthermore, the favourable side effect profile of ARB suggests that it may be possible to employ higher doses. Preliminary data have shown that doubling the dose of an ARB may result in greater lowering of proteinuria without a further reduction in blood pressure.[66] Finally, the differing effects of ACEI and ARB on the RAS imply that in combination they may have additive or even synergistic effects. Among 8 patients with IgA nephropathy treated consecutively with an ACEI, ARB and combination therapy, the combination was associated with greater antiproteinuric effects than either treatment alone without significant additional antihypertensive effects.[72] Addition of an ARB to prior ACEI therapy in 11 patients with CRD was associated with a 6mmHg fall in MAP and a further 30% reduction in proteinuria.[73] Among type 2 diabetic patients with microalbuminuria, combination ACEI and ARB therapy afforded greater reductions in blood pressure and albuminuria than either treatment alone.[74] Although more data are required before firm recommendations can be made, evidence is accumulating that ARB will offer clinical renoprotection and may represent a useful addition to the use of ACEI.

Vasopeptidase Inhibitors

Vasopeptidase inhibitors (VPI) are a new class of drugs comprising single molecules that simultaneously inhibit both ACE and neutral endopeptidase (NEP). This latter ecto-enzyme is localized principally in the brush border membrane of renal tubule cells and catabolizes several vasodilator molecules including the natriuretic peptides, adrenomedullin and bradykinin.[75-6] Thus VPI treatment is associated with reduced production of the vasoconstrictor, AngII, and accumulation of the above vasodilators. In experimental[77-8] and clinical studies,[76] VPI have been shown to be effective antihypertensive agents in both low and high renin states. Recently, we reported that, in rats subjected to 5/6 nephrectomy, the VPI Omapatrilat produced greater lowering of P_{GC} than an ACEI. Furthermore, VPI treatment of rats with established renal injury after 5/6 nephrectomy almost doubled the delay in progression of CRD achieved with an ACEI despite equivalent control of systemic blood pressure.[79] If clinical studies produce similar results, this new class of drugs may have a major impact in reducing the number of CRD patients progressing to end-stage renal failure.

Anti-Inflammatory Therapies

In recent years, attention has focused on the role of cytokines and other inflammatory molecules in mediating the cellular events involved in progressive renal injury.[80] In the 5/6 nephrectomy model and in human CRD, glomerular and interstitial infiltration by macrophages is characteristically present.[81-3] Furthermore, several studies have observed the apparently coordinated upregulation of a number of cytokines, cell adhesion molecules and profibrotic and profibrotic growth factors in the 5/6 nephrectomy model.[84-6] If these inflammatory elements do, in fact, play a role in progressive renal injury in CRD, anti-inflammatory therapies or interventions directed at inhibiting specific inflammatory or fibrotic molecules may result in additional renoprotection. Interestingly, several studies have now shown that treatment of 5/6 nephrectomized rats with the immunosuppressive agent mycophenolate mofetil was associated with substantial renoprotection.[87-9] Clearly, the potential benefits of this approach must be weighed against the obvious risks of immunosuppression. It is likely that a wide range of specific inhibitors of cytokines and profibrotic growth factors will soon be available, providing new tools for investigating this emerging field.

A Strategy for Maximal Renoprotection

In this review, we have considered individually a variety of interventions that have been shown to slow the rate of progression of CRD. At best, however, each intervention slows the rate of progression by

Table 1. A comprehensive strategy and therapeutic goals for achieving maximal renoprotection in non-diabetic chronic renal disease.

Intervention	Goal
1. Dietary protein restriction	0.6g/kg/day
2. ACEI therapy (or ARB if not tolerated)	Proteinuria <1g/day
	GFR decline <1ml/min/month
3. Antihypertensive therapy	<125/75 if proteinuria >1g/d
	<130/80 if proteinuria <1g/d
4. Smoking Cessation	
5. Lipid lowering therapy	

50%. We therefore suggest that in order to achieve more effective long-term renoprotection, a comprehensive strategy employing all of these elements is required. Moreover, once treatments have been introduced, close monitoring of blood pressure, proteinuria and GFR is essential so that therapy can be escalated until therapeutic goals have been achieved (**Table 1**). In this regard, our approach is analogous to that applied in modern chemotherapeutic strategies where multiple agents are used and treatment is directed towards correcting all signs of disease activity until the patient is said to be in "remission". It should be noted that these recommendations are based on currently available interventions, and the measurements required for monitoring are already widely used. Thus, a comprehensive approach to renoprotection is an achievable goal for all patients with CRD. If widely applied, this strategy may substantially reduce the number of CRD patients progressing to ESRD and provide a means to address the global problem of rapidly increasing demand for renal replacement therapy.

References

1. Mitch WE, Walser M, Buffington GA, Leman, Jr J: A simple method for estimating progression of chronic renal failure. Lancet 2:1326-8, 1976
2. Rutherford WE, Blondin J, Miller JP, Greenwalt AS, Vavra JD: Chronic progressive renal disease: rate of change of serum creatinine. Kidney Int 11:62-70, 1977
3. Shimamura T, Ashton B, Morrison MD: A progressive glomerulosclerosis occurring in partial five-sixths nephrectomized rats. Am J Pathol 79:95-106, 1975
4. Hostetter TH, Olson JL, Rennke HG, Venkatachalam MA, Brenner BM: Hyperfiltration in remnant nephrons: a potentially adverse response to renal ablation. Am J Physiol 241:F85-93, 1981
5. Brenner BM, Meyer TW, Hostetter TH: Dietary protein intake and the progressive nature of kidney disease: the role of hemodynamically mediated glomerular injury in the pathogenesis of progressive glomerular sclerosis in aging, renal ablation, and intrinsic renal disease. N Engl J Med 307:652-9, 1982
6. Hostetter TH, Meyer TW, Rennke HG, Brenner BM: Chronic effects of dietary protein in the rat with intact and reduced renal mass. Kidney Int 30:509-17, 1986
7. Anderson S, Meyer TW, Rennke HG, Brenner BM: Control of glomerular hypertension limits glomerular injury in rats with reduced renal mass. J Clin Invest 76:612-9, 1985
8. Anderson S, Rennke HG, Brenner BM: Therapeutic advantage of converting enzyme inhibitors in arresting progressive renal disease associated with systemic hypertension in the rat. J Clin Invest 77:1993-2000, 1986
9. Kagami S, Border WA, Miller DE, Noble NA: Angiotensin II stimulates extracellular matrix protein synthesis through induction of transforming growth factor-beta expression in rat glomerular mesangial cells. J Clin Invest 93:2431-7, 1994
10. van Leeuwen RT, Kol A, Andreotti F, Kluft C, Maseri A, Sperti G: Angiotensin II increases plasminogen activator inhibitor type 1 and tissue-type plasminogen activator messenger RNA in cultured rat aortic smooth muscle cells. Circulation 90:362-8, 1994
11. Vaughan DE, Lazos SA, Tong K: Angiotensin II regulates the expression of plasminogen activator inhibitor-1 in cultured endothelial cells. A potential link between the renin-angiotensin system and thrombosis. J Clin Invest 95:995-1001, 1995
12. Foris G, Dezso B, Medgyesi GA, Fust G: Effect of angiotensin II on macrophage functions. Immunology 48:529-35, 1983
13. Hahn AW, Jonas U, Buhler FR, Resink TJ: Activation of human peripheral monocytes by angiotensin II. FEBS Lett 347:178-80, 1994
14. Greene EL, Kren S, Hostetter TH: Role of aldosterone in the remnant kidney model in the rat. J Clin Invest 98:1063-8, 1996
15. Lewis EJ, Hunsicker LG, Bain RP, Rohde RD: The effect of angiotensin-converting-enzyme inhibition on diabetic nephropathy. N Engl J Med 329:1456-62, 1993
16. Maschio G, Alberti D, Janin G, Locatelli F, Mann JF, Motolese M, Ponticelli C, Ritz E, Zuchelli P: Effect of angiotensin-converting-enzyme inhibitor benazepril on the progression of chronic renal insufficiency. The Angiotensin-Converting-Enzyme Inhibition in Progressive Renal Insufficiency Study Group. N Eng J Med 334:939-45, 1996
17. GISEN (Gruppo Italiano di Studi Epidemiologici in Nefrologia): Randomised placebo-controlled trial of effect of ramipril on decline in glomerular filtration rate and risk of terminal renal failure in proteinuric, non-diabetic nephropathy. Lancet 349:1857-63, 1997
18. Ruggenenti P, Perna A, Gherardi G, Gaspari F, Benini R, Remuzzi G: Renal function and requirement for dialysis in chronic nephropathy patients on long-term ramipril: REIN follow-up trial. Gruppo Italiano di Studi Epidemiologici in Nefrologia (GISEN). Ramipril Efficacy in Nephropathy. Lancet 352:1252-6, 1998
19. Ruggenenti P, Perna A, Benini R, Bertani T, Zoccali C, Maggiore Q, Salvadori M, Remuzzi G: In chronic nephropathies prolonged ACE inhibition can induce remission: dynamics of time-dependent changes in GFR. Investigators of the GISEN Group. Gruppo Italiano Studi Epidemiologici in Nefrologia. J Am Soc Nephrol 10:997-1006, 1999

20. Ruggenenti P, Perna A, Gherardi G, Garini G, Zoccali C, Salvadori M, Scolari F, Schena FP, Remuzzi G: Renoprotective properties of ACE-inhibition in non-diabetic nephropathies with non-nephrotic proteinuria. Lancet 354:359-64, 1999
21. HOPE (The Heart Outcomes Prevention Evaluation Study Investigators): Effects of an angiotensin-converting-enzyme inhibitor, ramipril on cardiovascular events in high-risk patients. N Engl J Med 342:145-53, 2000
22. Mogensen CE: Progression of nephropathy in long-term diabetics with proteinuria and effect of initial anti-hypertensive treatment. Scand J Clin Lab Invest 36:383-8, 1976
23. Parving HH, Andersen AR, Smidt UM, Svendsen PA: Early aggressive antihypertensive treatment reduces rate of decline in kidney function in diabetic nephropathy. Lancet 1:1175-9, 1983
24. Klag MJ, Whelton PK, Randall BL, Neaton JD, Brancati FL, Ford CE, Shulman NB, Stamler J: Blood pressure and end-stage renal disease in men. N Engl J Med 334:13-8, 1996
25. Klahr S, Levey AS, Beck GJ, Caggiula AW, Hunsicker L, Kusek JW, Striker G: The effects of dietary protein restriction and blood-pressure control on the progression of chronic renal disease. Modification of Diet in Renal Disease Study Group. N Engl J Med 330:877-84, 1994
26. Peterson JC, Adler S, Burkart JM, Greene T, Hebert LA, Hunsicker LG, King AJ, Klahr S, Massry SG, Seifter JL: Blood pressure control, proteinuria, and the progression of renal disease. The Modification of Diet in Renal Disease Study. Ann Intern Med 123:754-62, 1995
27. Taal MW, Chertow GM, Rennke HR, Gurnani A, Jiang T, Shahsafaei A, Troy JL, Brenner BM, Mackenzie HS: Mechanisms underlying renoprotection during renin-angiotensin system blockade. Am J Physiol 280:F343-55, 2001
28. Lewis JB, Berl T, Bain RP, Rohde RD, Lewis EJ: Effect of intensive blood pressure control on the course of type 1 diabetic nephropathy. Collaborative Study Group. Am J Kidney Dis 34:809-17, 1999
29. Levey AS, Adler S, Greene T, Hunsicker LG, Kusek JW, Rogers NL, Teschan PE: Effects of dietary protein restriction on the progression of moderate renal disease in the Modification of Diet in Renal Disease Study. J Am Soc Nephrol 7:2616-26, 1996
30. Levey AS, Adler S, Caggiula AW, England BK, Greene T, Hunsicker LG, Kusek JW, Rogers NL, Teschan PE: Effects of dietary protein restriction on the progression of advanced renal disease in the Modification of Diet in Renal Disease Study. Am J Kidney Dis 27:652-63, 1996
31. Pedrini MT, Levey AS, Lau J, Chalmers TC, Wang PH: The effect of dietary protein restriction on the progression of diabetic and nondiabetic renal diseases: a meta-analysis. Ann Intern Med 124:627-32, 1996
32. Remuzzi G, Bertani T: Pathophysiology of progressive nephropathies. N Engl J Med 339:1448-56, 1998
33. Zoja C, Morigi M, Figliuzzi M, Bruzzi I, Oldroyd S, Benigni A, Ronco P, Remuzzi G: Proximal tubular cell synthesis and secretion of endothelin-1 on challenge with albumin and other proteins. Am J Kidney Dis 26:934-41, 1995
34. Wang Y, Chen J, Chen L, Tay YC, Rangan GK, Harris DC: Induction of monocyte chemoattractant protein-1 in proximal tubule cells by urinary protein. J Am Soc Nephrol 8:1537-45, 1997
35. Zoja C, Donadelli R, Colleoni S, Figliuzzi M, Bonazzola S, Morigi M, Remuzzi G: Protein overload stimulates RANTES production by proximal tubular cells depending on NF-kappa B activation. Kidney Int 53:1608-15, 1998
36. Abbate M, Zoja C, Corna D, Capitanio M, Bertani T, Remuzzi G: In progressive nephropathies, overload of tubular cells with filtered proteins translates glomerular permeability dysfunction into cellular signals of interstitial inflammation. J Am Soc Nephrol 9:1213-24, 1998
37. Eddy AA, Giachelli CM: Renal expression of genes that promote interstitial inflammation and fibrosis in rats with protein-overload proteinuria. Kidney Int 47:1546-57, 1995
38. Monzani G, Bergesio F, Ciuti R, Rosati A, Frizzi V, Serruto A, Vitali D, Benucci A, Tosi PL, Bandini S, Salvadori M: Lipoprotein abnormalities in chronic renal failure and dialysis patients. Blood Purif 14:262-72, 1996
39. Hunsicker LG, Adler S, Caggiulia A, England BK, Greene T, Kusek JW, Rogers NL, Teschan PE: Predictors of progression of renal disease in the Modification of Diet in Renal Disease Study. Kidney Int 51:1908-19, 1997
40. Samuelsson O, Aurell M, Knight-Gibson C, Alaupovic P, Attman P-O: Apolipoprotein-B-containing lipoproteins and the progression of renal insufficiency. Nephron 63:279-85, 1993
41. Krolewski AS, Warram JH, Christlieb AR: Hypercholesterolemia- a determinant of renal function loss and deaths in IDDM patients with nephropathy. Kidney Int 45:S-125-31, 1994
42. Ravid M, Brosh D, Ravid-Safran D, Levy Z, Rachmani R: Main risk factors for nephropathy in type 2 diabetes mellitus are plasma cholesterol levels, mean blood pressure, and hyperglycemia. Arch Intern Med 158:998-1004, 1998
43. Mulec H, Johnson S-A, Bjorck S: Relation between serum cholesterol and diabetic nephropathy. Lancet 335:1537-8, 1990
44. Maschio G, Oldrizzi L, Rugiu C, Loschiavo C: Serum lipids in patients with chronic renal failure on long-term, protein-restricted diets. Am J Med 87:51N-4N, 1989
45. Grone EF, Abboud HE, Hohne M, Walli AK, Grone HJ, Stuker D, Robenek H, Wieland E, Seidel D: Actions of lipoproteins in cultured human mesangial cells: modulation by mitogenic vasoconstrictors. Am J Physiol 263:F686-96, 1992
46. Rovin BH, Tan LC: LDL stimulates mesangial fibronectin production and chemoattractant expression. Kidney Int 43:218-25, 1993
47. Wheeler DC, Chana RS, Topley N, Petersen MM, Davies M, Williams JD: Oxidation of low density lipoprotein by mesangial cells may promote glomerular injury. Kidney Int 45:1628-36, 1994
48. Kasiske B, O'Donnell MP, Schmitz PG, Kim Y, Keane WF: Renal injury of diet-induced hypercholesterolemia in rats. Kidney Int 37:880-91, 1990
49. Kasiske BL, O'Donnel MP, Garvis WJ, Keane WF: Pharmacologic treatment of hyperlipidemia reduces injury in rat 5/6 nephrectomy model of chronic renal failure. Circ Res 62:367-74, 1988
50. Kasiske BL, O'Donnell MP, Cleary MP, Keane WF: Treatment of hyperlipidemia reduces glomerular injury in obese Zucker rats. Kidney Int 33:667-72, 1988
51. O'Donell MP, Kasiske BL, Kim Y, Schmitz PG, Keane WF: Lovastatin retards the progression of established glomerular disease in obese Zucker rats. Am J Kidney Dis 22:83-9, 1993
52. Park Y-S, Guijarro C, Kim Y, Massy ZA, Kasiske BL, Keane WF, O'Donnell MP: Lovastatin reduces glomerular macrophage influx and monocyte chemoattractant protein-1 mRNA in nephrotic rats. Am J Kidney Dis 31:190-4, 1998
53. D'Amico G, Gentile MG: Pharmacological and dietary treatment of lipid abnormalities in nephrotic patients. Kidney Int 39:S-65-9, 1991
54. Maschio G, Oldrizzi L, Rugiu C, De Base V, Loschiavo C: Effect of dietary manipulation on the lipid abnormalities in patients with chronic renal failure. Kidney Int 39:S-70-2, 1991
55. Spitalewitz S, Porush JG, Cattran D, Wright N: Treatment of hyperlipidemia in the nephrotic syndrome: the effects of pravastatin therapy. Am J kidney Dis 22:143-50, 1993
56. Thomas ME, Harris KPG, Ramaswamy C, Hattersley JM, Wheeler DC, Varghese Z, Williams JD, Walls J, Moorhead JF: Simvastatin therapy for hypercholesterolemic patients with

nephrotic syndrome or significant proteinuria. Kidney Int 44:1124-9, 1993

57. Muhlhauser I, Sawicki P, Berger M: Cigarette-smoking as a risk factor for macroproteinuria and proliferative retinopathy in Type I (insulin-dependent) diabetes. Diabetologia 29:500-2, 1986
58. Chase HP, Garg SK, Marshall G, Berg CL, Harris S, Jackson WE, Hamman RE: Cigarette smoking increases the risk of albuminuria among subjects with type I diabetes. JAMA 265:614-7, 1991
59. McKenna K, Thompson C: Microalbuminuria: a marker to increased renal and cardiovascular risk in diabetes mellitus. Scott Med J 42:99-104, 1997
60. Orth SR, Stockmann A, Conradt C, Ritz E, Ferro M, Kreusser W, Piccoli G, Rambausek M, Roccatello D, Schafer K, Sieberth HG, Wanner C, Watschinger B, Zucchelli P: Smoking as a risk factor for end-stage renal failure in men with primary renal disease. Kidney International 54:926-31, 1998
61. Ward MM, Studenski S: Clinical prognostic factors in lupus nephritis. The importance of hypertension and smoking. Arch Intern Med 152:2082-8, 1992
62. Stengel B, Couchoud C, Cenee S, Hemon D: Age, blood pressure and smoking effects on chronic renal failure in primary glomerular nephropathies. Kidney International 57:2519-26, 2000
63. Arakawa K: Serine protease angiotensin II systems. J Hypertens Suppl 5:S3-7, 1996
64. Taal MW, Brenner BM: Renoprotective benefits of RAS inhibition: from ACEI to angiotensin II antagonists. Kidney Int 57:1803-17, 2000
65. Nielsen S, Dollerup J, Nielsen B, Jensen HA, Mogensen CE: Losartan reduces albuminuria in patients with essential hypertension. An enalapril controlled 3 months study. Nephrol Dial Transplant 2:19-23, 1997
66. Gansevoort RT, de Zeeuw D, de Jong PE: Is the antiproteinuric effect of ACE inhibition mediated by interference in the renin-angiotensin system? Kidney Int 45:861-7, 1994
67. Lacourciere Y, Belanger A, Godin C, Halle JP, Ross S, Wright N, Marion J: Long-term comparison of losartan and enalapril on kidney function in hypertensive type 2 diabetics with early nephropathy. Kidney International 58:762-9, 2000
68. Goldberg AI, Dunlay MC, Sweet CS: Safety and tolerability of losartan potassium, an angiotensin II receptor antagonist, compared with hydrochlorothiazide, atenolol, felodipine ER, and angiotensin-converting enzyme inhibitors for the treatment of systemic hypertension. Am J Cardiol 75:793-5, 1995
69. Weber M: Clinical safety and tolerability of losartan. Clin Ther 19:604-16, 1997
70. Lacourciere Y, Brunner H, Irwin R, Karlberg BE, Ramsay LE, Snavely DB, Dobbins TW, Faison EP, Nelson EB: Effects of modulators of the renin-angiotensin-aldosterone system on cough. Losartan Cough Study Group. J Hypertens 12:1387-93, 1994
71. Benz J, Oshrain C, Henry D, Avery C, Chiang YT, Gatlin M: Valsartan, a new angiotensin II receptor antagonist: a double-blind study comparing the incidence of cough with lisinopril and hydrochlorothiazide. J Clin Pharmacol 37:101-7, 1997
72. Russo D, Pisani A, Balletta MM, De Nicola L, Savino FA, Andreucci M, Minutolo R: Additive antiproteinuric effect of converting enzyme inhibitor and losartan in normotensive patients with IgA nephropathy. American Journal of Kidney Diseases 33:851-6, 1999
73. Zoccali C, Valvo E, Russo D, Panichi V, Zuccala A: Antiproteinuric effect of Losartan in patients with chronic renal diseases (Letter). Nephrol Dial Transplant 12:234-5, 1997
74. Mogensen CE, Noltham S, Tikkanen I, Oren S, Viskoper R, Watts RW, Cooper ME: Randomised controlled trial of dual blockade of renin-angiotensin system in pateints with hypertension, microalbuminuria, and non-insulin dependent diabetes: the candesartan and lisinopril microalbuminuria (CALM) study. BMJ 321:1440-4, 2000
75. Burnett JC, Jr.: Vasopeptidase inhibition: a new concept in blood pressure management. J Hypertension 17 (suppl 1):S37-43, 1999
76. Weber M: Emerging treatments for hypertension: potential role for vasopeptidase inhibition. Am J Hypertension 12:139S-47S, 1999
77. Trippodo NC, Robl JA, Asaad MM, Fox M, Panchal BC, Schaeffer TR: Effects of omapatrilat in low, normal, and high renin experimental hypertension. Am J Hypertension 11:363-72, 1998
78. Intengan HD, Schiffrin EL: Vasopeptidase inhibition has potent effects on blood pressure and resistance arteries in stroke-prone spontaneously hypertensive rats. Hypertension 35:1221-5, 2000
79. Taal MW, Nenov VD, Wong W, Satyal SR, Sakharova O, Hoon Choi J, Troy JL, Brenner BM: Vasopeptidase inhibition affords greater renoprotection than angiotensin-converting enzyme inhibition alone in rats with established nephropathy after 5/6 nephrectomy. (Abstract). J Am Soc Nephrol 11, 2000
80. Taal MW, Omer SA, Nadim MK, Mackenzie HS: Cellular and molecular mediators in common pathway mechanisms of chronic renal disease progression. Curr Opin Nephrol Hypertens 9:323-31, 2000
81. van Goor H, Fidler V, Weening JJ, Grond J: Determinants of focal and segmental glomerulosclerosis in the rat after renal ablation. Evidence for involvement of macrophages and lipids. Lab Invest 64:754-65, 1991
82. Floege J, Burns MW, Alpers CE, Yoshimura A, Pritzl P, Gordon K, Seifert RA, Bowen-Pope DF, Couser WG, Johnson RJ: Glomerular cell proliferation and PDGF expression precede glomerulosclerosis in the remnant kidney model. Kidney Int 41:297-309, 1992
83. Wu LL, Yang N, Roe CJ, Cooper ME, Gilbert RE, Atkins RC, Lan HY: Macrophage and myofibroblast proliferation in remnant kidney: role of angiotensin II. Kidney Int Suppl 63:S221-5, 1997
84. Schiller B, Moran J: Focal glomerulosclerosis in the remnant kidney model--an inflammatory disease mediated by cytokines. Nephrol Dial Transplant 12:430-7, 1997
85. Wu LL, Cox A, Roe CJ, Dziadek M, Cooper ME, Gilbert RE: Transforming growth factor beta 1 and renal injury following subtotal nephrectomy in the rat: role of the renin-angiotensin system. Kidney Int 51:1553-67, 1997
86. Taal MW, Zandi-Nejad Z, Weening B, Shahsafaei A, Kato S, Lee K-W, Ziai F, Jiang T, Brenner BM, Mackenzie HS: Pro-inflammatory gene expression and macrophage recruitment in the rat remnant kidney. Kidney Int 58:1664-76, 2000
87. Fujihara CK, Malheiros DM, Zatz R, Noronha ID: Mycophenolate mofetil attenuates renal injury in the rat remnant kidney. Kidney International 54:1510-9, 1998
88. Romero F, Rodriguez-Iturbe B, Parra G, Gonzalez L, Herrera-Acosta J, Tapia E: Mycophenolate mofetil prevents the progressive renal failure induced by 5/6 renal ablation in rats. Kidney Int 55:945-55, 1999
89. Remuzzi G, Zoja C, Gagliardini E, Corna D, Abbate M, Benigni A: Combining an antiproteinuric approach with mycophenolate mofetil fully suppresses progressive nephropathy of experimental animals. J Am Soc Nephrol 10:1542-9, 1999.

2 Anemia of Chronic Kidney Disease and its Management with Recombinant Human Erythropoietin and Darbepoetin Alfa

ALLEN R. NISSENSON, MD AND ERIC M. TONG, MD

Introduction

Chronic kidney disease (CKD) encompasses the full continuum of renal insufficiency and often goes undetected for months, even years. Patients with CKD may go on to develop end-stage renal disease (ESRD), at which point renal replacement therapy – dialysis or transplantation – becomes necessary to sustain life.[1]

There is a high prevalence of CKD in the United States (US). Based on serum creatinine (SCr) values obtained from a representative sample (18,723 participants) of the US population, the Third National Health and Nutrition Examination Survey estimated a prevalence of CKD (SCr ≥1.5 mg/dL) as high as 6.2 million people.[2,3] In our study of patients in a large US health maintenance organization (HMO), we estimated – by applying the 1990 age- and sex-specific prevalence rates in the HMO to the US population – that approximately 9.1 million Americans overall had at least one stet elevated sex-specific SCr value.[4] CKD is an important public health problem; and early identification and management of patients with CKD could potentially slow the progression to ESRD, improve patient outcomes, and constrain the growth in costs of patients entering dialysis programs.

Anemia is a major and persistent manifestation of CKD[5] and develops as renal function falls below 50% of normal.[1] Studies indicate that approximately 40% of patients with CKD (SCr ≥2.0 mg/dL for males and ≥1.5 mg/dL for females) are anemic,[6] with the prevalence of anemia directly correlated with the severity of renal insufficiency. An analysis of anemic patients with CKD beginning dialysis in the US found that 67% had a hematocrit of less than 30%, and 51% had a hematocrit of less than 28%.[2]

Patients with anemia may present with various symptoms, including lethargy, weakness, angina and shortness of breath. When untreated, anemia causes or contributes to fatigue, insomnia, depression, cognitive dysfunction, decreased libido and left ventricular hypertrophy.[7,8] These patients have an impaired quality of life, greater need for red blood cell transfusions, increased hospitalizations and increased risk of death.[7,9]

Anemia in CKD is caused primarily by a deficiency in endogenous erythropoietin (EPO).[10] The term 'erythropoietin' was not used until nearly 100 years following Bright's recognition of renal anemia in 1836.[11] In 1953, Erslev and colleagues confirmed the presence of EPO in the blood of anemic animals.[12] Subsequent studies by Goldwasser and colleagues demonstrated that the kidneys were the source of this hormone, which was produced in response to a fall in oxygen delivery to the renal parenchyma.

Diseases destroying the tubulo-interstitial cells of the kidney, which are responsible for EPO production, are major causes of hypoproliferative anemia. In addition to the relative lack of EPO, increased red blood cell destruction and loss must be considered as possible contributing causes to renal anemia.[5]

Endogenous EPO deficiency can be effectively corrected by the administration of recombinant human erythropoietin (rHuEPO, epoetin alfa), which was developed following the breakthrough in the isolation and cloning of the EPO gene by Lin and colleagues.[13] rHuEPO was approved for use in the US by the Food and Drug Administration (FDA) in 1989.[14,15] Prior to that, management of anemia in patients with CKD was poor; and treatment with regular blood transfusions and administration of androgenic steroids was required, often with significant resultant side effects and complications. Even with these therapies, most patients remained severely anemic, with hemoglobin values generally 10 g/dL or less.

rHuEPO has now become the standard of care for renal anemia.[16,17] In addition to dramatically improving the clinical outcomes and quality of life for patients with ESRD, rHuEPO has provided a key tool for investigators to better understand the normal and abnormal physiology associated with anemia in a variety of disease states. It is through such basic and translational research that biomedical and scientific knowledge, in general, advances and leads to improvements in patient care.

M.M. Avram.(ed.), Improving Prognosis for Kidney Disorders, 9-27.

The biomedical research into the structure of rHuEPO led to the development of a novel erythropoiesis stimulating protein, darbepoetin alfa (Aranesp^{TM}, Amgen Inc., Thousand Oaks, CA). Darbepoetin alfa, also known as NESP (novel erythropoiesis-stimulating protein), is a longer-acting erythropoietic agent that allows less frequent dosing to treat anemia, compared with rHuEPO.[18] Decreased dosing frequency should result in enhanced patient compliance and convenience and minimize the burden that frequent administration places on patients and healthcare staff.

This chapter reviews our current knowledge and understanding of anemia in CKD and highlights its management with the currently established therapy, rHuEPO. In addition, this chapter provides data on the use of the novel erythropoiesis stimulating protein, darbepoetin alfa.

Physiology of EPO

Structure of Endogenous EPO

The gene for EPO was isolated in 1985.[13] It is located on chromosome 7 and consists of five exons and four introns. EPO is a 166-amino acid peptide that has two sulfide bridges, four sites of carbohydrate attachment and a molecular weight of 30,000 daltons.[19] In order to be secreted and to have significant biological activity, the protein molecule must be glycosylated. This is accomplished with four complex carbohydrate chains containing sialic acid molecules.[20] It is the sialic acid moieties that allow EPO to circulate in the blood for a sufficient time to reach the bone marrow and stimulate EPO receptors.[21]

Physiology of Erythropoiesis

Synthesis and Stimulus

EPO is synthesized by fibroblast-derived interstitial cells in proximity to proximal tubular cells of the cortex and outer medulla of the kidney.[22,23] Because expression of the EPO gene *in vitro* in isolated renal cell lines has not yet been accomplished, it is difficult to study the cellular mechanisms that control the renal production of this hormone. Normal plasma levels of EPO are 8-24 mU/mL, requiring daily continuous synthesis of 2-3 U/kg body weight.[24] It is known that the production of EPO is regulated by oxygen availability and increases when arterial pO_2 is decreased or in conditions of anemia or increased hemoglobin affinity.[25] It has also been established that activation of EPO gene expression requires specific transcription factors, including hypoxia-inducible factor-1, a DNA-binding transcriptional complex that is essential for the enhancer function of this gene.[26]

In the adult, EPO synthesis also takes place in hepatocytes[27,28] and the Ito cells[29] of the liver,[30] although to a lesser degree than in the kidney. In addition, EPO gene expression has been found in the lung, spleen,[31,32] brain, testes and ovaries.[23] Although it is known that EPO regulates the growth and development of erythroid progenitor cells, this hormone may have other physiological functions because functional EPO receptors have been discovered on human, rat and mouse kidney cells.[33]

The EPO receptor is a 55,000 dalton transmembrane protein.[34] This protein is a 507-amino acid polypeptide having a single membrane-spanning domain, the extracellular N-terminal region containing the EPO-binding domain and the C-terminal intracellular region participating in signal transduction.[35] The process of signal transduction involves the activation of tyrosine kinase, which phosphorylates a set of intracellular proteins, resulting in the release of second messengers.[36] It is unclear how these second messengers act, but it is thought that the signals prevent apoptosis of the progenitor cells.[37]

Life Cycle of Erythropoiesis

The development of an erythrocyte begins with the differentiation of a pool of pluripotent stem cells from a stochastic differentiation of bipotential or multipotential progenitors in the bone marrow (**Figure 1**).[38] These committed progenitor cells are stimulated from the G0 to G1 cell cycle stage by interleukin-1, interleukin-6 and granulocyte-macrophage colony-stimulating factor (GM-CSF).[39] From G1, the progenitor cells differentiate into the burst-forming unit-erythroid (BFU-E), stimulated by interleukin-3 and GM-CSF. The BFU-E is different from the previous cell type because, although it has EPO receptors, it has lost the ability of self-renewal. The BFU-E differentiates into a colony forming unit-erythroid (CFU-E). The number of CFU-Es is proportional to the EPO level.[40,41] The CFU-E is more sensitive and dependent on EPO for survival and differentiation into a proerythroblast,[42] although it cannot be distinguished from the BFU-E by specific morphological features. The proerythroblast, which is unaffected by EPO, then continues to develop into a normoblast. The normoblast goes on to form a reticulocyte and then finally matures into an erythrocyte (**Figure 1**). Although erythropoiesis is mainly controlled by EPO, it is also influenced by cytokines and other growth factors. Interleukin-9 and GM-CSF have been shown to have burst-promoting effects.[43,44] In addition, a subset of BFU-Es is able to survive without

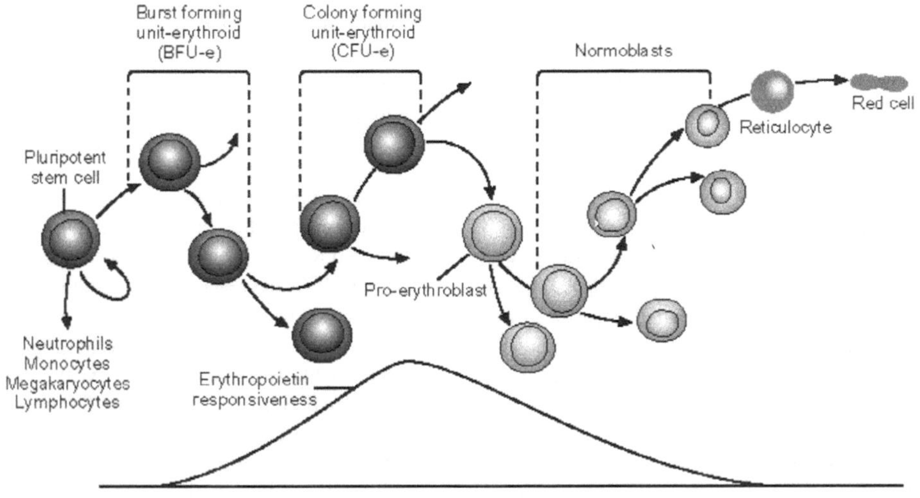

Figure 1. The involvement of EPO in cellular differentiation during erythropoiesis. Reproduced with the permission of McGraw-Hill.[216]

EPO if interleukin-3 or GM-CSF is present.[45] Steel factor (SF, also called c-kit ligand), interleukin-3 or GM-CSF, along with EPO, are required by BFU-Es to increase the number of cells and mature to form CFU-Es.[46-50] Insulin, or insulin-like growth factor I, is also needed for optimal transformation of a CFU-E to an erythroblast.[51] Other factors, such as androgens, thyroxine, somatomedin and catecholamines, appear to increase the growth of CFU-E but are not considered to be essential.[52] In addition, vitamin A has been shown to increase the concentration of EPO when added to hepatoma cell lines in medium and thus may influence erythropoiesis.[53] Cytokines that have a negative effect on erythropoiesis include interleukin-1α and -1β, interleukin-2, tumor necrosis factor-α (TNF-α) and transforming growth factor-β (TGF-β).[54-56]

Although the erythroblast does not require EPO for maturation, EPO continues to have an influence at this stage of erythropoiesis. For example, it appears to be involved in preventing neocytolysis, which is a process of selective hemolysis of the youngest circulating erythrocytes when there is an over-abundance of red blood cells.[57] This effect has been documented in astronauts and in individuals who have been living at high altitude and who then descend to sea level.[58-60] Studies in patients on hemodialysis have shown that neocytolysis contributes to the anemia of renal disease[61] and can be prevented with low doses of subcutaneous (SC) EPO.[60]

rHuEPO

Available Forms

Currently there are two forms of rHuEPO – epoetin alfa and epoetin beta – in clinical use worldwide, and an additional form – epoetin omega – is currently under evaluation.[62] At the present time, epoetin alfa is the only form of rHuEPO available in the US; while epoetin beta, with a similar efficacy and safety profile, is available in other countries. Because of the need for glycosylation, epoetin alfa is manufactured in mammalian (Chinese hamster ovary) cells. The novel erythropoiesis stimulating protein, darbepoetin alfa, has also become available in Europe and Australia for the management of anemia in patients with CKD and is currently awaiting FDA approval in the US.

Pharmacology of rHuEPO

The metabolism of rHuEPO does not appear to depend on the kidney or liver; it is thought to be metabolized by a compartment known as the 'erythron', which is the total mass of cells in the erythropoietic pathway that is EPO-dependent.[2] Animal studies have shown that removal of the kidneys or liver does not affect the volume of distribution, mean residence time or half-life of I^{125}-labeled rHuEPO.[63] The pharmacokinetics of rHuEPO are nonlinear.[64-65] The half-life of intravenous (IV) rHuEPO is 4–9 hours and greater than 24 hours when given by SC injection.[66] The distribution volume is similar in uremic and normal individuals after IV dosing.[67] However, the termination elimination half-life is longer; and the whole body clearance is reduced in uremic patients. After SC dosing, the bioavailability of rHuEPO is lower in uremic patients compared to normal individuals, with a lower and delayed peak concentration.

Route of Administration

rHuEPO can be given either by the IV, SC or intraperitoneal route, with the IV route being favored in the US. The intraperitoneal administration of rHuEPO is generally not recommended because of low bioavailability (2–12%) compared with IV and SC dosing.[68-69] If intraperitoneal rHuEPO must be utilized, it should be administered when there is no dialysate in the peritoneal cavity.[70] SC injection frequently gives a plasma level that is 10% of that seen with IV dosing. The time to peak concentration after SC administration is usually greater than 10 hours, while the bioavailability ranges from 16% to 50%.[68,71–75] The bioavailability of rHuEPO has also been shown to vary depending on where the SC injection is given, with greater bioavailability seen when it is given in the thigh compared with the abdomen or arm.[76] The amount of skinfold thickness of the patient has also been shown to inversely influence the effectiveness of a given dose of SC rHuEPO.[77]

Target Hemoglobin

There is continued debate about the appropriate target hemoglobin level in renal patients treated with rHuEPO. When the planning for the Phase 3 trial for rHuEPO was undertaken, hematologists proposed a normal hemoglobin target (14 g/dL), whereas nephrologists recommended a lower level because of concern about potential vascular complications of higher hemoglobin levels.[78] A compromise was reached, and a target hematocrit of 32–38% was used. Subsequently, the National Kidney Foundation Dialysis Outcomes Quality Initiative guidelines recommended a target hemoglobin of 11-12 g/dL (hematocrit 33-36%), which is supported by a large body of evidence.[79] A number of nephrologists, in fact, consider that an even lower hemoglobin level may be adequate to achieve sufficient clinical benefits.[80]

There is increasing evidence to suggest that normalization of hemoglobin may be beneficial in some patients. The greatest amount of data in this regard relates to brain function. There is clear evidence that brain electrophysiology improves when hemoglobin is normalized compared with when hemoglobin levels are below normal.[81] Further studies in dialysis-dependent patients have confirmed that normalization of hemoglobin level improves brain circulation, metabolism and oxygen delivery.[82-3] Physical performance as well as sleep disorders, which are common in dialysis-dependent patients, improve significantly when hemoglobin is normalized.[84-85]

However, the Normal Hematocrit Cardiac Trial in hemodialysis-dependent patients with coronary artery disease and/or symptomatic heart failure was discontinued because the group of patients who were randomized to the normal hematocrit group were found to have a 30% increased risk of death or myocardial infarction when compared with the control group.[86] Although the safety of raising the hemoglobin to normal levels needs to be confirmed, particularly in light of the Normal Hematocrit Cardiac Trial,[86] clinicians must exercise clinical judgment and try to aim for an appropriate target hemoglobin for each patient. Results of additional studies in this area should provide further guidance on the target hemoglobin level.[87-89]

Dosing of rHuEPO

The initial IV dose of rHuEPO should be 120–180 U/kg/week, given in three divided doses.[79] When the SC route is used in adult patients with ESRD, rHuEPO is generally initiated at 80–120 U/kg/week, given in two to three doses. Pediatric patients less than 5 years of age commonly require higher doses (300 U/kg/week) than older pediatric patients[90-91] and adults.

The dose that is initially selected should achieve the target hemoglobin (11–12 g/dL) or hematocrit (33–36%) within a 2- to 4-month period. During dose titration of rHuEPO, hemoglobin or hematocrit should be measured every 1–2 weeks until a stable target level is achieved. Frequent monitoring is needed initially to detect a poor or overly rapid response to rHuEPO. After a stable target hemoglobin or hematocrit is achieved, hemoglobin or hematocrit should be monitored every 2–4 weeks.[79] The maintenance dose varies tremendously among patients, from 1000 U to over 10,000 U per treatment;[64-65,68] although the average dose in the US is currently around 17,000 U per week.[92] In general, doses of rHuEPO should not be changed by more than 25%. Such dosage modifications are generally not necessary or effective more frequently than every 2–4 weeks.[79] Withdrawal of rHuEPO to permit a fall in hemoglobin that is higher than the upper target limit is rarely necessary and should be discouraged.

Refractoriness to rHuEPO

An IV dose of 450 U/kg/week or SC dose of 300 U/kg/week will achieve the target hemoglobin level in 96% of patients within 4–6 months, as long as there are adequate iron stores.[78,93] rHuEPO resistance should be considered in patients with sufficient iron stores who do not achieve the target hemoglobin level within this time frame and in those who fail to maintain the hemoglobin level at the previously effective dose.

Iron deficiency is the most common cause of initial or acquired resistance to rHuEPO and is still highly prevalent, despite the availability of parenteral iron compounds.[94-95] Functional iron deficiency develops when the demand for iron exceeds availability.[96] It is common in hemodialysis-dependent patients because of the chronic blood loss (as much as 4500 mL on an annual basis) that results from laboratory tests and blood remaining in the dialyzer and tubing. In addition, rHuEPO, by accelerating erythropoiesis, further increases the demand for iron. The best way to replenish iron stores in hemodialysis-dependent patients is by IV iron infusion. However, patients on peritoneal dialysis and patients with CKD but not yet on dialysis may be able to maintain iron stores with oral iron, although gastrointestinal side effects may limit the effectiveness of this therapy.[97] In addition, as transferrin saturation rises above 15%, intestinal iron absorption becomes impaired, thus decreasing the bioavailability of oral iron.[98]

Inflammatory states are also frequently the cause of poor response to rHuEPO. These may result from chronic infections, post-surgery, rheumatologic diseases or the dialysis process itself, particularly if bioincompatible dialysis membranes or pyrogen-containing water are used. The inflammatory state is usually associated with inflammatory cytokines, such as interleukin-1β and TNF-α, which decrease bone marrow responsiveness to rHuEPO.[99-100] The presence of inflammation is also associated with an impairment of iron release from the reticuloendothelial system ('reticuloendothelial blockade').[101] An elevated C-reactive protein level may be a useful diagnostic indicator when chronic inflammation is suspected as a cause of resistance to rHuEPO.[102-103]

Activation of the renin-angiotensin system is thought to increase endogenous EPO production.[104] Angiotensin-converting enzyme inhibitors (ACEIs) may also contribute to a decrease in rHuEPO responsiveness; and indeed, EPO production has been shown to decrease in patients with CKD who are treated with ACEI.[105] In addition, post-renal transplant erythrocytosis has been effectively treated with ACEI.[106] The exact mechanism of how ACEI may decrease erythropoiesis in patients receiving exogenous EPO is unknown. Some hypotheses for this phenomenon include a reduction in production of interleukin-12, which is known to stimulate erythropoiesis,[107] and a decrease in angiotensin II-stimulated erythroid progenitor cell maturation, an effect that has been demonstrated *in vitro*.[108] The data are conflicting as to whether ACEIs inhibit erythropoiesis in dialysis patients receiving rHuEPO because many of the studies have been uncontrolled or had small numbers of patients.[109-112]

Blood loss through the gastrointestinal tract, repeated episodes of dialyzer clotting or hemolysis should also be considered in the evaluation of rHuEPO resistance. Recently, hemolysis of erythrocytes has been demonstrated in hemodialysis patients due to high levels of chloramine present in the water used to prepare dialysate.[113-115]

L-carnitine deficiency has been suggested by some to contribute to refractoriness to rHuEPO. Dialysis patients may have decreased predialytic serum concentrations of free L-carnitine, and low muscle carnitine content.[116-118] Some studies have shown that L-carnitine may increase reticulocyte count[119] or improve mechanical stability of erythrocytes.[120] However, the majority of studies designed to evaluate the benefit of L-carnitine in this setting have yielded conflicting results.[121-124]

Severe hyperparathyroidism, resulting in osteitis fibrosa cystica with bone marrow fibrosis, has also been shown to cause rHuEPO resistance.[125] Other explanations for the relationship between parathyroid hormone (PTH) and rHuEPO resistance include a direct toxic effect of PTH on erythroid precursors, PTH-induced hemolysis or PTH inhibition of endogenous EPO production.[126,127] Although there is little *in vivo* evidence that any of these mechanisms are active, other than bone marrow fibrosis, it has been shown that medical treatment or surgical parathyroidectomy is effective in reducing rHuEPO resistance.[128-132]

Clinical Effects of Partial Anemia Correction

Quality of Life

Anemia of renal disease manifests by a variety of symptoms that differ from patient to patient. Symptoms related to quality of life include alterations in psychosocial function, poor physical and mental function, sexual dysfunction and a high incidence of depression.

Improvements in a variety of these symptoms after partial correction of anemia with rHuEPO have been demonstrated using the Kidney Disease Quality of Life-Short Form (KDQOL-SF 36), the Karnofsky index, the Sickness Impact Profile and many other indexes.[133-137] A greater improvement in quality of life on the Sickness Impact Profile was achieved with the correction of anemia to hemoglobin levels of more than 12 g/dL.[138] In another study, correcting anemia resulted in an improvement in sexual function, which may be secondary to increased serum testosterone or decreased lutenizing hormone.[139] Exercise capacity improves significantly in patients treated with rHuEPO, including those patients with coronary artery disease and rest angina.[140,141]

Sensitization is associated with multiple blood transfusions and may be avoided with rHuEPO, increasing the chances of acceptance of renal transplantation and indirectly improving quality of life.[142]

Brain and Cognitive Function

Despite adequate dialysis, patients with ESRD still have mild neurobehavioral impairments, with abnormalities persisting on cognitive function and electrophysiological testing.[143–145] Although there are many factors contributing to these abnormalities, it is clear that anemia is one of the most important factors impacting on brain function in these patients.[146] The impairment in cognitive function may be due to alterations in cerebral oxygen delivery that occur in the presence of anemia.[147] Cognitive function in these patients improves when the hematocrit is increased to 36%.[148–151] Normalizing the hematocrit to 40–45% may lead to even further improvement in neurocognitive function, shown using quantitative electroencephalographic techniques.[81]

Cardiovascular Disease

Cardiovascular disease still accounts for over 50% of total deaths in patients on dialysis,[152] with significant cardiac disease often present prior to starting on dialysis.[153] The anemia of renal failure causes hypoxic vasodilatation, increased sympathetic stimulation and decreased blood viscosity.[154] The latter exacerbates peripheral vasodilatation and contributes to decreased total systemic vascular resistance.[155] Cardiac output increases in a compensatory fashion to maintain adequate perfusion to tissues.[156]

Serial echocardiographic studies performed in ESRD patients following the initiation of chronic dialysis have shown that left ventricular dilatation with compensatory hypertrophy is the major pattern of disease progression.[89] Patients with left ventricular dilatation and normal systolic function have a poor prognosis, with a high mortality rate at 2 years. The prognosis in patients with left ventricular hypertrophy with normal systolic function, on the other hand, is better.[157] Anemia is an important risk factor for these cardiac abnormalities and a predictor of mortality in patients with ESRD.[158] Patients with anemia of renal failure have a higher risk of developing cardiomyopathy, which increases the risk of congestive heart failure and death.

In numerous studies, partial correction of anemia with rHuEPO was shown to decrease hypoxic vasodilatation, increase systemic vascular resistance and reduce cardiac output.[156,159–165] In addition, partial correction of anemia with rHuEPO may result in decreased left ventricular mass and volume.[156,159,160,166–168] The Canadian randomized controlled trial of hemoglobin normalization with rHuEPO showed that there was no significant regression of left ventricular mass index in patients with left ventricular hypertrophy, but there was slowed progression in patients with left ventricular dilation.[89] However, it is less clear whether such changes will result in improved mortality or regression of cardiomyopathy. The Normal Hematocrit Cardiac Trial in hemodialysis patients with coronary artery disease and/or symptomatic heart failure was discontinued before differences reached statistical significance after it was found that the patients who were randomized to the normal hematocrit group had a 30% increased risk of death or myocardial infarction when compared with the control group.[86] The effect that normalizing hemoglobin with rHuEPO had on cardiomyopathy progression was recently examined in hemodialysis patients with concentric left ventricular hypertrophy or left ventricular dilatation.[169] Study results showed that normalizing the hemoglobin did not cause regression of the concentric left ventricular hypertrophy or left ventricular dilatation.

Mortality

Several epidemiological studies have demonstrated the survival benefits of partial correction of anemia with rHuEPO. Madore and colleagues retrospectively studied 21,899 patients who were on hemodialysis throughout the US from October 1 through December 31, 1992.[170] Compared with patients with a hemoglobin concentration of 10–11 g/dL, those with a hemoglobin concentration of 8 g/dL or less had a two-fold increase in the odds ratio of death. There was no decrease in the odds ratio of death in patients with a hemoglobin concentration greater than 11 g/dL. Other patient characteristics and laboratory data, however, were not adjusted for in this analysis.

Ma and colleagues retrospectively studied Medicare patients on hemodialysis and included in the analysis comorbidity ('severity of disease') adjustment and data on hospitalizations.[171] The group of patients with hematocrit levels less than 30% had an overall relative risk of death that was 12–33% higher than that of patients with hematocrit levels in the range of 30–33%, even after adjusting for the severity of disease.

In an additional report using United States Renal Data System (USRDS) data, Collins and colleagues evaluated whether changes in hematocrit level, rather than just a single or average value, would affect mortality rates over a 6-month period.[172–174] As had been shown in the previous studies, patients with the lowest hematocrits had the highest risk of death. Lower hematocrit levels were more likely for those patients who were younger, female and African-American, as well as for those with more comorbidities, hospital days, blood transfusions and vascular access procedures. Patients who started with a low hematocrit that then rose had a risk of death that was equivalent to the group of patients whose hematocrit had been stable at the higher level for the full year. This study showed that a patient with a low hematocrit that is responsive to rHuEPO has a good prognosis, while refractoriness to rHuEPO in a patient with a low hematocrit is a poor prognostic sign.

Hospitalizations

There are only a small number of studies that have assessed the relationship between the level of anemia and hospitalizations in rHuEPO-treated patients. In a case-controlled study by Churchill and colleagues, patients treated with rHuEPO had fewer hospitalizations and decreased length of stay compared with a matched group of patients who did not receive rHuEPO, but the differences were not statistically significant.[175] Xia and coworkers analyzed the data from the mortality analysis of Ma and colleagues[171] and found that patients with hematocrit levels less than 30% had a 14–30% increased risk of hospitalization without disease severity adjustment; this increased risk fell somewhat to 7–8% with disease severity adjustment.[176] Patients with hematocrit levels in the 33–36% range had the lowest risk of hospitalization.

Side Effects of rHuEPO

Hypertension

rHuEPO is known to be associated with the development or worsening of pre-existing hypertension within weeks to months of initiation in approximately 25% of treated patients.[177–180] However, this was not confirmed in a recent study of the effects of normalizing the hemoglobin level on ambulatory blood pressure in patients with cardiac disease.[181]

The specific mechanism of rHuEPO-related hypertension is unknown, but there are many theories based on animal and human studies, which focus mostly on the possible role of stimulation of endothelin by rHuEPO.[182–185] One study demonstrated that endothelin antagonists were able to inhibit rHuEPO-induced hypertension.[186] It has also been shown that EPO induces nitric oxide synthase activity without affecting endothelin-1 release, suggesting that the mechanism of rHuEPO-related hypertension is not a direct effect on endothelial cells.[187] In contrast, animal studies have suggested that rHuEPO-related hypertension may be caused by resistance to the vasodilatory action of nitric oxide.[188,189] An increase in calcium uptake, which has been demonstrated *in vitro* with endothelial cells treated with rHuEPO, may also play a part in the development of hypertension.[190,191]

Research has shown that the increase in hemoglobin and hematocrit are not themselves responsible for the rise in blood pressure.[188,189,192,193] rHuEPO-induced hypertension can easily be treated by initiating or increasing anti-hypertensive medications or by increasing the amount of ultrafiltration during dialysis. Withholding or decreasing the dose of rHuEPO has not been shown to be effective or necessary, although this may be tried if the hypertension is refractory to anti-hypertensive medication.

Other Adverse Effects

Although initial concern existed about the possibility of various other side effects associated with rHuEPO treatment, none of these have proven to be clinically manifested at the currently achieved target hemoglobin levels. Seizures were initially thought to occur with a higher frequency in patients receiving rHuEPO,[78] but a controlled study did not show this correlation.[194] In addition, an increase in vascular access thrombosis has not been convincingly demonstrated.[195] The Normal Hematocrit Cardiac Trial did, however, show an increased risk of vascular access thrombosis in the high hematocrit group (39% versus 29%)[86] in native fistulas as well as grafts, suggesting that this issue requires further investigation. Hyperkalemia was also initially observed with early use of rHuEPO,[15] but more recent data suggest that significant hyperkalemia is not a serious rHuEPO-related problem.[195–198] There is a recent report that EPO stimulates the proliferation of human renal cell carcinoma cells *in vitro.*[199] To date, however, there is no indication that renal cell carcinoma has become more prevalent since the widespread use of rHuEPO began.

Public Policy Issues

There is little debate about the clinical value of treating anemic renal patients with rHuEPO and correcting anemia to the currently recommended target levels. It is clear, however, that this treatment is costly; and the Health Care Financing Administration (HCFA), now called the Center for Medicare and Medicaid Services

(CMS), in the US is concerned about the benefits of further expenditures in this area. If one looks only at the change in hematocrit and the cost of the rHuEPO used to achieve this change over the past 5 years, it would appear that considerably more rHuEPO is being used with only a small improvement in hematocrit.[200] This should not be surprising, however, because there is not a linear dose–response relationship between dose of rHuEPO and resultant hematocrit. Two recently published studies on normalizing hematocrit in patients on hemodialysis both showed that a three- to four-fold increase in rHuEPO dose is necessary to raise the hematocrit from the low 30s to the low 40s.[81,86]

A recent study by Collins and coworkers looked not only at the direct cost of rHuEPO but all Medicare expenditures in a cohort of patients receiving rHu EPO.[201] This comprehensive analysis showed that, although the direct costs for rHuEPO rose between 1991 and 1995, total Medicare expenditures were significantly lower for patients with a hematocrit of 33–36%. It is hypothesized that patients with higher hematocrits are more likely to be healthier and to require less rHu EPO and, thus, consume fewer health resources overall and cost less; but this remains to be validated.

At the present time, clinicians must provide medical justification if they feel that a patient would benefit from a hematocrit level maintained above 36.5%. While the benefits of normal hematocrits have not been conclusively proven, it is clear that they are real in some patients.

The most vexing policy issue involving rHuEPO relates to the current pricing, cost and reimbursement system. Dialysis facilities negotiate the per-unit cost of rHuEPO with the only available supplier in the US, Amgen. Large dialysis chains are able to negotiate discounts and obtain further discounts based on hitting specific anemia management targets. However, this results in the increasing reliance of dialysis facilities on profits from rHuEPO to support the overall operation of their facilities. This payment fills in the gap between the cost of providing dialysis services and the payment per treatment (the composite rate), which has remained static for many years and is no longer adequate to cover the costs of services. This shortfall makes facilities, especially those in under-served and rural areas, vulnerable to uncontrollable events, like drug price increases, as recently occurred with rHu EPO. For dialysis to continue to be available as needed, policymakers must re-examine the structure of the entire payment system for outpatient dialysis, including the method of payment of pharmaceuticals such as rHuEPO.

Darbepoetin Alfa – Preclinical and Clinical Development

Following the introduction of rHuEPO over 10 years ago, epoetin alfa has become the standard of care for renal anemia.[16,17] However, the pharmacodynamic efficacy of rHuEPO has been limited by its relatively short half-life (4–8 hours)[64] and by its requirement for repeated administration. The current standard of care is to administer rHuEPO two to three times per week, which may require patients on home dialysis or those with CKD but not yet on dialysis having to make special trips to the physician or clinic for their rHuEPO injection.

In order to simplify the management of anemia, darbepoetin alfa was developed.[18] This created the potential for dosing once weekly and once every other week to treat renal anemia in patients with CKD[202] and dialysis-dependent patients.[18]

The Development, Structure and Mechanism of Action of Darbepoetin Alfa

The discovery and development of darbepoetin alfa arose from research into the structural features of EPO. To create a molecule with enhanced biological activity and to allow less frequent dosing, research was initially directed towards elucidating those factors and structural features that control the *in vivo* activity of EPO.[203]

Studies of EPO carbohydrate isoforms in animals demonstrated a direct relationship between the sialyated carbohydrate content of EPO and its half-life and *in vivo* biological activity. In addition, the sialyated carbohydrate content correlated inversely with its receptor-binding affinity (determined by radioreceptor assay).[204] The experiments showed that, for EPO, serum clearance has a stronger influence on *in vivo* activity than receptor-binding affinity.[203]

These observations led to the hypothesis that increasing the carbohydrate content of EPO would lead to a molecule with increased serum half-life and hence enhanced biological activity. Darbepoetin alfa was developed to test this hypothesis. By combining the carbohydrate addition sites of two successfully glycosylated four-chain analogs into one molecule, an analog with five N-linked chains, darbepoetin alfa, was created.[203]

Darbepoetin alfa is biochemically distinct from rHuEPO, having an increased molecular weight and greater negative charge (**Figure 2**).

Darbepoetin alfa binds to the same receptor and has the same mechanism of action and intracellular

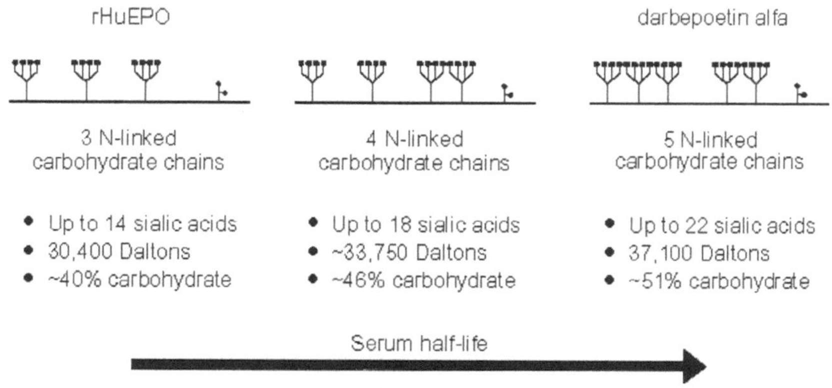

Figure 2. Comparison of the structure and biochemical properties of rHuEPO and erythropoietic proteins containing four and five N-linked carbohydrate chains.[203]

signaling mechanism (involving receptor tyrosine kinase phosphorylation) as EPO.[18] It stimulates the proliferation and differentiation of red blood cell pre-cursors in the bone marrow and prolongs their survival by inhibiting apoptosis. This serves to increase the blood hemoglobin concentration, hence correcting anemia.

Pharmacokinetics and Biological Activity of Darbepoetin Alfa in Animals

The pharmacokinetic profile and biological activity of darbepoetin alfa, relative to rHuEPO, were determined in rats, dogs and mice.[203] To confirm that the mechanism of increased activity was due to an increase in the circulating half-life, the pharmacokinetics of rHuEPO, a molecule with one additional carbohydrate chain and a molecule with two additional carbohydrate chains (darbepoetin alfa) were compared. Results showed that the greater the sialic acid-containing content of the molecule, the longer its circulating half-life.[203]

These results confirmed the hypothesis that increasing the sialic acid-containing carbohydrate content beyond the theoretical maximum of EPO could extend the serum half-life of an erythropoietic protein, and that the longer serum half-life would lead to an increase of *in vivo* biological activity. This was confirmed by dose-dependent increases in the hemoglobin levels in normal mice injected with darbepoetin alfa by the IV, intraperitoneal and SC routes.[203] Darbepoetin alfa was approximately 3.6-fold more potent than rHuEPO when each molecule was administered three times per week. However, when each molecule was administered once-weekly, darbepoetin alfa was found to be 13- to 14-fold more potent.[203]

Pharmacokinetic Profile of Darbepoetin Alfa in Humans

A clinical program was initiated to verify that darbepoetin alfa (due to its increased sialyated carbohydrate content) had a longer serum half-life in patients, so that it could be administered less frequently than rHuEPO.

In a double-blind, randomized crossover study, the single-dose pharmacokinetics of rHuEPO (100 U/kg) and an equivalent peptide mass of darbepoetin alfa administered by the IV route were compared in 11 patients receiving peritoneal dialysis.[69] Serum levels of rHuEPO and darbepoetin alfa were determined by immunoassay at regular time points for up to 96 hours after dosing. In all patients, darbepoetin alfa had a longer terminal half-life than rHuEPO (**Figure 3**). The mean terminal half-life for darbepoetin alfa following IV injection was 25.3 hours, approximately three-fold longer than that determined for rHuEPO (8.5 hours). Darbepoetin alfa had a significantly greater area under serum concentration-time curve, and clearance was lower compared with similar doses of rHuEPO (**Table 1**). The volume of distribution of darbepoetin alfa was similar to that of rHuEPO (52.4 mL/kg versus 48.7 mL/kg).[69] This first study in humans confirmed that darbepoetin alfa has a longer serum half-life than rHuEPO.

Pharmacokinetic investigation following SC administration in six of these patients showed that the mean terminal elimination half-life for darbepoetin alfa was 48.8 hours, which was twice as long as that for IV darbepoetin alfa (**Table 1**).

A longer half-life was expected because of the slower absorption into the circulation from the SC injection site. The mean bioavailability of SC

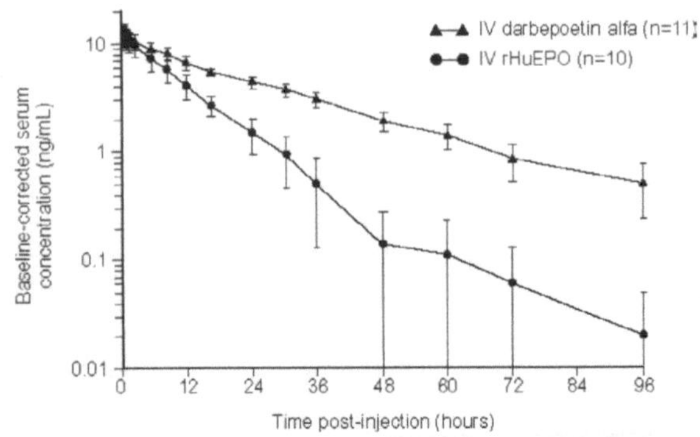

Figure 3. Comparative pharmacokinetics of darbepoetin alfa and epoetin alfa in anemic dialysis patients. Results are expressed as the mean (±SD). Reproduced with the permission of Lippincott Williams and Wilkins.[69]

darbepoetin alfa was 36.9%,[69] which was similar to that reported for SC rHuEPO.[73]

The pharmacokinetics of darbepoetin alfa have also been determined following chronic IV[205] and SC[206] administration. Darbepoetin alfa administered by the IV route three times a week or once a week was compared with IV administration of rHuEPO three times weekly. The elimination half-life of darbepoetin alfa was again approximately three-fold longer than that of rHuEPO. The pharmacokinetics of chronic IV therapy were both dose- and time-linear, and there was no evidence of accumulation during 48 weeks of treatment.[205] The pharmacokinetic profile of SC darbepoetin alfa given once weekly was also investigated over 7 days during weeks 1 and 8 of a long-term maintenance study. The results suggested that there was no evidence of dose- or time-dependence with chronic SC administration and no accumulation of darbepoetin alfa over time.[206]

The pharmacokinetics of IV and SC darbepoetin alfa were also evaluated in a small number of pediatric patients with CKD and were found to be similar to those in adults.[207] There was evidence from the time to maximum serum concentration (t_{max}) that SC darbepoetin alfa may be absorbed more rapidly in children (mean t_{max}, 36.2 hours in children versus 54.1 hours in adults),[207] an effect that has been documented with rHuEPO.[208]

Clinical Trials of Darbepoetin Alfa in Dialysis Patients with Anemia

The clinical study program for darbepoetin alfa in the nephrology setting has, to date, involved over 1500 patients in studies conducted across the US, Europe, Australia and Canada. The clinical program examined the efficacy and safety of darbepoetin alfa in three phases of anemia management in CKD: correction in rHuEPO-naive patients, conversion from rHuEPO to darbepoetin alfa, and long-term maintenance of hemoglobin concentrations.

Correction of Anemia in rHuEPO-Naive Patients

Two multicenter studies were initiated using an open-label, dose-escalation protocol to find the optimal darbepoetin alfa dose.[209] The study designs were very similar: one study involving hemodialysis patients treated with IV darbepoetin alfa and the other involving peritoneal dialysis patients receiving SC darbepoetin alfa. Patients received darbepoetin alfa once-weekly at a dose range of 0.075–0.75 µg/kg or three times weekly at a dose range of 0.025–0.25 µg/kg.[209]

There was a dose-dependent increase in hemoglobin in both studies (**Figure 4**). These dose-finding studies suggested that an appropriate starting dose for the treatment of anemia with darbepoetin alfa was in the range of 0.45–0.75 µg/kg administered IV or SC once-weekly.

Table 1. Comparison of the mean pharmacokinetic parameters of IV rHuEPO with IV and SC darbepoetin alfa.[69]

Parameter	IV rHuEPO (n = 10)	IV Darbepoetin Alfa (n = 11)	SC Darbepoetin Alfa (n = 6)
$t_{½z}$ (h)	8.5	25.3	48.8
T_{max} (h)	–	–	54.1
C_{max} (mg/L)	–	–	0.9
AUC (mg/h/L)*	131.9	291.0	108.2
CL (mL/h/kg)	4.0	1.6	–
V_d (mL/kg)	48.7	52.4	–
F (%)	–	–	36.9

Abbreviations: $t_{½z}$, terminal phase elimination half-life; T_{max}, time to maximum serum concentration; C_{max}, maximum serum concentration; AUC, area under serum concentration–time curve: CL, clearance; V_d, volume of distribution at steady state; F, bioavailability.
*$AUC_{(0-96)}$ IV; $AUC_{(0-\infty)}$ SC.

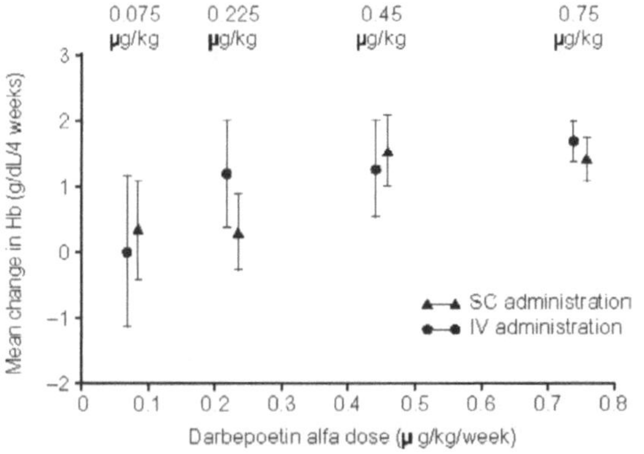

Figure 4. Mean rise in hemoglobin concentration (95% CI) over the first 4 weeks of SC darbepoetin alfa administration in patients on peritoneal dialysis (▲) and IV darbepoetin alfa administration in patients on hemodialysis (•). Reproduced with the permission of Oxford University Press.[18]

Switching Patients from rHuEPO to Darbepoetin Alfa Therapy

Dialysis-dependent patients who were successfully maintained on rHuEPO were switched to darbepoetin alfa therapy in two studies to determine whether darbepoetin alfa was as effective and safe in maintaining hemoglobin levels when administered at a reduced dosing frequency compared with rHuEPO.[210,211] Patients were clinically stable and had a hemoglobin concentration of 9.5–12.5 g/dL during a 4-week screening and baseline period. Patients were then randomized to darbepoetin alfa or rHuEPO, with the darbepoetin alfa-treated patients switching to an equivalent total weekly dose but with a reduced frequency of administration; and the rHuEPO-treated patients continuing with the same dose and frequency of administration. The route of administration remained the same. The primary endpoint for these studies was the change in hemoglobin concentration between the baseline period on rHuEPO and the evaluation period (i.e. following 20–24 weeks of darbepoetin alfa therapy).

In the first study — a multicenter, double-blind study — 507 hemodialysis patients in North America were randomized either to receive IV darbepoetin alfa once-weekly plus placebo twice-weekly ($n = 169$) or to continue on IV rHuEPO three times weekly ($n = 338$). The mean hemoglobin concentration remained stable in both treatment groups from baseline to evaluation period. The mean change in hemoglobin level was +0.16 g/dL for darbepoetin alfa and 0.00 g/dL for rHuEPO, which was neither a statistically nor clinically significant difference.[210]

The second study was a large, multicenter study, in which 522 patients receiving hemodialysis or peritoneal dialysis were randomized to darbepoetin alfa ($n = 347$) or rHuEPO ($n = 175$).[211] Patients on rHuEPO two or three times a week converted to once-weekly darbepoetin alfa. Patients on once-weekly rHuEPO converted to darbepoetin alfa once every 2 weeks. The mean hemoglobin concentration remained stable from the baseline to the evaluation period for both treatment groups, with a change in hemoglobin of –0.03 g/dL for darbepoetin alfa and –0.06 g/dL for rHuEPO. The between-group difference in the mean change in hemoglobin concentration from baseline to the evaluation period was neither statistically or clinically significant. At the end of the evaluation period (weeks 24–32), 97% of darbepoetin alfa patients assigned to once-weekly dosing and 95% of patients assigned to once every other week dosing were successfully managed at these reduced dose frequencies.[211]

The conclusion from both these studies is that darbepoetin alfa is as effective as rHuEPO for maintaining hemoglobin levels with the advantage of less frequent dosing.

Maintenance of Hemoglobin Levels with Darbepoetin Alfa

The ability of darbepoetin alfa to safely maintain hemoglobin levels for up to 1 year was evaluated in an open-label, multicenter study conducted in Europe and Australia.[206] A total of 703 patients on hemodialysis or peritoneal dialysis with a stable baseline hemoglobin concentration of 9.5–12.5 g/dL were switched from rHuEPO to darbepoetin alfa therapy. The frequency of darbepoetin alfa was reduced to once every other week in patients receiving rHuEPO once-weekly ($n = 157$) and to once-weekly in patients receiving rHuEPO twice ($n = 203$) or three times ($n = 343$) weekly. The darbepoetin alfa dose was titrated to maintain the hemoglobin level within –1.0 and +1.5 g/dL of the patient's baseline hemoglobin, and within a range of 9.0–13.0 g/dL.

The mean change in hemoglobin concentration from baseline to week 36 was –0.08 g/dL. The median weekly dose of darbepoetin alfa during the study was equivalent to the weekly dose of rHuEPO at study enrollment, and 96% of patients were managed at the reduced dosing frequency, including 89% (139/157) of patients on once every other week dosing.[206] These results confirm that darbepoetin alfa is as effective as rHuEPO, with the added benefit of less frequent dosing.

Clinical Trials of Darbepoetin Alfa in Patients with CKD Not Yet on Dialysis

A multicenter, randomized, open-label, parallel-group study was conducted in Europe to evaluate the efficacy and safety of darbepoetin alfa for the correction of anemia in rHuEPO-naive patients with CKD.[202] Patients who were not yet on dialysis were included in the CKD study if they were anemic (hemoglobin < 11 g/dL) and had a creatinine clearance of less than 30 mL/min. Of the 166 patients recruited into the study, 129 received 0.45 µg/kg SC darbepoetin alfa once-weekly, and 37 received 50 U/kg SC rHuEPO twice-weekly. The rHuEPO dose was approximately 10% higher than the total weekly dose of darbepoetin alfa.

A similar proportion of patients achieved a hemoglobin response in the darbepoetin alfa (93%) and rHuEPO (92%) treatment groups. The mean rise in hemoglobin of 1.38 g/dL after 4 weeks of darbepoetin alfa treatment was similar to that after rHuEPO therapy (1.40 g/dL). The median time to achieve a hemoglobin response was 7 weeks in both groups. At the time of the peak hemoglobin response, the median weekly dose was 0.46 µg/kg for darbepoetin alfa and 100 U/kg for rHuEPO.[202] After correction of anemia, target hemoglobin concentrations were maintained with a median darbepoetin alfa dose of 0.34 µg/kg.[202] The study shows that darbepoetin alfa administered once weekly by the SC route at a starting dose of 0.45 µg/kg is safe and effective for the correction of anemia in rHuEPO-naive patients with CKD.

A smaller, single-center study evaluated the effectiveness of fixed doses of darbepoetin alfa given SC once every other week for the treatment of anemia in patients with CKD not yet on dialysis.[212] The starting dose of darbepoetin alfa was 0.75 µg/kg. The dose was titrated to achieve and maintain the hemoglobin level within the target range of 11–13 g/dL. An analysis was conducted of the initial 23 patients enrolled into the study who had completed at least 10 weeks of darbepoetin alfa treatment. The median time to achieve a hemoglobin response was 6 weeks (range 0–17 weeks), and 91% of patients reached the target hemoglobin range within 10 weeks of initiating darbepoetin alfa therapy (95% CI, 73.2% to 97.6%). The median darbepoetin alfa dose at the time of hemoglobin response was 50 µg every other week (range, 30–130 µg). This study supports the use of fixed doses of darbepoetin alfa once every other week for the treatment of anemia in rHuEPO-naive patients with CKD.[212]

Further studies are ongoing to provide further clinical information on the use of darbepoetin alfa in patients with CKD.

Safety Profile of Darbepoetin Alfa

The safety and tolerability of darbepoetin alfa were evaluated based on an integrated safety database of 1598 patients who received darbepoetin alfa and 600 patients who received rHuEPO.[213] Safety information was available for up to 1 year for most patients, and a long-term safety study was used to collect safety information beyond 1 year.

The overall safety profile of darbepoetin alfa was similar to that of rHuEPO when assessed by the incidence of adverse events, relationship of events to study drug, withdrawals due to adverse events and deaths during studies. Analyses of laboratory results showed no trends indicative of a treatment-related effect.[213]

Treatment was discontinued due to adverse events in 3% of patients on darbepoetin alfa and in 4% of patients on rHuEPO. The percentage of deaths during the study period was 6% in both treatment groups. Cardiac-related events were the most common cause of death (3% for darbepoetin alfa, 5% for rHuEPO),[213] as would be expected overall in patients with ESRD.[214] The incidence of deaths in the darbepoetin alfa clinical program was low relative to the dialysis population as a whole, and the most common causes of death were as would be expected for patients with CKD.[214]

Adverse events reported in clinical trials of darbepoetin alfa in anemic patients with CKD were similar to those reported with rHuEPO. The most common adverse events were hypertension, hypotension, myalgia and headache (**Table 2**). These events are characteristic of patients with CKD and are not necessarily attributable to darbepoetin alfa. The adverse events most commonly considered to be treatment-related by investigators were hypertension (9% for darbepoetin alfa, 7% for rHuEPO) and injection site pain (7% for darbepoetin alfa, 1% for rHuEPO). Injection site pain was generally mild and transient in nature. All other adverse events were reported with a similar incidence in both treatment groups.[213]

All patients in the darbepoetin alfa clinical trial program were tested for antibodies to darbepoetin alfa (and rHuEPO). To date, there have been no reports of antibody formation associated with darbepoetin alfa in clinical trials of more than 1500 patients.[213]

Darbepoetin alfa can be safely withdrawn in patients whose hemoglobin concentration exceeds the desired upper target level. In patients with CKD and dialysis-dependent patients whose hemoglobin concentration reached more than 14 g/dL, cessation of treatment resulted in a progressive reduction in hemoglobin concentration at a similar rate for both darbepoetin alfa and rHuEPO (**Figure 5**).[215]

Table 2. Proportion of patients reporting adverse events (incidence >10%).[213]

Adverse events*	Incidence (%)	
	Darbepoetin alfa (n = 1598)	rHuEPO (n = 600)
Hypertension	23	26
Hypotension	22	24
Myalgia	21	27
Headache	16	18
Diarrhea	16	21
Vomiting	15	20
Upper respiratory infection	14	23
Nausea	14	24
Dyspnea	12	18
Abdominal pain	12	17
Peripheral edema	11	17
Arthralgia	11	14

*The total proportion of patients reporting adverse events was 90% in the darbepoetin alfa group and 95% in the rHuEPO group.

Discussion and Conclusions

The availability of rHuEPO is certainly one of the milestones in nephrology in the past 20 years. rHuEPO has revolutionized the treatment of anemia of CKD and has improved the lives of hundreds of thousands of patients since the drug's approval in 1989. Increased survival, decreased hospitalizations, improved brain and cognitive function, and improved quality of life for renal patients are some of the benefits of this biotechnology product. Remaining clinical issues related to this remarkable compound include predicting and overcoming resistance, avoiding iron deficiency and determining appropriate target hemoglobin level.

Much has been learned since the development of rHuEPO regarding the physiology of endogenous EPO and the pathophysiology of anemia, as well as of the structure and mechanism of action of rHuEPO. Research into the factors and structural features that control the *in vivo* activity of EPO have led to the development of the analog containing five N-linked carbohydrate chains, darbepoetin alfa.[203]

Darbepoetin alfa, a novel erythropoiesis stimulating protein, represents a new generation of long-acting erythropoietic proteins. It is biochemically distinct from rHuEPO, having an increased sialyated carbohydrate content, which results in enhanced biological activity and a prolonged half-life. This allows less frequent dosing, compared with rHuEPO, for the treatment of renal anemia.[69] Less frequent administration may improve compliance and decrease administration costs.

The preclinical and clinical data on darbepoetin alfa enable several conclusions to be drawn regarding its clinical use in treating the anemia associated with CKD. Darbepoetin alfa administered once-weekly by either the IV or SC route, at a starting dose of 0.45 µg/kg, is effective in increasing hemoglobin levels. In rHuEPO-naive patients with CKD, darbepoetin alfa produces an improvement in hemoglobin concentration similar to that obtained with rHuEPO, with the advantage of less frequent dosing. Furthermore, patients who are being maintained on rHuEPO treatment can be safely and effectively switched to darbepoetin alfa at a reduced frequency of dosing compared with rHuEPO. Patients receiving rHuEPO two or three

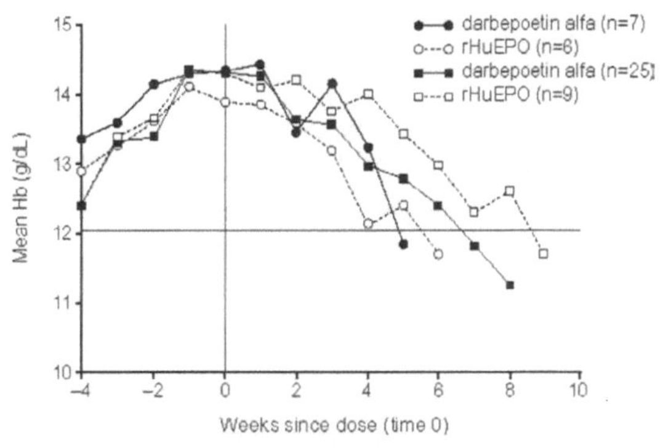

Figure 5. Change in hemoglobin after withholding darbepoetin alfa or rHuEPO treatment. Reproduced with the permission of Oxford University Press.[215]

times a week can be changed to darbepoetin alfa given once-weekly, and patients receiving rHuEPO once-weekly can be switched to darbepoetin alfa given once every other week. After switching patients from rHu EPO to darbepoetin alfa therapy, darbepoetin alfa can maintain hemoglobin levels as effectively as rHuEPO yet with less frequent dosing. In addition, darbepoetin alfa is well tolerated and has a safety profile comparable to that of rHuEPO.

The nephrology clinical trial program continues to explore the efficacy and safety of darbepoetin alfa in alleviating anemia and improving patient outcomes, such as quality of life, when administered at a reduced dosing frequency compared with rHuEPO.

Currently, rHuEPO is the established treatment for anemia; but its use may be hampered by the need for administration two or three times a week, particularly in patients not on hemodialysis. Darbepoetin alfa has been shown to be as effective as rHuEPO with the added benefit of less frequent dosing (once-weekly or once every other week) and, thus, potentially represents a new standard of care in anemia management. Darbepoetin alfa is likely to simplify anemia management in CKD and offers clinical advantages for patients and healthcare providers.

References

1. National Institute of Diabetes and Digestive and Kidney Diseases. Healthy people 2010: chronic kidney disease 2000. Bethesda (MD): National Institutes of Health, 2000.
2. Besarab A. Physiological & pharmacodynamic considerations for route of EPO administration. *Semin Nephrol* 2000;20:364–74.
3. Jones CA, McQuillan G, Kusek J. Serum creatinine levels in the US population: Third National Health and Nutrition Examination Survey [published erratum appears in *Am J Kidney* Dis 2000;35:178]. *Am J Kidney Dis* 1998;32:992-9.
4. Nissenson AR, Pereira BJ, Collins AJ, Steinberg EP. Prevalence and characteristics of individuals with chronic kidney disease in a large health maintenance organization. *Am J Kidney Dis* 2001;37:1177-83.
5. Eckardt KU. Pathophysiology of renal anemia. *Clin Nephrol* 2000;53:S2–8.
6. Kausz AT, Khan SS, Abichandani R, et al. Management of patients with chronic renal insufficiency in the Northeastern United States. *J Am Soc Nephrol* 2001;12:1501–7.
7. Pereira BJ. Optimization of pre-ESRD care: the key to improved dialysis outcomes. *Kidney Int* 2000;57:351–65.
8. Kuriyama S, Tomonari H, Yoshida H, Hashimoto T, Kawaguchi Y, Sakai O. Reversal of anemia by erythropoietin therapy retards the progression of chronic renal failure, especially in nondiabetic patients. *Nephron* 1997;77:176–85.
9. Klang B, Bjorvell H, Clyne N. Quality of life in predialytic uremic patients. *Qual Life Res* 1996;5:109–16.
10. Caro J, Brown S, Miller O, Murray T, Erslev AJ. Erythropoietin levels in uremic nephric and anephric patients. *J Lab Clin Med* 1979;93:449–58.
11. Bright R. Cases and observations, illustrative of renal disease accompanied with the secretion of albuminous urine. *Guys Hosp Rep* 1836;1:338-79.
12. Erslev AJ. Humoral regulation of red cell production. *Blood* 1953;8:349-57.
13. Lin F-K, Suggs S, Lin CH, et al. Cloning and expression of the human erythropoietin gene. *Proc Natl Acad Sci USA* 1985; 82:7580-4.
14. Winearls CG, Oliver DO, Peppard MJ, Reid C, Downing MR, Cotes PM. Effect of human erythropoietin derived from recombinant DNA on the anaemia of patients maintained by chronic hemodialysis. *Lancet* 1986;2:1175-8.
15. Eschbach JW, Egrie JC, Downing MR, Browne JK, Adamson JW. Correction of the anemia of end-stage renal disease with recombinant human erythropoietin. Results of a combined phase I and phase II clinical trial. *N Engl J Med* 1987;316:73-8.
16. Eschbach JW. The anemia of chronic renal failure: pathophysiology and the effects of recombinant erythropoietin [clinical conference]. *Kidney Int* 1989;35:134-48.
17. Sundal E, Kaeser U. Correction of anemia of chronic renal failure with recombinant human erythropoietin: safety and effi-cacy of one year's treatment in a European multicentre study of 150 haemodialysis-dependent patients. *Nephrol Dial Transplant* 1989;4:979-87.
18. Macdougall IC. Novel erythropoiesis stimulating protein. *Semin Nephrol* 2000;20:375-81.
19. Recny MA, Scoble HA, Kim Y. Structural characterization of natural human urinary and recombinant DNA-derived erythropoietin. Identification of des-arginine 166 erythropoietin. *J Biol Chem* 1987;262:17156-63.
20. Wang FF, Kung CK, Goldwasser E. Some chemical properties of human erythropoietin. *Endocrinology* 1985;116:2286-92.
21. Dube S, Fisher JW, Powell JS. Glycosylation at specific sites of erythropoietin is essential for biosynthesis, secretion, and biological function. *J Biol Chem* 1988;263:17516–21.
22. Bachmann S, Le Hir M, Eckardt K-U. Co-localization of erythropoietin mRNA and ecto-5'-nucleotidase immunoreactivity in peritubular cells of rat renal cortex indicates that fibroblasts produce erythropoietin. *J Histochem Cytochem* 1993; 41:335–41.
23. Maxwell PH, Osmond MK, Pugh CW, et al. Identification of the renal erythropoietin-producing cells using transgenic mice. *Kidney Int* 1993;44:1149–62.
24. Erslev AJ. Erythropoietin. *N Engl J Med* 1991;324:1339–44.
25. Jelkmann W. Erythropoietin: structure, control of production, and function. *Physiol Rev* 1992;72:449–89.
26. Semenza GL, Wang GL. A nuclear factor induced by hypoxia via de novo protein synthesis binds to the human erythropoietin gene enhancer at a site required for transcriptional activation. *Mol Cell Biol* 1992;12:5447–54.
27. Koury ST, Bondurant MC, Koury MJ, Semenza GL. Localization of cells producing erythropoietin in murine liver by *in situ* hybridization. *Blood* 1991;77:2497–503.
28. Schuster SJ, Koury ST, Bohrer M, Salceda S, Caro J. Cellular sites of extrarenal and renal erythropoietin production in anaemic rats. *Br J Haematol* 1992;81:153–9.
29. Maxwell PH, Ferguson DJ, Osmond MK, et al. Expression of a homologously recombined erythopoietin-SV40 T antigen fusion gene in mouse liver: evidence for erythropoietin production by Ito cells. *Blood* 1994;84:1823–30.
30. Fried W. The liver as a source of extrarenal erythropoietin production. *Blood* 1972;40:671–7.

31. Tan CC, Eckardt KU, Ratcliffe PJ. Organ distribution of erythropoietin messenger RNA in normal and uremic rats. *Kidney Int* 1991;40:69–76.
32. Fandrey J, Bunn HF. *In vivo* and *in vitro* regulation of the EPO mRNA: measurement by competitive polymerase chain reaction. *Blood* 1993;81:617–23.
33. Westenfelder C, Biddle DL, Baranowski RL. Human, rat, and mouse kidney cells express functional erythropoietin receptors. *Kidney Int* 1999;55:808–20.
34. D'Andrea AD, Lodish HF, Wong GG. Expression cloning of the murine erythropoietin receptor. *Cell* 1989;57:277–85.
35. Wong GG, Jones SS, D'Andrea AD. The molecular biology of erythropoietin receptors. In: Erslev AJ, Adamson JW, Eschbach JW, Winearls GC, editors. *Erythropoietin: molecular, cellular, and clinical biology*. Baltimore: John Hopkins University Press, 1991. p. 133–61.
36. Klingmuller U, Lorenz U, Cantley LC, Neel BG, Lodish HF. Specific recruitment of SH-PTP1 to the erythropoietin receptor causes inactivation of JAK2 and termination of proliferative signals. *Cell* 1995;80:729–38.
37. Koury MJ, Bondurant MC. Erythropoietin retards DNA breakdown and prevents programmed death in erythroid progenitor cells. *Science* 1990;248:378–81.
38. Suda T, Suda J, Ogawa M. Disparate differentiation in mouse hematopoietic colonies derived from paired progenitors. *Proc Natl Acad Sci USA* 1984;81:2520–4.
39. Spivak JL. The mechanism of action of erythropoietin. *Int J Cell Cloning* 1986;4:139–66.
40. Hara H, Ogawa M. Erythropoietic precursors in mice under erythropoietic stimulation and suppresion. *Exp Hematol* 1977; 5:141-8.
41. Schuster SJ, Cao J. Erythropoietin: physiologic basis for clinical applications. *Vox Sang* 1993;65:169-79.
42. Stephenson JR, Axelrad AA, McLeod DL, Shreeve MM. Induction of colonies of hemoglobin-synthesizing cells by erythropoietin *in vitro*. *Proc Natl Acad Sci USA* 1971;68:1542-6.
43. Sonada Y, Maekawa T, Kuzuyama Yea. Human interleukin-9 supports formation of a subpopulation of erythroid bursts that are responsive to interleukin-3. *Am J Hematol* 1992;20:418-24.
44. Lu L, Leemhuis T, Srour EF. Human interleukin-9 specifically stimulates proliferation of CD34++ DR++ CD33- erythroid progenitors in normal human bone marrow in the absence of serum. *Exp Hematol* 1992;21:418-24.
45. Sieff CA, Ekern SC, Nathan DG, Anderson JW. Combinations of recombinant colony-stimulating factors are required for optimal hematopoietic differentiation in serum-deprived culture. *Blood* 1989;73:688-93.
46. Galli SJ, Zsebo KM, Geissler EN. The kit ligand, stem cell factor. *Adv Immunol* 1994;55:1-96.
47. Abkowitz JL, Sabo KM, Nakamoto B, et al. Diamond-Blackfan anemia: *in vitro* response of erythroid progenitors to the ligand for c-kit. *Blood* 1991;78:2198-202.
48. Bagnara GP, Zauli G, Vitale L, et al. *In vitro* growth and regulation of bone marrow enriched CD34+ hematopoietic progenitors in Diamond-Blackfan anemia. *Blood* 1991;78:2203-10.
49. Oliveri NF, Grunberger T, Ben-David Y. Diamond-Blackfan anemia: heterogeneous response of hematopoietic progenitor cells *in vitro* to the protein product of the Steel locus. *Blood* 1991;78:2211-5.
50. Axelrad A, McLeod D, et al. Properties of cells that produce erythrocytic colonies *in vitro*. In: Robinson WA, editor. *Hematopoiesis in culture*. Bethesda, MD: National Institutes of Health, 1974. p. 226.
51. Sawada K, Krantz SB, Dessypris EN, Koury ST, Sawyer ST. Human colony-forming units-erythroid do not require accessory cells, but do require direct interaction with insulin-like growth factor I and/or insulin for erythroid development. *J Clin Invest* 1989;83:1701-9.
52. Krantz SB. Erythropoietin. *Blood* 1991;77:419-34.
53. Jelkmann W, Pagel H, Hellwig T, Fandrey J. Effects of antioxidant vitamins on renal and hepatic erythropoietin production. *Kidney Int* 1997;51:497-501.
54. Means RT Jr, Krantz SB. Inhibition of human erythroid colony-forming units by tumor necrosis factor requires beta interferon. *J Clin Invest* 1993;91:416-9.
55. Faquin WC, Schneider TJ, Goldberg MA. Effect of inflammatory cytokines on hypoxia-induced erythropoietin production. *Blood* 1992;79:1987-94.
56. Roodman GD, Bird A, Hutzler D, Montgomery W. Tumor necrosis factor-alpha and hematopoietic progenitors: effects of tumor necrosis factor on the growth of erythroid progenitors CFU-E and BFU-E and the hematopoietic cell lines K562, HL60, and HEL cells. *Exp Hematol* 1987;15:928-35.
57. Alfrey CP, Rice L, Udden MM, Driscoll TB. Neocytolysis: physiological down-regulator of red-cell mass. *Lancet* 1997;349:1389-90.
58. Alfrey CP, Udden MM, Leach-Huntoon C, Driscoll T, Pickett MH. Control of red blood cell mass in spaceflight. *J Appl Physiol* 1996;81:98-104.
59. Rice L, Udden MM, Driscoll T, et al. Neocytolysis in the adaptation of red cell mass on descent from altitude. *Acta Andina* 1997;6:17-20.
60. Rice L, Alfrey C, Ruiz W, Driscoll T, Whitley C, Gonzales G. Neocytolysis on descent from altitude. *Blood* 1997;90:8b.
61. Rice L, Alfrey CP, Driscoll T, Whitley CE, Hachey DL, Suki W. Neocytolysis contributes to the anemia of renal disease. *Am J Kidney Dis* 1999;33:59-62.
62. Bren AF. Personal communication, 2000.
63. Widness JA, Veng-Pedersen P, Schmidt RL, Lowe LS, Kisthard JA, Peters C. *In vivo* ^{125}I-erythropoietin pharmacokinetics are unchanged after anesthesia, nephrectomy and hepatectomy in sheep. *J Pharmacol Exp Ther* 1996;279:1205-10.
64. Besarab A, Flaharty KK, Erslev AJ, et al. Clinical pharmacology and economics of recombinant human erythropoietin in end-stage renal disease: the case for subcutaneous administration. *J Am Soc Nephrol* 1992;2:1405-16.
65. Halstenson CE, Macres M, Katz SA, et al. Comparative pharmacokinetics and pharmacodynamics of epoetin alfa and epoetin beta. *Clin Pharmacol Ther* 1991;50:702-12.
66. Egrie J, Eschbach JW, McGuire T, et al. Pharmacokinetics of recombinant human erythropoietin administered in hemodialysis patients. *Kidney Int* 1988;33:262.
67. Jensen JD, Madsen JK, Jensen LW, Pedersen EB. Reduced production, absorption, and elimination of erythropoietin in uremia compared with healthy volunteers. *J Am Soc Nephrol* 1994; 5:177-85.
68. Kampf D, Kahl A, Passlick J, et al. Single-dose kinetics of recombinant human erythropoietin after intravenous, subcutaneous and intraperitoneal administration. Preliminary results. *Contrib Nephrol* 1989;76:106-10.
69. Macdougall IC, Gray SJ, Elston O, et al. Pharmacokinetics of novel erythropoiesis stimulating protein compared with epoetin alfa in dialysis patients. *J Am Soc Nephrol* 1999;10:2392-5.
70. Bargman JM, Jones JE, Petro JM. The pharmacokinetics of intraperitoneal erythropoietin administered undiluted or diluted in dialysate. *Perit Dial Int* 1992;12:369-72.
71. Flaherty KK, Caro J, Erslev A, et al. Pharmacokinetics and erythropoietic response to human recombinant erythropoietin in healthy men. *Clin Pharmacol Ther* 1991;50:702-12.
72. Nielsen OJ. Pharmacokinetics of recombinant human erythropoietin in chronic haemodialysis patients. *Pharmacol Toxicol* 1990;66:83-6.
73. Boelaert JR, Schurgers ML, Matthys EG, et al. Comparative pharmacokinetics of recombinant erythropoietin administered by the intravenous, subcutaneous, and intraperitoneal routes in

continuous ambulatory peritoneal dialysis (CAPD) patients. *Perit Dial Int* 1989;9:95-8.
74. Macdougall IC, Roberts DE, Neubert P, Dharmasena AD, Coles GA, Williams JD. Pharmacokinetics of intravenous, intraperitoneal, and subcutaneous recombinant erythropoietin in patients on CAPD. A rationale for treatment. *Contrib Nephrol* 1989; 76:112-21.
75. Neumayer HH, Brockmoller J, Fritschka E, Roots I, Scigalla P, Wattenberg M. Pharmacokinetics of recombinant human erythropoietin after SC administration and in long-term IV treatment in patients on maintenance hemodialysis. *Contrib Nephrol* 1989;76:131-42.
76. Horl WH. Optimal route of administration of erythropoietin in chronic renal failure patients: intravenous versus subcutaneous. *Acta Haematol* 1992;87:16-9.
77. Brahm M. Subcutaneous treatment with recombinant human erythropoietin - the influence of injection frequency and skinfold thickness. *Scand J Urol Nephrol* 1999;33:192-6.
78. Eschbach JW, Abdulhadi MH, Browne JK, et al. Recombinant human erythropoietin in anemic patients with end-stage renal disease. Results of a phase III multicenter clinical trial. *Ann Intern Med* 1989;111:992-1000.
79. Eschbach J, De Oreo P, Adamson J, et al. rHuEPO clinical practice guidelines for the treatment of anemia of chronic renal failure. *Am J Kidney Dis* 1997;30:S192-240.
80. Walls J. Haemoglobin - is more better? *Nephrol Dial Transplant* 1995;10:56-61.
81. Pickett JL, Theberge DC, Brown WS, Schweitzer SU, Nissenson AR. Normalizing hematocrit in dialysis patients improves brain function. *Am J Kidney Dis* 1999;33:1122-30.
82. Metry G, Wikstrom B, Valind S, et al. Effect of normalization of hematocrit on brain circulation and metabolism in hemodialysis patients. *J Am Soc Nephrol* 1999;10:854-63.
83. Hirakata H, Kanai H, Fukuda K, et al. Optimal hematocrit for the maximum oxygen delivery to the brain with recombinant human erythropoietin in hemodialysis patients. *Clin Nephrol* 2000;53:354-61.
84. McMahon L, McKenna MR, Hovick ET, Peterson DD. Physical performance and associated electrolyte changes after haemoglobin normalization: a comparative study in haemodialysis patients. *Nephrol Dial Transplant* 1999;14:1182-7.
85. Benz RL, Pressman MR, Hovick ET, Peterson DD. A preliminary study of the effects of correction of anemia with recombinant human erythropoietin therapy on sleep, sleep disorders, and daytime sleepiness in hemodialysis patients. *Am J Kidney Dis* 1999;34:1089-95.
86. Besarab A, Bolton W, Browne J, et al. The effects of normal as compared with low hematocrit values in patients with cardiac disease who are receiving hemodialysis and epoetin. *N Engl J Med* 1998;339:584-90.
87. Furuland H, Linde T, Danielson BG. Cardiac function in patients with end-stage renal disease after normalization of hemoglobin with erythropoietin. American Society of Nephrology 31st Annual Meeting and Scientific Exposition, October 25-28, 1998.
88. Furuland H, Linde T, Danielson BG. Physical exercise capacity in patients with end-stage renal disease after normalization of hemoglobin with erythropoietin. American Society of Nephrology 31st Annual Meeting and Scientific Exposition October 25-28, 1998.
89. Foley RN, Parfrey PS, Morgan J. A randomized controlled trial of complete vs partial correction of anemia in hemodialysis patients with asymptomatic LV hypertrophy or LV dilation. American Society of Nephrology 31st Annual Meeting and Scientific Exposition October 25-28, 1998.
90. Jabs K, Alexander S, McCabe D, Lerner G. Primary results from the US multicenter pediatric recombinant erythropoietin study. *J Am Soc Nephrol* 1994;5:456.
91. Scigalla P. Effect of recombinant human erythropoietin treatment on renal anemia and body growth of children with end-stage renal disease. The European Multicenter Study Group. *Contrib Nephrol* 1991;88:201–11.
92. Collins A. Personal communication, 2000.
93. Eschbach JW, Kelly MR, Haley NR, Abels RI, Adamson JW. Treatment of the anemia of progressive renal failure with recombinant human erythropoietin. *N Engl J Med* 1989;321:158–63.
94. National Institute of Diabetes and Digestive and Kidney Diseases. The USRDS dialysis, morbidity, and mortality study (wave 1). In: *US Renal Data System Annual Data Report 4*. Bethesda, MD: National Institutes of Health, 1996. p. 45-67.
95. Macdougall IC, Hutton RD, Cavill I, Coles GA, Williams JD. Poor response to treatment in renal anaemia with erythropoietin corrected by iron given intravenously. *BMJ* 1989;299:157–8.
96. Eschbach J. Current concepts of anemia management in chronic renal failure: impact of NKF-DOQI. *Semin Nephrol* 2000; 20:320–9.
97. Horl WH. How to get the best out of r-HuEPO. *Nephrol Dial Transplant* 1995;10:92–5.
98. Van Wyck D. Efficacy and adverse effects of oral iron supplements. *Semin Dial* 1999;12:235–6.
99. Clibon U, Bonewald L, Caro J, Roodman GD. Erythropoietin fails to reverse the anemia in mice continuously exposed to tumor necrosis factor-alpha *in vivo*. *Exp Hematol* 1990;18:438–41.
100. Macdougall IC, Allen DA, Cavill I, Baker LRI, Raine AEG. Poor response to erythropoietin in inflammatory conditions may be mediated by interleukin-gamma. *Nephrol Dial Transplant* 1994;9:1033.
101. Douglas SW, Adamson JW. The anemia of chronic disorders: studies of marrow regulation and iron metabolism. *Blood* 1975;45:55–65.
102. Barany P, Divino Filho JC, Bergstrom J. High C-reactive protein is a strong predictor of resistance to erythropoietin in hemodialysis patients. *Am J Kidney Dis* 1997;29:565–8.
103. Gunnell J, Yeun JY, Depner TA, Kaysen GA. Acute-phase response predicts erythropoietin resistance in hemodialysis and peritoneal dialysis patients. *Am J Kidney Dis* 1999;33:63–72.
104. Vlahakos DV, Balodimos C, Papachristopoulos V, Vassilakos P, Hinari E, Vlachojannis JG. Renin–angiotensin system stimulates erythropoietin secretion in chronic hemodialysis patients. *Clin Nephrol* 1995;43:53–9.
105. Kamper AL, Nielsen OJ. Effect of enalapril on haemoglobin and serum erythropoietin in patients with chronic nephropathy. *Scand J Clin Lab Invest* 1990;50:611–8.
106. Gaston RS, Julian BA, Curtis JJ. Posttransplant erythrocytosis: an enigma revisited. *Am J Kidney Dis* 1994;24:1–11.
107. Constantinescu CS, Goodman DB, Ventura ES. Captopril and lisinopril suppress production of interleukin-12 by human peripheral blood mononuclear cells. *Immunol Lett* 1998;62:25–31.
108. Mrug M, Stopka T, Julian BA, Prchal JF, Prchal JT. Angiotensin II stimulates proliferation of normal early erythroid progenitors. *J Clin Invest* 1997;100:2310–4.
109. Dhondt AW, Vanholder RC, Ringoir SM. Angiotensin-converting enzyme inhibitors and higher erythropoietin requirement in chronic haemodialysis patients. *Nephrol Dial Transplant* 1995;10:2107–9.
110. Abu-Alfa AK, Cruz D, Perazella MA, Mahnensmith RL, Simon D, Bia MJ. ACE inhibitors do not induce recombinant human erythropoietin resistance in hemodialysis patients. *Am J Kidney Dis* 2000;35:1076–82.
111. Erturk S, Ates K, Duman N, Karatan O, Erbay B, Ertug E. Unresponsiveness to recombinant human erythropoietin in haemodialysis patients: possible implications of angiotensin-converting enzyme inhibitors. *Nephrol Dial Transplant* 1996;11:396–7.

112. Albitar S, Genin R, Fen-Chong M, Serveaux MO, Bourgeon B. High dose enalapril impairs the response to erythropoietin treatment in haemodialysis patients. *Nephrol Dial Transplant* 1998;13:1206–10.
113. Fluck S, McKane W, Cairns T, et al. Chloramine-induced haemolysis presenting as erythropoietin resistance. *Nephrol Dial Transplant* 1999;14:1687–91.
114. Richardson D, Bartlett C, Goutcher E, Jones CH, Davison AM, Will EJ. Erythropoietin resistance due to dialysate chloramine: the two-way traffic of solutes in haemodialysis. *Nephrol Dial Transplant* 1999;14:2625–7.
115. Beck JJ. Chloramines in municipal water: considerations for dialysis facilities. *Nephrol News Issues* 1997;11:19–22.
116. Wanner C, Horl WH. Carnitine abnormalities in patients with renal insufficiency. Pathophysiological and therapeutical aspects. *Nephron* 1988;50:89–102.
117. Minigardi G, Bizzi A, Cini M, Licini R, Mecca G, Garatini S. Carnitine balance in hemodialyzed patients. *Clin Nephrol* 1980; 13:269-70.
118. Bahmer T, Rydning A, Solberg HE. Carnitine levels in human serum in health and disease. *Clin Chim Acta* 1974;57:55–61.
119. Trovato GM, Ginardi V, DiMarco V, et al. Long-term L-carnitine treatment of chronic anemia of patients with end-stage renal failure. *Curr Ther Res* 1982;31:1042-79.
120. Arduini A, Rossi M, Mancinelli G, et al. Effect of L-carnitine and acetyl-L-carnitine on the human erythrocyte membrane stability and deformability. *Life Sci* 1990;47:2395-400.
121. Kooistra MP, Struyvenberg A, van Es A. The response to recombinant human erythropoietin in patients with the anemia of end-stage renal disease is correlated with serum carnitine levels. *Nephron* 1991;57:127-8.
122. Berard E, Iordache A. Effect of low doses of L-carnitine on the response to recombinant human erythropoietin in hemodialyzed children: about two cases. *Nephron* 1992;62:368-9.
123. Labonia WD. L-carnitine effects on anemia in hemodialyzed patients treated with erythropoietin. *Am J Kidney Dis* 1995; 26:757-64.
124. Kletzmayr J, Mayer G, Legenstein E, et al. Anemia and carnitine supplementation in hemodialyzed patients. *Kidney Int Suppl* 1999;69:S93-106.
125. Rao DS, Shih MS, Mohini R. Effect of serum parathyroid hormone and bone marrow fibrosis on the response to erythropoietin in uremia. *N Engl J Med* 1993;328:171-5.
126. Urena P, Eckardt KU, Sarfati E, et al. Serum erythropoietin and erythropoiesis in primary and secondary hyperparathyroidism: effect of parathyroidectomy. *Nephron* 1991;59:384-93.
127. Washio M, Iseki K, Onoyama K, et al. Elevation of serum erythropoietin after subtotal parathyroidectomy in chronic hemodialysis patients. *Nephrol Dial Transplant* 1992;7:121-4.
128. Barbour GL. Effect of parathyroidectomy on anemia in chronic renal failure. *Arch Intern Med* 1979;139:889-91.
129. Zingraff J, Drueke T, Marie P, Man NK, Jungers P, Bordier P. Anemia and secondary hyperparathyroidism. *Arch Intern Med* 1978;138:1650-2.
130. Goicoechea M, Gomez-Campdera F, Polo JR, et al. Secondary hyperparathyroidism as cause of resistance to treatment with erythropoietin: effect of parathyroidectomy. *Clin Nephrol* 1996; 45:420-1.
131. Goicoechea M, Vazquez MI, Ruiz MA, Gomez-Campdera F, Perez-Garcia R, Valderrabano F. Intravenous calcitriol improves anaemia and reduces the need for erythropoietin in haemodialysis patients. *Nephron* 1998;78:23-7.
132. Taccone-Gallucci M, Marca di Villahermosa A, et al. Control of secondary hyperparathyroidism with 'pulse' oral calcitriol improves anemia in haemodialysis patients under maintenance erythropoietin therapy. *J Am Soc Nephrol* 1998;9:571.
133. Canadian Erythropoietin Study Group. Association between recombinant human erythropoietin and quality of life and exercise capacity of patients receiving hemodialysis. *BMJ* 1990;300:573-8.
134. McMahon L, Dawborn J. Changes in quality of life at comparative levels of hemoglobin after long-term treatment with erythropoietin. *Am J Nephrol* 1992;12:358-62.
135. Evans RW, Rader B, Manninen DL. The quality of life of hemodialysis recipients treated with recombinant human erythropoietin. Cooperative Multicenter EPO Clinical Trial Group. *JAMA* 1990;263:825-30.
136. Karnofsky DA, Burchenal JH. The clinical evaluation of chemotherapeutic agents in cancer. In: Maleod CM, editor. *Evaluation of chemotherapeutic agents*. New York: Columbia University Press, 1949. p. 191-205.
137. Bergner M, Bobbitt RA, Carter WB, Gilson BS. The Sickness Impact Profile: development and final revision of a health status measure. *Med Care* 1981;19:787-805.
138. Moreno F, Lopez Gomez JM, Sanz-Guajardo D, Jofre R, Valderrabano F. Quality of life in dialysis patients. A Spanish multicentre study. Spanish Cooperative Renal Patients Quality of Life Study Group. *Nephrol Dial Transplant* 1996;11:125-9.
139. Valderrabano F. Quality of life benefits of early anaemia treatment. *Nephrol Dial Transplant* 2000;15(Suppl 3):23-8.
140. Barany P, Freyschuss U, Pettersson E, Bergstrom J. Treatment of anaemia in haemodialysis patients with erythropoietin. *Kidney Int* 1990;38:480-6.
141. Nagao K, Tsuchihashi K, Ura N, Nakata T, Shimamoto K. Appropriate hematocrit levels of erythropoietin supplementary therapy in end-stage renal failure complicated by coronary artery disease. *Can J Cardiol* 1997;13:747-53.
142. Vella JP, O'Neill D, Atkins N, Donohoe JF, Walshe JJ. Sensitization to human leukocyte antigen before and after the introduction of erythropoietin. *Nephrol Dial Transplant* 1998;13:2027-32.
143. Wolcott DL, Marsh JT, La Rue A, Carr C, Nissenson AR. Recombinant human erythropoietin treatment may improve quality of life and cognitive function in chronic hemodialysis patients. *Am J Kidney Dis* 1989;14:478-85.
144. Nissenson AR. Recombinant human erythropoietin: impact on brain and cognitive function, exercise tolerance, sexual potency, and quality of life. *Semin Nephrol* 1989;9:S25-31.
145. Nissenson AR, Marsh JT, Brown WS, Wolcott D. Central nervous system function in dialysis patients: a practical approach. *Semin Dial* 1991;4:115-23.
146. Nissenson AR. Epoetin and cognitive function. *Am J Kidney Dis* 1992;20:21-4.
147. Grotta JC, Manner C, Pettigrew LC, Yatsu FM. Red blood cell disorders and stroke. *Stroke* 1986;17:811-7.
148. Grimm G, Stockenhuber F, Schneeweiss B, Madl C, Zeitlhofer J, Schneider B. Improvement of brain function in hemodialysis patients treated with erythropoietin. *Kidney Int* 1990;38:480-6.
149. Marsh JT, Brown WS, Wolcott D, et al. rHuEPO treatment improves brain and cognitive function of anemic dialysis patients. *Kidney Int* 1991;39:155-63.
150. Sagales T, Gimeno V, Planella MJ, Raguer N, Bartolome J. Effects of rHuEPO on Q-EEG and event-related potentials in chronic renal failure. *Kidney Int* 1993;44:1109-15.
151. Brown WS, Marsh JT, Wolcott D, et al. Cognitive function, mood and P3 latency: effects of the amelioration of anemia in dialysis patients. *Neuropsychologia* 1991;29:35-45.
152. National Institute of Diabetes and Digestive and Kidney Diseases. *US Renal Data System Annual Report*. Bethesda, MD: National Institutes of Health, 1990.
153. Foley RN, Parfrey PS. *Complications of long-term dialysis: cardiovascular complications and cardiac risk factor interventions*. Oxford: Oxford University Press, 1999.
154. London GM, Parfrey PS. Cardiac disease in chronic uremia: pathogenesis. *Adv Ren Replace Ther* 1997;4:194-211.

155. Mann JF. What are the short-term and long-term consequences of anaemia in CRF patients? *Nephrol Dial Transplant* 1999; 14:29-36.
156. London GM, Zins B, Pannier B, et al. Vascular changes in hemodialysis patients in response to recombinant human erythropoietin. *Kidney Int* 1989;36:878-82.
157. Foley RN, Parfrey PS, Harnett JD, Kent GM, Murray DC, Barre PE. The prognostic importance of left ventricular geometry in uremic cardiomyopathy. *J Am Soc Nephrol* 1995;5:2024-31.
158. Foley RN, Parfrey PS, Harnett JD, Kent GM, Murray DC, Barre PE. The impact of anemia on cardiomyopathy, morbidity, and mortality in end-stage renal disease. *Am J Kidney Dis* 1996;28:53-61.
159. Low-Fredrich I, Gruntzmacher P, Marz W, et al. Therapy with recombinant human erythropoietin reduces cardiac size and improves cardiac function in chronic hemodialysis patients. *Am J Nephrol* 1991;11:54-60.
160. Martinez-Vea A, Bardaji A, Garcia Cea. Long term myocardial effects of correction of anemia with recombinant erythropoietin in aged patients on hemodialysis. *Am J Kidney Dis* 1992;14:353-7.
161. Schwartz AB, Prior JE, Mintz GS, Kim KE, Kahn SB. Cardiovascular hemodynamic effects of correction of anemia of chronic renal failure with recombinant-human erythropoietin. *Transplant Proc* 1991;23:1827-30.
162. Cannella G, La Canna G, Sandrini M. Renormalization of high cardiac output and of left ventricular size following long-term recombinant human erythropoietin treatment of anemic dialyzed uremic patients. *Clin Nephrol* 1990;34:272-8.
163. Teruel JL, Pascual J, Jimenez M, et al. Hemodynamic changes in hemodialyzed patients during treatment with recombinant human erythropoietin. *Nephron* 1991;58:135-7.
164. Low I, Gruntzmacher P, Bergmann M. Echocardiographic findings in patients on maintenance hemodialysis substituted with recombinant human erythropoietin. *Clin Nephrol* 1989; 31:26-30.
165. Onoyama K, Hori K, Osato S, Fujishima M. Haemodynamic effect of recombinant human erythropoietin on hypotensive haemodialysis patients. *Nephrol Dial Transplant* 1991;6:562-5.
166. Silverberg J, Racine N, Barre P, Sniderman AD. Regression of left ventricular hypertrophy in dialysis patients following correction of anemia with recombinant human erythropoietin. *Can J Cardiol* 1990;6:1-4.
167. Goldberg N, Lundin AP, Delano B, Friedman EA, Stein RA. Changes in left ventricular size, wall thickness, and function in anemic patients treated with recombinant human erythropoietin. *Am Heart J* 1992;124:424-7.
168. Pascual J, Teruel JL, Moya JL, Liano F, Jimenez-Mena M, Ortuno J. Regression of left ventricular hypertrophy after partial correction of anemia with erythropoietin in patients on hemodialysis: a prospective study. *Clin Nephrol* 1991;35:280-7.
169. Foley RN, Parfrey PS, Morgan AG, et al. Effect of hemoglobin levels in hemodialysis patients with asymptomatic cardiomyopathy. *Kidney Int* 2000;58:1325-38.
170. Madore F, Lowrie EG, Brugnara C, et al. Anemia in hemodialysis patients: variables affecting this outcome predictor. *J Am Soc Nephrol* 1997;8:1921-9.
171. Ma JZ, Ebben J, Xia H, Collins AJ. Haematocrit level and associated mortality in hemodialysis patients. *J Am Soc Nephrol* 1999;10:1309-16.
172. Collins M, Hsieh A, Ohazama CJ, et al. Assessment of regional wall motion abnormalities with real-time 3-dimensional echocardiography. *J Am Soc Echocardiogr* 1999;12:7-14.
173. Collins A, Xia H, Ebben J. Change in hematocrit and risk of mortality. *J Am Soc Nephrol* 1998;9:204A.
174. Collins AJ, Xia H, Ebben J. Change in hematocrit and risk of hospitalizations. *J Am Soc Nephrol* 1998;9:204A.
175. Churchill DN, Muirhead N, Goldstein M, et al. Effect of recombinant human erythropoietin on hospitalization of hemodialysis patients. *Clin Nephrol* 1995;43:184-8.
176. Xia H, Ebben J, Ma JZ, Collins AJ. Hematocrit levels and hospitalization risks in hemodialysis patients. *J Am Soc Nephrol* 1999;10:1309-6.
177. Abraham PA, Macres MG. Blood pressure in hemodialysis patients during amelioration of anemia with erythropoietin. *J Am Soc Nephrol* 1991;2:927-36.
178. Buckner FS, Eschbach JW, Haley NR, Davidson RC, Adamson JW. Hypertension following erythropoietin therapy in anemic hemodialysis patients. *Am J Hypertens* 1990;3:947-55.
179. Raine AE, Roger SD. Effects of erythropoietin on blood pressure. *Am J Kidney Dis* 1991;18:76-83.
180. Vaziri ND. Mechanism of erythropoietin-induced hypertension. *Am J Kidney Dis* 1999;33:821-8.
181. Berns JS, Rudnick MR, Cohen RM, Bower JD, Wood BC. Effects of normal hematocrit on ambulatory blood pressure in epoetin-treated hemodialysis patients with cardiac disease. *Kidney Int* 1999;56:253-60.
182. Carlini R, Obialo CI, Rothstein M. Intravenous erythropoietin (rHuEPO) administration increases plasma endothelin and blood pressure in hemodialysis patients. *Am J Hypertens* 1993;6:103-7.
183. Takahashi K, Totsune K, Imai Y, et al. Plasma concentrations of immunoreactive-endothelin in patients with chronic renal failure treated with recombinant human erythropoietin. *Clin Sci (Colch)* 1993;84:47-50.
184. Zhou XJ, Pandian D, Wang XQ, Vaziri ND. Erythropoietin-induced hypertension in rat is not mediated by alterations of plasma endothelin, vasopressin, or atrial natriuretic peptide levels. *J Am Soc Nephrol* 1997;8:901-5.
185. Hon G, Vaziri ND, Kaupke CJ, Tehranzadeh A, Barton C. Lack of a fast-acting effect of erythropoietin on arterial blood pressure and endothelin level. *Artif Organs* 1995;19:188-91.
186. Brochu E, Lacasse S, Lariviere R, Kingma I, Grose JH, Lebel M. Differential effects of endothelin-1 antagonists on erythropoietin-induced hypertension in renal failure. *J Am Soc Nephrol* 1999;10:1440-6.
187. Banerjee D, Rodriguez M, Nag M, Adamson JW. Exposure of endothelial cells to recombinant human erythropoietin induces nitric oxide synthase activity. *Kidney Int* 2000;57:1895-904.
188. Vaziri ND, Zhou XJ, Smith J, Oveisi F, Baldwin K, Purdy RE. *In vivo* and *in vitro* pressor effects of erythropoietin in rats. *Am J Physiol* 1995;269:F838-45.
189. Kaupke CJ, Kim S, Vaziri ND. Effect of erythrocyte mass on arterial blood pressure in dialysis patients receiving maintenance erythropoietin therapy. *J Am Soc Nephrol* 1994;4:1874-8.
190. Tepel M, Wischniowski H, Zidek W. Erythropoietin increases cytosolic free calcium concentration and thrombin induced changes in cytosolic free calcium in platelets from spontaneously hypertensive rats. *Biochem Biophys Res Commun* 1991; 177:991-7.
191. Miller BA, Bell LL, Lynch CJ, Cheung JY. Erythropoietin modulation of intracellular calcium: a role for tyrosine phosphorylation. *Cell Calcium* 1994;16:481-90.
192. Samtleben W, Baldamus CA, Brommer J. Blood pressure changes during treatment with recombinant human erythropoietin. *Contrib Nephrol* 1988;66:114-22.
193. Vaziri ND, Zhou XJ, Naqvi F, et al. Role of nitric oxide resistance in erythropoietin-induced hypertension in rats with chronic renal failure. *Am J Physiol* 1996;271:E113-22.
194. Laupacis A. Changes in quality of life and functional capacity in hemodialysis patients treated with recombinant human erythropoietin. The Canadian Erythropoietin Study Group. *Semin Nephrol* 1990;10:11-9.
195. Bahlmann J, Schoter KH, Scigalla P, et al. Morbidity and mortality in hemodialysis patients with and without

erythropoietin treatment: a controlled study. *Contrib Nephrol* 1991;88:90-106.
196. Buccianti G, Colombi L, Battistel V. Use of recombinant human erythropoietin (rh-EPO) in the treatment of anemia in hemodialysis patients: a multicenter Italian experience. *Haematologica* 1993;78:111-7.
197. Stevens ME, Summerfield GP, Hall AA, et al. Cost benefits of low dose subcutaneous erythropoietin in patients with anaemia of end stage renal disease. *BMJ* 1992;304:474-7.
198. Klinkmann H, Wieczorek L, Scigalla P. Adverse events of subcutaneous recombinant human erythropoietin therapy: results of a controlled multicenter European study. *Artif Organs* 1993; 17:219-25.
199. Westenfelder C, Baranowski RL. Erythropoietin stimulates proliferation of human renal carcinoma cells. *Kidney Int* 2000; 58:647-57.
200. Cotter DJ, Thamer M, Kimmel PL, Sadler JH. Secular trends in recombinant erythropoietin therapy among the US hemodialysis population: 1990-1996. *Kidney Int* 1998;54:2129-39.
201. Collins AJ, Li S, Ebben J, Ma JZ, Manning W. Hematocrit levels and associated Medicare expenditures. *Am J Kidney Dis* 2000;36:282-93.
202. Locatelli F, Olivares J, Walker R, Wilkie M, Group EANS. Novel Erythropoiesis Stimulating Protein (NESP) administered subcutaneously corrects anemia in subjects with chronic renal insufficiency (CRI) when administered at a reduced frequency compared with recombinant human erythropoietin (r-HuEPO). *J Am Soc Nephrol* 2000;11:A1486.
203. Egrie JC, Browne JK. Development and characterization of novel erythropoiesis stimulating protein (NESP). *Br J Cancer* 2001;84:3-10.
204. Dordal MS, Wang FF, Goldwasser E. The role of carbohydrate in erythropoietin action. *Endocrinology* 1985;116:2293-9.
205. Allon M, Kleinman K, Walczyk M, et al. The pharmacokinetics of novel erythropoiesis stimulating protein (NESP) following chronic intravenous administration is time- and dose-linear. 33rd Annual Meeting and Exposition of the American Society of Nephrology, Toronto, Canada, October 13-16, 2000.
206. Graf H, Lacombe J-L, Braun J, Gomes da Costa AA. Novel erythropoiesis stimulating protein (NESP) effectively maintains hemoglobin (Hgb) when administered at a reduced dose frequency compared with recombinant human erythropoietin (r-HuEPO) in ESRD patients. 33rd Annual Meeting and Exposition of the American Society of Nephrology, Toronto, Canada, October 13-16, 2000
207. Lerner GR, Kale AS, Warady BA, et al. The pharmacokinetics of novel erythropoiesis stimulating protein (NESP) in pediatric patients with chronic renal failure (CRF) or end-stage renal disease. 33rd Annual Meeting and Exposition of the American Society of Nephrology, Toronto, Canada, October 13-16, 2000
208. Evans JH, Brocklebank JT, Bowmer CJ, Ng PC. Pharmacokinetics of recombinant human erythropoietin in children with renal failure. *Nephrol Dial Transplant* 1991;6:709-14.
209. Macdougall IC. Novel erythropoiesis stimulating protein (NESP) for the treatment of renal anaemia. *J Am Soc Nephrol* 1998;9:258a-9a.
210. Nissenson AR, Swan SK, Lindberg JS, et al. Novel erythropoiesis stimulating protein (NESP) safely maintains hemoglobin concentration levels in hemodialysis patients as effectively as r-HuEPO when administered once-weekly. 33rd Annual Meeting and Exposition of the American Society of Nephrology, Toronto, Canada, October 13-16, 2000.
211. Vanrenterghem Y, Barany P, Mann J. Novel erythropoiesis stimulating protein (NESP) maintains hemoglobin in ESRD patients when administered once weekly or once every other week. *J Am Soc Nephrol* 1999;10:270A.
212. Suranyi M, Jackson L, Lubina J, McDermott-Vitak AD. Novel erythropoiesis stimulating protein (NESP) administered once every other week corrects anemia in patients with chronic renal insufficiency. National Kidney Foundation 50th Annual Meeting, San Francisco, USA, October 11–14, 2001.
213. Amgen Inc. Integrated summary of safety. Data on file.
214. National Institute of Diabetes and Digestive and Kidney Diseases. *US Renal Data System 2000 Annual Report*. Bethesda, MD: National Institutes of Health, 2000.
215. Macdougall IC. An overview of the efficacy and safety of novel erythropoiesis stimulating protein (NESP). *Nephrol Dial Transplant* 2001;16:14-21.
216. Bunn H. Pathophysiology of the anemias. In: Braunwald E, editor. *Harrison's principles of internal medicine*. New York: McGraw-Hill, 1987. p. 1489-93.

3 Cardiovascular Disease in Patients with Chronic Kidney Disease: The Causes and Effects

Adeera Levin, MD, Ognjenka Djurdjev, Brendan Barrett, MD, Ellen Burgess, MD, Euan Carlisle, MD, Jean Ethier, MD, Kailash Jindal, MD, David Mendelssohn, MD, Sheldon Tobe, MD, Joel Singer, MD and Christopher Thompson, MD

Abstract

The high prevalence of cardiovascular disease in patients with kidney disease is well described. This Canadian, multi-centre, observational cohort study reports the prevalence and risk factors of CVD associated with kidney disease in a cohort of patients with established chronic kidney disease (CKD) who are followed by nephrologists. This analysis sought to answer 2 questions:

(1) in patients with established CKD, are the prevalence and progression of CVD accounted for by conventional or uremia related risk factors?

(2) to what extent can progression to RRT be explained by CVD versus 'traditional risk factors' for kidney disease?

This study population consists of 313, predominantly male patients who had a mean age of 56 years and a mean creatinine clearance of 36 ml/min. Thirty percent were diabetic. The overall prevalence of CVD was 46% and was independent of severity of kidney dysfunction (p=0.700). The median follow up time was 23 months, for a total of 462 patient years. We note the overall incidence of CVD events (new CVD or worsening of CVD) was 47/244 (20%). The best predictors of new CVD events among those without pre-existing CVD were diabetes (OR=5.35, p=0.018) and age (OR= 1.26, p=0.08). In those with pre-existing CVD, low DP (OR=0.72, p=0.004) and high triglycerides (OR=1.48, p=0.019) at baseline were independent predictors of progression of CVD. We could not determine an independent impact of kidney function on CVD in the overall cohort. Furthermore, we determined that the presence of CVD itself confers an increased risk of progression to RRT (RR= 1.58, p=0.047), adjusted for kidney function.

This is the first in-depth analysis of CVD in a cohort of patients with established chronic kidney disease who are not on dialysis. The question regarding the impact of the altered biology of uremia in contributing to CVD progression remains unanswered and clearly needs further study. However, the findings do raise the issue of whether aggressive treatment of CVD and risk factors might, in fact, reduce progression to RRT. Further large scale observational studies as well as interventional studies are needed to more clearly understand the complex biology of cardiovascular and kidney disease progression.

Introduction

The high prevalence and incidence of cardiovascular disease (CVD) in both dialysis patients and transplant patients is well described,[1-5] as is the adverse impact of CVD on long-term outcomes.[6-8] Risk factors recognized to contribute to CVD in the general population, hypertension and diabetes, are present in patients with chronic kidney disease (CKD). Numerous studies to date have shown an independent effect of kidney disease itself on CVD outcomes.[7-11]

Contribution of kidney dysfunction itself, and of other factors associated with kidney disease, to the poor outcomes is unknown. In chronic kidney disease populations, both on and not on dialysis, there are specific 'uremia' related risk factors that have been associated with CVD outcomes: most notable is the consistent association of anemia and LVH and CHF.[6,12-14] Abnormal calcium phosphate metabolism and hyperparathryoidism have also been associated with myocardial fibrosis, hypertrophy and vascular calcification.[15-18] However, there is limited understanding of the differential impact of each risk factor on kidney function and cardiovascular function and the interaction between established cardiovascular disease and kidney disease. The issue of reverse causality and survival bias confounds most analyses performed to date.[19]

We report here the results of data collected for the Canadian Multi-centre Study in Patients with Renal

M.M. Avram (ed.), Improving Prognosis for Kidney Disorders, 29-38.

Insufficiency, commenced in 1994. This study is an observational cohort study funded by the Kidney Foundation of Canada. We have previously reported on the risk factors associated with Left Ventricular growth and LVH.[12] We identified the increased prevalence of LVH at each level of creatinine clearance. Further, we found that anemia and systolic blood pressure were independent risk factors for cardiac growth and hypertrophy in patients with varying degrees of kidney dysfunction. In this same group of patients with established chronic kidney disease, this study attempts to answer additional questions:

(1) Is there an independent impact of 'uremia associated' risk factors, such as Hgb, iPTH, and calcium phosphate product, after correcting for the level of kidney function, on the prevalence and incidence of CVD in patients with chronic kidney disease?

(2) Is there an independent impact of the presence of CVD on the progression of kidney disease, in addition to established risk factors such as hypertension, proteinuria, age and gender?

Materials and Methods

Study Population and Design

This Canadian multi-centre cohort study enrolled patients who had been identified by nephrologists as having chronic kidney disease. The details of the study have been reported elsewhere.[12] Consecutive patients in 7 different geographical locations across Canada, who had calculated creatinine clearances between 75 and 10 ml/min (calculated using the Cockcroft-Gault formula), who were expected by their physicians to live and to be off dialysis for at least 12 months of follow-up were entered. Informed consent was obtained from all patients, and the ethics board of each institution approved the study. There were no attempts to modify therapy during the study. All patients had clinical, laboratory and CV symptoms reviewed at one-year intervals. Hospitalization events, and medication use were also evaluated. The data was captured using standardized data collection sheets, and was then entered into a central database for analysis.

Definitions of Cardiovascular Disease

CV disease was defined by both history of CV event or condition and/or current symptoms according to NYHA and CCS classifications for heart failure and angina respectively. CV event history included history of MI, angina, CABG or angioplasty, TIA or CVA, PVD, and CHF. Research assistants administered standardized questionnaires that describe symptoms associated with each class of heart failure or angina to each patient, and symptoms were graded using conventional NYHA and CCS classifications. Change in cardiovascular status was defined as either change in NYHA or CCS classification or a cardiac-related hospitalization.

Chronic Kidney Disease: Calculations and Definitions

Serum creatinine was measured in each patient's own laboratory, which was maintained through the study period. Calculations using the formula of Cockcroft Gault[12] were used to determine level of creatinine clearance. Four categories of kidney function were identified: mild (>50<75ml/min), moderate (35-49ml/min), moderate severe (25-34 ml/min), or severe (10-24 ml/min). Renal replacement therapy was defined as the need for either dialysis or transplantation.

Outcomes of Interest

The major outcomes of interest for this analysis included kidney survival (time to RRT) and change in CVD status.

Statistical Analysis

The baseline clinical characteristics of patients were compared using the ANOVA or Kruskal-Wallis test for continuous variables, depending on distribution, and the Chi square test for categorical variables.

We used the Chi square test for discrete variables and *t* test or Wilcoxon rank-sum test, where appropriate, for continuous variables to compare patients with and without CVD at baseline, as well as patients with change and without change of CVD status. Univariate odds ratios were adjusted for degree of kidney function by using logistic regression. The logistic regression was used to determine the association between patient baseline characteristics and presence of CVD at baseline and then to predict change in CVD status.

Time to RRT therapy was calculated based on the time from study enrollment to the dialysis start or transplantation date. Renal survival was estimated using the Kaplan-Meier method. The survival curves by presence of CVD were compared using the log-rank test. We used proportional hazards regression models to assess the effect of baseline patient characteristics on time to RRT after controlling for baseline kidney function. The Cox regression model was used to identify independent and significant predictors of time to RRT. All multivariate models were developed by using a backward elimination technique, including the following variables: patient age, sex, diabetes status, creatinine

Table 1. Baseline Characteristics by Level of Renal Function

Characteristic	All *n=313*	>50 *ml/min* *n=62*	35 – 49 *ml/min* *n=83*	25 – 34 *ml/min* *n=74*	10 – 24 *ml/min* *n=94*	*P* Value
Age *yrs*	56.3 ± 14.5	53.5 ± 13.4	54.9 ± 15.3	56.5 ± 14.7	59.3 ± 14.1	.0604
Gender *% Male*	211 (67.4%)	54 (87%)	64 (77%)	47 (64%)	46 (49%)	.001
Race *% Caucasian*	267 (87.0%)	54 (88%)	74 (91%)	59 (81%)	80 (87%)	.268
Diabetes	91 (29.1%)	21 (34%)	24 (29%)	16 (22%)	30 (32%)	.383
CrCl *ml/min*	36.2 ± 16.8	62.6 ± 10.5	41.9 ± 4.3	29.9 ± 3.0	18.8 ± 3.8	.0001
24hr Urine Protein *g/L*	1.04 ± 1.36	0.96 ± 1.24	0.97 ± 1.22	1.03 ± 1.75	1.22 ± 1.25	.7165
Systolic BP *mm Hg*	144.4 ± 23.4	143.9 ± 20.9	142.7 ± 21.6	141.0 ± 24.7	149.3 ± 24.4	.0847
Diastolic BP *mm Hg*	85.4 ± 11.6	87.3 ± 11.8	85.1 ± 11.3	84.8 ± 12.7	84.9 ± 10.9	.5519
Pulse Pressure *mm Hg*	58.9 ± 20.8	56.5 ± 19.1	57.0 ± 21.8	56.1 ± 21.8	64.4 ± 21.2	.0242
Total Cholesterol *g/L*	5.70 ± 1.34	5.76 ± 1.19	5.58 ± 1.16	5.98 ± 1.64	5.56 ± 1.30	.1592
HDL *mmol/L*	1.15 ± 0.51	1.04 ± 0.54	1.06 ± 0.31	1.26 ± 0.65	1.22 ± 0.48	.0166
Triglycerides *mmol/L*	2.36 ± 1.69	2.57 ± 1.44	2.46 ± 2.27	2.45 ± 1.53	2.07 ± 1.29	.2424
Hemoglobin *g/L*	128.1 ± 19.5	141.5 ± 16.6	134.3 ± 19.3	125.7 ± 16.6	115.6 ± 15.3	.0001
Ca*PO4 *mmol/L *mmol/L*	2.78 ± 0.62	2.50 ± 0.49	2.66 ± 0.56	2.73 ± 0.54	3.12 ± 0.65	.0001
Log PTH *pmol/L*	2.22 ± 0.85	1.64 ± 0.58	1.88 ± 0.67	2.34 ± 0.79	2.80 ± 0.81	.0001
LVMI g/m^2	111.3 ± 35.3	110.0 ± 35.2	106.8 ± 28.8	106.1 ± 34.7	120.2 ± 39.8	.0474
ACEi alone or in comb.	155 (49.7%)	37 (59.7%)	47 (56.6%)	37 (50.0%)	34 (36.6%)	.002
Beta blockers alone or in comb.	74 (23.7%)	15 (24.2%)	20 (24.1%)	16 (21.6%)	23 (24.7%)	.970
Any lipid lowering agent	42 (13.5%)	10 (16.1%)	10 (12.1%)	12 (16.2%)	10 (10.9%)	.676
Any Hx or Sx of CVD	143 (45.7%)	27 (43.5%)	41 (49.4%)	29 (39.2%)	46 (48.9%)	.788
Hx of Any CVD	120 (38.3%)	22 (35.5%)	32 (38.6%)	26 (35.14%)	40 (42.6%)	.743
Hx of Angina	52 (16.7%)	11 (18.0%)	16 (19.5%)	8 (10.8%)	17 (18.1%)	.472
Hx of CHF	23 (7.6%)	5 (8.3%)	6 (7.5%)	3 (4.2%)	9 (9.8%)	.596
Hx of MI	39 (12.7%)	10 (16.4%)	10 (12.2%)	10 (13.7%)	9 (9.9%)	.686
Hx of PVD	38 (12.4%)	8 (13.1%)	9 (11.0%)	10 (13.9%)	11 (12.1%)	.953
NYHA: I-II	76 (24.3%)	15 (24.2%)	25 (30.1%)	13 (17.6%)	23 (24.5%)	.331
III-IV	7 (2.2%)	1 (1.6%)	0 (0%)	2 (2.7%)	4 (4.3%)	
CCS: I-II	70 (22.4%)	16 (25.8%)	20 (24.1%)	13 (17.6%)	21 (22.3%)	.712
III-IV	6 (1.9%)	1 (1.6%)	1 (1.2%)	3 (4.1%)	1 (1.1%)	

clearance, systolic and diastolic blood pressure, total cholesterol, triglycerides, hemoglobin, phosphate-calcium product, iPTH, and presence of CVD at baseline.

A p value of less than 0.05 for two-sided univariate tests was considered statistically significant.We set the p-value for multivariate analyses to 0.10 to account for the hypothesis generating purpose of this analysis. Statistical analyses were performed using SAS software, version 6.12 (SAS Institute, Cary, NC).

Results

Baseline Characteristics

The original study enrolled 447 patients, of whom 417 had initial evaluation of cardiac status. We excluded 104 patients from this analysis due to missing baseline values for key variables of interest. Thus, this analysis includes 313 predominantly male (67%) and Caucasian (87%) patients, who had a mean age of 56 years (**Table 1**). The mean calculated creatinine clearance (Ccr) was 36.2±16.8 ml/min. Twenty nine percent of the group were diabetic; and the prevalence of the causes of kidney disease paralleled those in national registries: hypertension (27%), glomerulonephritis (18%), and diabetes (25%), PCKD (8%).

Table 1 demonstrates the baseline demographics of the whole cohort and compares a number of pertinent variables relative to baseline kidney function. Gender, hemoglobin, pulse pressure, calcium-phosphate product, iPTH, HDL, LVMI were different between groups with different kidney function. The use of ACEi therapy was the lowest in those with the worst kidney function. The prevalence of CVD was similar at each level of kidney function.

Table 2. Conventional and Uremia Associated Risk Factors in Patients with and without CVD at Baseline

Variables	CVD (-) N=170	CVD (+) N=143	*P* Value
Age *yrs*	53.5 ± 14.9	59.6 ± 13.4	.0002
Gender *% Male*	108 (63.5%)	103 (72.0%)	.110
Diabetes	37 (21.8%)	54 (37.8%)	.002
CrCl (Calculated) *ml/min*	35.9 ± 16.2	36.6 ± 17.5	.7000
24hr urine Protein *g/L*	1.08 ± 1.48	1.01 ± 1.24	.6945
Systolic BP *mm Hg*	143.5 ± 23.2	145.3 ± 23.7	.4950
Diastolic BP *mm Hg*	87.2 ± 11.7	83.3 ± 11.2	.0029
Pulse Pressure *mm Hg*	56.3 ± 20.4	62.0 ± 21.0	.0154
Total Cholesterol *mmol/L*	5.77 ± 1.54	5.62 ± 1.06	.3209
HDL *mmol/L*	1.19 ± 0.55	1.09 ± 0.46	.1168
Triglycerides *mmol/L*	2.36 ± 1.39	2.36 ± 1.99	.9808
Hemoglobin *g/L*	128.0 ± 19.3	128.2 ± 19.9	.9196
PO4*Ca *mmol/L *mmol/L*	2.78 ± 0.61	2.80 ± 0.63	.7663
log PTH *pmol/L*	2.27 ± 0.88	2.16 ± 0.82	.2246
LVMI g/m^2	105.59 ± 31.83	117.94 ± 37.95	.0034
ACEi alone or in comb.	88 (51.8%)	67 (47.2%)	.420
Beta blockers alone or in comb.	34 (20.0%)	40 (28.2%)	.091
Any lipid lowering agent	17 (10.0)	25 (17.7%)	.047

Prevalence of Cardiovascular Disease at Baseline

A Comparison of Conventional and Uremia Related Risk Factors

Comparisons between patients with and without CVD at baseline are presented in **Table 2**. Those with CVD at baseline were likely to be older, diabetic, have lower diastolic blood pressures, higher pulse pressures, and larger values for LVMI. However, in this cohort, the presence or absence of CVD at baseline is not different with respect to creatinine clearance (35.9 ml/min vs. 36.6 ml/min, p= .700). Again, the use of ACEi was not different as a function of presence or absence of CVD, but lipid lowering agents were used more often in those with CVD than those without (18% vs. 10% p=.047).

After adjustment for the level of renal function, the same risk factors, i.e. age (OR=1.17, p=.0002), diabetes (OR=2.18, p=.0022), diastolic BP (OR=0.81, p=.0002), pulse pressure (OR=1.07, p=.013) and LVMI (OR=1.11, p=.0033), were associated with presence or absence of CVD at baseline . We used the multivariate analysis, adjusted for severity of kidney disease, to identify older age, diabetes and low diastolic blood pressure as factors associated with increasing the probability of the CVD presence at baseline (**Table 3**).

Cardiovascular Disease – Change in CVD Status during Follow-up

Impact of Pre-existing CVD

Of the original 313 patients included in this analysis, 36 patients were lost or refused further follow-up, 8

Table 3. Multivariate Analysis of Risk Factors Associated with the Presence of CVD at Baseline

Variables	**Odds Ratio**	**95% CI**	***P* Value**
Age *5 years*	1.143	1.047-1.248	.0028
Male Gender	1.355	0.793-2.313	.2663
Diabetes	2.024	1.206-3.397	.0076
CrCl *5 ml/min*	1.025	0.952-1.103	.5169
Diastolic BP *5 mm Hg*	0.898	0.808-0.998	.0464

Table 4. Patient Characteristics Associated with CVD Status in Patients with and Those without CVD at Baseline

Variables	No Preexisting CVD N=135			Preexisting CVD n=109		
	No CVD n=125	CVD n=10	*P* Value	Stable n=71	Worsening n=38	*P* Value
Age *yrs*	52.3 ± 15.4	61.8 ± 13.1	.0592	58.4 ± 13.3	63.2 ± 10.7	.0564
Gender *% Male*	80 (64.0%)	5 (50.0%)	.499	51 (71.8%)	26 (68.42%)	.709
Diabetes	21 (16.8%)	5 (50.0%)	.023	19 (26.8%)	17 (44.7%)	.057
CrCl *ml/min*	37.8 ± 16.3	33.7 ± 16.1	.4440	37.8 ± 17.3	32.8 ± 13.1	.1224
24hr Urine Protein *g/L*	0.84 ± 1.01	1.08 ± 1.29	.5246	0.75 ± 1.05	1.48 ± 1.53	.0278
Systolic BP *mm Hg*	141.2 ± 23.8	149.8 ± 27.9	.2808	147.0 ± 24.8	141.8 ± 24.3	.2980
Diastolic BP *mm Hg*	86.2 ± 11.8	87.0 ± 14.1	.8492	85.8 ± 10.7	78.3 ± 11.1	.0008
Pulse Pressure *mm Hg*	55.0 ± 20.7	62.8 ± 22.8	.2562	61.2 ± 22.9	63.5 ± 19.79	.5950
Total Cholesterol *mmol/L*	5.66 ± 1.27	6.34 ± 1.44	.1102	5.57 ± 0.90	5.89 ± 1.19	.1228
HDL *mmol/L*	1.21± 0.60	1.11± 0.30	.3604	1.16±0.43	1.04±0.60	.5958
Triglycerides *mmol/L*	2.36 ± 1.32	2.54 ± 1.22	.6816	2.03 ± 1.30	3.04 ± 3.09	.0183
Hemoglobin *g/L*	130.6 ± 19.3	121.8 ± 17.1	.1659	127.5 ± 19.0	129.0 ± 18.2	.6867
Ca*PO4 *mmol/L *mmol/L*	2.70 ± 0.61	2.87 ± 0.37	.3926	2.77 ± 0.59	2.83 ± 0.48	.5827
Log PTH *pmol/l*	2.24± 0.84	1.97± 0.76	.3339	2.06±0.79	2.26±0.78	.1957
LVMI g/m^2	103.28± 32.17	115.61±34.95	.2738	115.7±37.35	125.38±42.64	.2414

patients died, 24 patients started dialysis and one patient was transplanted before at least one cardiovascular follow-up evaluation. Hence, 244 patients had evaluable cardiovascular follow-up: median duration of follow-up was 23 months, with a total of 5547 months or 462 patient years of follow-up. During the follow up period, 48/244 (20%) of patients developed new or worsening cardiac symptoms or were hospitalized for cardiac disease. Of the 135 patients who had no pre-existing CVD, 10 (7.4%) developed new CVD; this is in contrast to the 109 patients with pre-existing cardiac disease, of which 38 (35%) developed a new event or worsening of CVD (p =. 001). Thus, 21% of the 48 patients with new or worsening cardiac disease had no previous CVD.

Table 4 describes the results of a univariate analysis comparing the association of conventional and

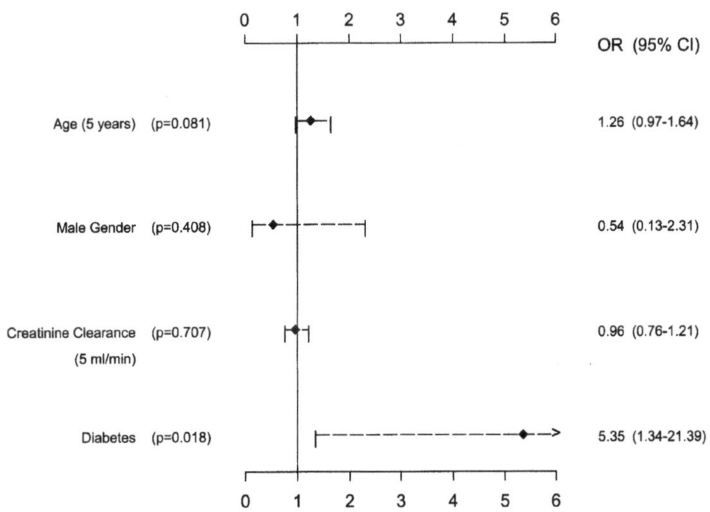

Figure 1. Factors Associated with Change of CVD Status in Patients without History or Symptoms of CVD at Baseline.

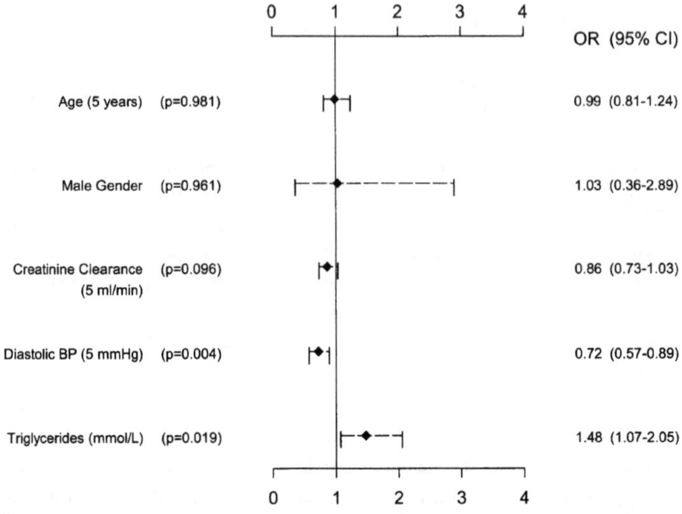

Figure 2. Factors Associated with Change of CVD Status in Patients with History or Symptoms of CVD at Baseline.

uremia related variables with change in CVD status in patients with and without pre-existing CVD. Note that age and diabetes at baseline predict change in CVD status in both groups of patients, while higher serum triglyceride levels and lower diastolic blood pressure predict worsening of CVD among patients with pre-existing CVD over the follow-up period. There were no apparent associations of 'uremia specific' factors such as hemoglobin, calcium phosphate product, iPTH level, nor of level of kidney dysfunction itself, with change of CVD status. The same baseline characteristics were associated with change in CVD status, depending on the presence or absence of CVD at baseline, after adjustment for level of kidney function.

A multivariate analysis revealed that diabetes increases the probability of change in CVD status in those without pre-existing CVD (**Figure 1**). Low diastolic blood pressure and high triglycerides were independent and significant predictors of change in CVD status in those with pre-existing CVD (**Figure 2**).

We performed a separate multivariate analysis for all patients who had change in NYHA class heart failure versus patients who had change in CCS class angina. The important predictors of NYHA class change were older age (OR=1.21 per 5 years; p=.0588), lower diastolic BP (OR=0.79 per 5 mm Hg; p=.0175), higher triglycerides (1.44 per mmol/L; p=.0118), and

Table 5. Associations of Baseline Characteristics, Adjusted for Kidney Function, with Time to RRT

Variables	Risk Ratio	95% C.I.	*P* Value
Age *5yr*	0.879	0.816-0.947	.0007
Gender *Male*	1.957	1.204-3.181	.0068
Diabetes	2.181	1.376-3.457	.0009
CrCl *5 ml/min*	0.708	0.639-0.785	.0001
24hr urine Protein *g/L*	1.550	1.377-1.746	.0001
Systolic BP *5 mm Hg*	0.990	0.942-1.041	.6991
Diastolic BP *5 mm Hg*	1.120	1.004-1.250	.0417
Pulse Pressure *5 mm Hg*	0.997	0.950-1.046	.9042
Total Cholesterol *mmol/L*	0.819	0.680-0.988	.0371
HDL *mmol/L*	0.614	0.351-1.074	.0876
Triglycerides *mmol/L*	0.935	0.790-1.106	.4315
Hemoglobin *5 g/L*	0.863	0.804-0.926	.0001
Ca*PO4 *mmol/L *mmol/L*	1.651	1.229-2.217	.0009
log PTH *pmol/L*	1.613	1.199-2.168	.0016
Hx. or Sx. of CVD	1.580	1.006-2.482	.0470

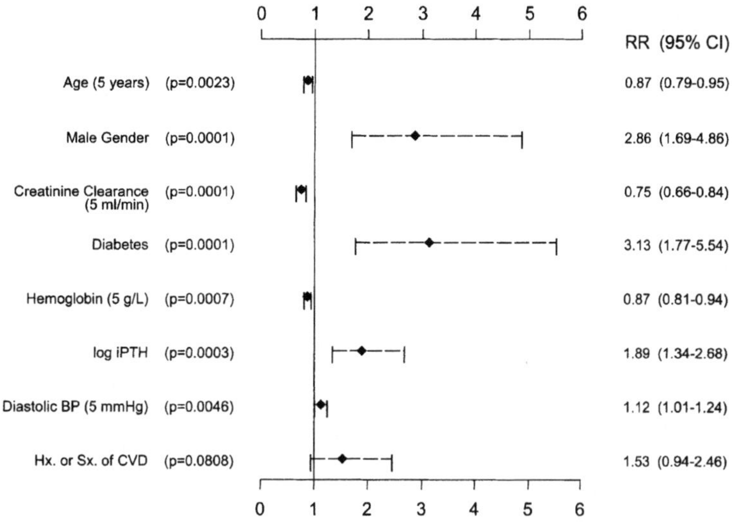

Figure 3. Independent Predictors of Time to RRT (Results of Cox Proportional Hazards Modeling).

presence of CVD at baseline (OR= 4.91; p=.0011). The change in CCS class was associated with lower baseline kidney function (OR=0.84 per 5 ml/min; p=.0624), diabetes (OR=3.96; p=.0035), lower diastolic BP (OR=0.79 per 5 mm Hg; p=.0284), and baseline CVD (OR= 3.88; p=.0111).

Loss of Kidney Function: Conventional and Other Predictors of Time to Renal Replacement Therapy

Table 5 describes risk factors associated with time to RRT, adjusted for baseline kidney function. In addition to known risk factors for progressive kidney function decline, (age, gender, diabetes, proteinuria, blood pressure and kidney function), there are 'uremia' specific factors - hemoglobin, iPTH, calcium phosphate product - which may also be associated with decline. Furthermore, the presence of CVD, as well as low HDL and cholesterol levels at baseline, are associated with increased risk of kidney failure leading to RRT. There were several factors that independently and significantly predicted decline of kidney function in multivariate analysis, shown in **Figure 3**: older age, male gender, diabetes, low baseline kidney function and hemoglobin, and high diastolic blood pressure and iPTH level. In terms of impact of CVD on time to RRT, there was only a trivial difference after adjustment for all of the above factors (univariate RR=1.58, multivariate RR=1.52), indicating the importance of this factor.

Figure 4 demonstrates the impact of CVD presence or absence at baseline on time to RRT.

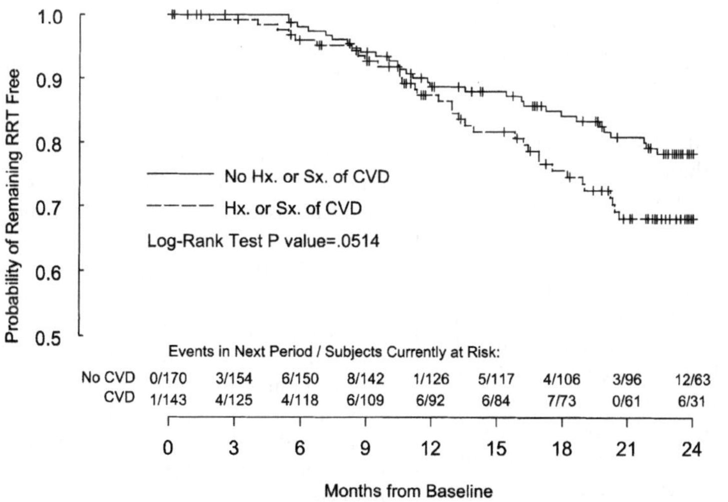

Figure 4. Kaplan-Meier Curves of Time to RRT by CVD Status at Baseline.

Discussion

This analysis of a cohort of patients with known chronic kidney disease describes the high prevalence of cardiac disease (46%) and of conventional cardiovascular risk factors. The analysis does not demonstrate that 'uremia' specific risk factors predict either the prevalence of CVD or the change in CVD status. Previous publications have described a similarly high prevalence of CVD risk factors and have determined that chronic kidney disease itself was a risk factor for CV outcome and mortality.[10,20,21] All of these studies compared patients with kidney disease to those without kidney disease, did not adjust for specific levels of kidney function, and did not measure specific variables associated with kidney disease - hemoglobin, iPTH, calcium, phosphate - that may mediate the impact of CKD on outcomes. Notably, Culleton et al reported findings similar to ours in the Framingham cohort[22]: despite a higher prevalence of CVD in patients with CKD at baseline, there was no impact of CKD on long term outcomes after controlling for conventional risk factors.

That uremia specific factors did not appear to exert an effect on CVD prevalence/incidence independent of conventional cardiac risk factors could be due to study limitations rather than to the absence of such an effect. Furthermore, the prevalence of ischemia related CVD (angina, CVA, MI, PVD) at baseline is similar in this population to that in other renal populations at later stages of disease (i.e. on dialysis and post transplant).[1,3,23,24] This finding supports the notion recently discussed in depth by Parfrey[25] in an editorial: cardiac function can be affected by processes different from simple atherosclerotic induced ischemia, and CVD with progressive kidney disease may be secondary to the influence of both atherogenic processes and factors which modulate cardiac muscle structure function. We did not measure left ventricular ejection fractions in this study; rather, we only have a measure of cardiac hypertrophy, LVMI, and pulse pressure. Pulse pressure, as an indicator of vascular stiffness, has recently been described as predicting morbidity and mortality and contributing to cardiac dysfunction[26,27] in cardiac populations. The current analysis shows that both LVMI and pulse pressure are significantly different between those patients with and without CVD at baseline.

Progressive cardiovascular disease and progressive decline of kidney function do have a number of risk factors in common, including hypertension and diabetes. There are some risk factors specific to each 'condition' and some that occur as a consequence of one of these impacting another. It may be that the purported 'uremic factors' exert their influence through affecting cardiac function, not the atherosclerotic process as previously thought. Interestingly, it is possible that these same factors that affect cardiac function may also accelerate decline of kidney function, both through activation of cytokines and growth factors; and that ongoing endothelial cell dysfunction may contribute simultaneously to both processes.[16,29-32] There is substantial animal and cellular data to support the impact of these factors on progressive kidney disease.[31] However, the current analysis is unable to determine the relative impact of each of these.

This study further demonstrates the association of conventional risk factors with kidney function decline and also demonstrates an additional association of CVD presence with 'kidney survival'. The data also suggest that anemia and hyperparathyroidism may contribute to progression of kidney disease, independent of kidney function level, gender, diabetes or age.[28] The presence of CVD at baseline confers a 50% increase in probability of renal replacement therapy. The explanation for this may be complex and multifactorial. Worsening cardiac function may lead to reduced blood flow to the kidney, thus adding a prerenal insult to kidneys with little reserve, and to activation of cellular mechanisms which lead to sclerosis and fibrosis. Alternatively, cardiac dysfunction may lead to the addition of medications/interventions that may further cause kidney injury or reduce function. These hypotheses are not mutually exclusive. Interestingly, a recent report by Silverberg and colleagues describes the treatment of heart failure and associated anemia with erythropoeiten. Importantly, the treatment group had significantly impaired kidney function (serum creatinine 2.3 mg/dl) prior to therapy. After correction of anemia and concomitant with improvement in cardiac status there was improvement of kidney function.[33]

The current analysis, demonstrating that CV disease and conventional risk factors for cardiac disease adversely affect the progression of kidney disease, provides hope that attention to CV health and risk factor modification might improve long-term outcomes for the progression of kidney disease. In this cohort, as in others,[34,8,35,36] there is sub-optimal use of cardiovascular medications such as angiotensin converting enzyme inhibitors, beta blockers and lipid lowering medications. It may be that both cardiologists and nephrologists caring for patients with established kidney disease actually practice 'therapeutic nihilism'.[35] This inadequate therapy of cardiac disease may accelerate the rate of kidney function decline in susceptible individuals. Thus, the high prevalence of those with established cardiac disease commencing dialysis may be the consequence of failure to institute treatment prior to dialysis.

This study is unique in that it describes the prevalence of CVD and its attendant risk factors in patients with kidney disease prior to dialysis known to nephrologists in Canada. Others have described unselected groups of general populations or used population databases or post hoc analyses of large studies to review the impact of kidney disease on CV outcomes.[7,9,10,22] These approaches suffer from a number of problems. There is a lack of uniformity in defining the presence and severity of kidney disease. There is little information about the stability of kidney dysfunction prior to study starts, and there is no documentation of the etiology of kidney dysfunction or of 'uremia' associated biochemical and hematological abnormalities. There is ample evidence to support the problems of use of serum creatinine alone as a marker for kidney disease.[37] The current analysis, in contrast, focuses on individuals with established, non-reversible kidney disease, using calculated estimates of kidney function. By examining those variables specifically associated with kidney disease, we are able to explore the hypothesis that there is an impact of these variables versus conventional risk factors versus kidney disease per se on CVD. This study also describes the complex interplay between CVD and progressive CKD. This is important if therapeutic strategies to treat one disease may actually be justified in terms of their impact on another aspect of this disease.

Our study, like all prospective observational studies, precludes the establishment of causality. Furthermore, due to missing values and loss of patients to follow-up, the true burden of illness in this population may be underestimated. This study did not capture events after RRT nor specific cardiac events. We believe, however, that the similarity of the prevalence of CVD in this cohort to that reported in other similar cohorts [34,38] makes it unlikely that there is significant underestimation of CVD. The issue of reverse causality, surviving off RRT to actually have a CVD event, and survival bias (i.e. those with worse CVD were put onto RRT as a means of controlling symptoms) cannot be addressed with this analysis, nor in this cohort. Importantly, this data can be used to generate hypotheses and develop interventional studies based on biologically plausible associations of specific risk factors. Ideally, we should establish follow-up in 2 distinct cohorts of patients: those with established kidney disease without CVD, and those with established cardiac disease without kidney dysfunction, and determine, through careful and systematic measurement of known risk factors, which of these are predisposed to developing into cardiac disease and to kidney disease respectively.

In summary, the prevalence of CVD in the population with CKD is high and is attributable to both ischemic disease and myocardial dysfunction. This study demonstrates an under-use of medications known to improve cardiac outcome in the general population. This may contribute to the poor cardiac outcomes seen in this group. Furthermore, the presence of CVD appears to predict an increased probability of RRT; thus the appropriate treatment of cardiac disease may, in fact, lead to delay of RRT and, thus, serve to lessen the burden of illness not only for the individual patients but also for health care systems.

Acknowledgments

The authors would like to acknowledge the support of the Kidney Foundation of Canada, the extensive assistance of Dr. Vadim Minster and Ms Cheyenne Reese for data organization and manuscript preparation, and all of the research assistants in each of the participating centers for their extensive data collection.

References

1. Foley RN, Parfrey PS, Harnett JD, Kent GM, Martin CJ, Murray DC, Barre PE: Clinical and echocardiographic disease in patients starting end-stage renal disease therapy. Kidney Int 47:186-192, 1995
2. Canadian Organ Replacement Registry, Canadian Institute for Health Information (CIHI), Don Mills, Ontario, Canada, 1999.
3. Parfrey PS: Cardiac disease in dialysis patients: diagnosis, burden of disease, prognosis, risk factors and management. Nephrol Dial Transplant 15:58-68, 2000
4. Sarnak MJ, Levey AS: Epidemiology, diagnosis, and management of cardiac disease in chronic renal disease. J Thromb Thrombolysis 10:169-180, 2000
5. Kasiske B, Guijarro C, Massy Z, Wiederkehr M, Ma J: Cardiovascular disease after renal transplantation. J Am Soc Nephrol 7:158-165, 1996
6. Foley RN, Parfrey PS, Harnett JD, Kent GM, Murray DC, Barre PE: The impact of anemia on cardiomyopathy, morbidity and mortality in end-stage renal disease. Am J Kidney Dis 28:53-61, 1996
7. Chertow GM, Normand S-LT, Silva LR, McNeil BJ: Survival after acute myocardial infarction in patients with end-stage renal disease: results from the Cooperative Cardiovascular Project. Am J Kidney Dis 35:1044-1051, 2000
8. Herzog CA: Poor long-term survival of dialysis patients after acute myocardial infarction: bad treatment or bad disease? Am J Kidney Dis 35:1217-1220, 2000
9. Mann J, Gerstein, HC, Pogue J, Baosch, Yusef, S: Renal insufficiency as a predictor of cardiovascular outcomes and the impact of ramipril: the HOPE randomized trial. Annals of Int Medicine 134:629-636, 2001
10. Hemmelgarn BR, Ghali WA, Quan H, Brant R, Norris CM, Taub KJ, Knudtson ML: Poor long-term survival after coronary angiography in patients with renal insufficiency. Am J Kidney Dis 37: 64-72, 2001
11. Beattie JN, Soman SS, Sandberg KR, Yee J, Borzak S, McCullough PA: Determinants of mortality after myocardial

infarction in patients with advanced renal dysfunction. Am J Kidney Disease 2001 (in press)

12. Levin A, Thompson CR, Ethier J, Carlisle EJ, Tobe S, Mendelssohn D, Burgess E, Jindal K, Barrett B, Singer J, Djurdjev O: Left ventricular mass index increase in early renal disease: impact of decline in hemoglobin. Am J Kidney Dis 34: 125-134, 1999
13. O'Riordan E, Foley RN: Effects of anaemia on cardiovascular status. Nephrol Dial Transplant 15:19-22, 2000
14. Levin A, Foley RN: Cardiovascular disease in chronic renal insufficiency. Am J Kidney Dis 36:24-30, 2000
15. Block GA, Port FK: Re-evaluation of risks associated with hyperphosphatemia and hyperparathyroidism in dialysis patients: recommendations for a change in management. Am J Kidney Dis 35:1226-1237, 2000
16. Pannier B, Guerin AP, Marchais SJ, Metivier F, Safar ME, London GM: Postischemic vasodilation, endothelial activation, and cardiovascular remodeling in end-stage renal disease. Kidney Int 57:1091-1099, 2000
17. Goodman WG, Goldin J, Kuizon BD, Yoon C, Gales B, Sider D, Wang Y, Chung J, Emerick A, Greaser L, Elashoff RM, Salusky IB: Coronary-artery calcification in young adults with end-stage renal disease who are undergoing dialysis. N Engl J Med 342:1478-1483, 2000
18. Amann K, Ritz E, Wiest G, Klaus G, Mall G: A role of parathyroid hormone for the activation of cardiac fibroblasts in uremia. J Am Soc Nephrol 4:1814-1819, 1994
19. Baigent C, Burbury K, Wheeler D: Premature cardiovascular disease in chronic renal failure. Lancet 356:147-152, 2000
20. Anderson RJ, O'Brien M, MaWhinney S, VillaNueva CB, Moritz TE, Sethi GK, Henderson, WG, Hammermeister KE, Grover, FL, Shroyer AL: Mild renal failure is associated with adverse outcome after cardiac valve surgery. Am J Kidney Dis 35:1127-1134, 2000
21. McCullough PA, Soman SS, Shah SS, Smith ST, Marks KR, Yee J, Steven Boržak S: Risks associated with renal dysfunction in coronary care unit patients. J Am Coll Cardiol 36:679-684, 2000
22. Culleton BF, Larson MG, Wilson PWF, Evans JC, Parfrey PS, Levy D: Cardiovascular disease and mortality in a community-based cohort with mild renal insufficiency: Kidney Int 56:2214-2219, 1999
23. Parfrey PS, Harnett JD, Foley RN: Heart failure and ischemic heart disease in chronic uremia. Curr Opin Nephrol Hypertens 4:105-110, 1995
24. Rigato C, Jeffery J, Foley R, Brown S, Tribula C, Negrijin C, Parfrey P: Risk factors for de novo ischaemic heart disease in renal transplant recipients. J Am Soc Nephrol, 11:705A-705A, 2000 (Abstract)
25. Parfrey, PS: Is renal insufficiency an atherogenic state? Reflection on prevalence, incidence and risk. Am J Kidney Dis 37:154-156, 2001
26. Mitchell GF: Pulse pressure, arterial compliance and cardiovascular morbidity and mortality. Curr Opin Nephrol Hypertens 8:335-342, 1999
27. Safar ME: Systolic blood pressure, pulse pressure and arterial stiffness as cardiovascular risk factors. Curr Opin Nephrol Hypertens 10:257-261, 2001
28. Hebert LA, Wilmer WA, Falkenhain ME, Ladson-Wofford SE, Nahman NS, Rovin BH: Renoprotection: One or many therapies? Kidney Int 59:1211-1226, 2001
29. Hunter JJ, Chien KR: Signaling pathways for cardiac hypertrophy and failure. N Engl J Med 341:1276-1283, 1999
30. Amann K, Kronenberg G, Gehlen F, Wessels S, Orth S, Munter K, Ehmke H, Mall G, Ritz E: Cardiac remodeling in experimental renal failure--an immunohistochemical study. Nephrol Dial Transplant 13:1958-1966, 1998
31. London GM, Fabiani F, Marchais SJ, et al: Uremic cardiomyopathy: an inadequate left ventricular hypertrophy. Kidney Int 31:973-980, 1987
32. Tonelli M, Bohm C, Pandeya S, Gill J, Levin A, Kiberd BA: Cardiac risk factors and the use of cardioprotective medications in patients with chronic renal insufficiency. Am J Kidney Dis 37:484-489, 2001
33. Silverberg D, Wexler D, Blum M, Keren G, Sheps D, Laibovitch E, Brosh D, Laniado S, Schwartz D, Yachnin T, Shapira I, Gavish D, Baruch R, Koifman B, Kaplan C, Steinbruch S, Iaina A: The use of subcutaneous erythropoietin and intravenous iron for the treatment of the anemia of severe, resistant congestive heart failure improves cardiac and renal function and functional cardiac class, and markedly reduces hospitalizations. J Am Coll Cardiol 35:1737-1744, 2000
34. Taal M, Omer SA, Nadim MK, McKenzie HS: Cellular and molecular mediators in common pathway mechanisms of chronic disease progression. Curr Opin Nephrol Hyperten 9:323-331, 2000
35. Levin, A, Stevens L, and McCullough P: Cardiovascular disease: the killer in chronic kidney disease. Postgraduate Medicine 2001 (in press)
36. Maschio G: How good are nephrologists at controlling blood pressure in renal patients? Nephrol Dial Transplant 14:2075-2077, 1999
37. Duncan L. Djurdjev O. Heathcote, J, Levin A: Screening for renal disease using serum creatinine : who are we missing? Nephrol Dial Transplant 2001 (in press)
38. Holland DC, Lam M: Predictors of hospitalization and death among pre-dialysis patients: a retrospective cohort study. Nephrol Dial Transplant 15: 650-658, 2000

4 Metabolic Pathogenesis of Cardio-Renal Disease

WILLIAM F. KEANE, MD

Abstract

Recent clinical data have established microalbuminuria/proteinuria as an independent risk factor for renal disease and for progression of renal disease in patients with diabetes and in those with essential hypertension. Moreover, changes in kidney function, even with modest as reductions in estimated creatinine clearance to approximately 60 ml/min/1.73m^2 or a serum creatinine of >1.4, is associated with increased cardiovascular risk. Treatment with angiotensin-converting enzyme inhibitors has been shown in clinical trials to delay or stabilize the rate of progression of renal disease. In addition, reduction in cardiovascular events such as stroke and myocardial infarctions, has been demonstrated in these high-risk individuals. These effects are both dependent and independent of blood pressure control suggesting a non-hemodynamic effect of blockade of the renin angiotensin system. In conjunction with other therapeutic interventions such as dietary modification and control of serum lipids, it appears that for at least a sub-group of patients it is possible to delay or prevent progression of kidney failure. There is frequently a clustering of risk factors in these individuals that includes insulin resistance, salt sensitivity, hypertension, and dyslipidemia. The mechanism of the relationship between albuminuria and cardiovascular disease is unclear but may be related to endothelial cell dysfunction. Nonetheless, the presence of this marker for cardiovascular disease has important implications for the identification and treatment of individuals at risk.

Introduction

During the past decade, a number of clinical trials and epidemiological studies have demonstrated a relationship between kidney disease and cardiovascular disease. Initially these studies focused on albuminuria as a risk for cardiovascular disease, but more recent evidence has indicated that subtle changes in serum creatinine also identify a group of individuals who have a potential increased risk for cardiovascular disease.[1] Numerous studies have demonstrated a relationship between the presence of elevated urinary albumin excretion and risk of progression of kidney disease in individuals with diabetes.[2-10] In patents with microalbuminuria and essential hypertension, a similar increased risk for cardio-renal disease has been suggested.

Reduction of albumin excretion with angiotensin-converting enzyme inhibitors and, more recently, angiotensin II receptor antagonists correlates with a plateau of or decrease in the rate of decline of renal function. This effect appears independent of the anti-hypertensive effect of these agents.[4;11-13] Microalbuminuria also has been implicated as an independent risk factor for cardiovascular disease and premature cardiovascular mortality for individuals with type 1[14;15] and type 2 diabetes mellitus,[16-18] and for patients with essential hypertension.[19-21] Epidemiological studies have demonstrated an association between microalbuminuria and insulin resistance, obesity, salt-sensitivity and dyslipidemia.[22] Also, it has been suggested that diffuse endothelial cell dysfunction makes these individuals particularly susceptible to cardiovascular disease.[23] In particular, the increased permeability to proteins may explain, in part, these deleterious vascular effects. The reversal of endothelial dysfunction with inhibitors or the renin angiotensin II system as well as with lipid lowering therapy, particularly with the statin class of agents, thus has important therapeutic implications. It is possible that improvement in endothelial function can be indirectly assessed by reductions in urine albumin excretion.

Metabolic Pathogenesis of Cardio-Renal Disease

Essential Hypertension

The prevalence of microalbuminuria in patients with essential hypertension ranges between five and thirty-seven per cent.[20;24-26] In a study of 11, 343 non-diabetic, hypertensive patients with a mean age of 57

M.M. Avram.(ed.), Improving Prognosis for Kidney Disorders, 39-43.

years, microalbuminuria was present in 32% of men and 28% of women and increased with severity and duration of hypertension and increasing patient age.[27] The magnitude of microalbuminuria tends to correlate with increasing blood pressure, particularly when 24 hour ambulatory measurements are performed.[20;24] Numerous clinical studies have demonstrated a positive correlation between microalbuminuria in patients with essential hypertension and increased cardiovascular events and/or mortality.[19] In addition, patients with essential hypertension and microalbuminuria have increased carotid artery wall thickness,[28] increased left ventricular hypertrophy, nonfatal myocardial in-farcts and peripheral vascular disease.[24] A secondary analysis of the Multiple Risk Factor Intervention Trial revealed that the presence of even 1+ proteinuria is associated with a 2.5 times greater risk of cardiovascular events, even after controlling for other cardiovascular risk factors.[29] A significant positive correlation between urinary albumin levels, fasting serum insulin levels and severity of angiographically demonstrated coronary artery disease has also been demonstrated. Hyperinsulinemia and microalbuminuria were both predictive for significantly increased risk of coronary artery disease.[30] Patients with newly diagnosed essential hypertension who also had microalbuminuria tended to be older, have a higher body mass index, and have a family history of essential hypertension, and were more likely to smoke and have a sedentary lifestyle than those without microalbuminuria.[31]

Many of these patients have been found to have insulin resistance, hyperinsulinemia, the loss of nocturnal dipping of blood pressure, and dyslipidemia.[24;32] Hypertensive patients with microalbuminuria have significantly higher plasma glucose levels, serum insulin levels and serum lipoprotein (a) levels compared with hypertensive patients without microalbuminuria and normotensive controls and have higher nocturnal blood pressure measurements. In addition, a significantly positive correlation exists among urinary albumin excretion, insulin area under the curve and 24 hour diastolic blood pressure.[32] Elevation of apolipoprotein B-containing lipids and decreased high-density lipoproteins are commonly seen in essential hypertension patients with microalbuminuria.[24] The relationship between this dyslipidemia and microalbuminuria is not well understood. It is not explained by obesity or increased body mass but may be secondary to the insulin resistance and hyperinsulinemia seen in these patients.[24;33] In 383 Caucasian patients with essential hypertension analyzed by albumin excretion rate: 55 per cent of patients excreted less than 11 μg/min; 18% 11-20 μg/min, and 27% more than 20 μg/min. The level of albumin excretion rate showed a significant positive correlation with systolic and diastolic blood pressure, left ventricular mass indexed for height, and creatinine clearance. There were no differences between the groups in age, body mass index, serum creatinine level and plasma renin activity; although when the group with highest excretion rate was compared with the group with the lowest rate, the prevalence of left ventricular hypertrophy and hypertensive retinopathy was significantly higher in the group that excreted more albumin; and they had higher values for 24 hour systolic, diastolic and mean blood pressures.[26]

Recent studies have shown that microalbuminuria is found in salt-sensitive patients and in those who cannot regulate their hemodynamic responses to a sodium load. Of particular interest is that both of these groups of patients share other metabolic abnormalities such as hyperinsulinemia and alterations of the Na^+/Li^+ countertransporter.[24] Salt-sensitive patients demonstrated increased insulin secretion compared to salt-resistant patients and, in addition, excreted a larger amount of urinary albumin and had higher levels of cholesterol and LDL cholesterol[33;34]

Gerber and co-workers looked at differences in urinary albumin excretion rate between normotensive and "mildly" hypertensive white and nonwhite, predominately Hispanic subjects. In mildly hypertensive Hispanic subjects with a diastolic blood pressure greater than 89 but less than 95 mmHg, urinary albumin excretion was increased in 31.1% of hypertensive subjects compared with 8.6% of normotensive subjects and in 39.5% of white hypertensive subjects compared to 17.4% of hypertensive nonwhites. Hypertensive white subjects were 5 times more likely than nonwhite hypertensive subjects to have increased urinary albumin excretion, and there was a 51% increase in risk of microalbuminuria for every 10 mmHg increase in systolic blood pressure.[20]

Diabetes Mellitus

Microalbuminuria in patients with type 1 and type 2 diabetes is a useful marker for those patients at greatest risk for the development of microvascular and macrovascular disease. For patients with insulin dependent diabetes mellitus (IDDM), the onset of microalbuminuria without overt proteinuria or decreased renal function is associated with the hyperfiltration of early diabetic nephropathy.[14;24] A number of studies have shown that microalbuminuria in IDDM appears to be an early marker of glomerular injury and presages macroalbuminuria and progressive renal disease.[24] The same is likely true for patients with non-insulin dependent diabetes mellitus (NIDDM)[24] As for patients with essential hypertension and microalbuminuria, a cluster of metabolic abnormalities, including hypertension, dyslipidemia, insulin resistance and coagulation abnormalities have been identified in diabetic patients with microalbuminuria. Since these are also cardiovascular risk factors, it is not surprising that these patients exhibit a higher incidence of coronary artery disease than patients without microalbuminuria or even non-diabetic patients who are also microalbuminuric.[24;30] The Scandinavian Simvastatin Survival Study found that patients with type 2 diabetes were 2.5 times more likely to have coronary artery disease than patients without diabetes. However, treatment of the dyslipidemia was associated with a significant decrease in coronary artery disease in diabetic patients that was greater than that seen for non-diabetic patients.[35;36] Microalbuminuria in patients with either type 1 or type 2 diabetes correlates strongly with cardiovascular morbidity and mortality.[15-18;37]

Endothelial Cell Dysfunction

A number of authors have suggested that microalbuminuria may be a marker of systemic vascular endothelial dysfunction.[10;23;38] McFarlane et al hypothesize that microalbuminuria may identify generalized cardiovascular/renal endothelial dysfunction and enhanced oxidative stress.[22] The vascular endothelium is intimately involved in hemostasis, fibrinolysis and vascular permeability. Indeed, microalbuminuria is the renal marker for a generalized increase in endothelial permeability that may promote enhanced cardiovascular risk by initiating the process leading to an atherosclerotic plaque. Von Willebrand Factor antigen is increased in patients with microalbuminuria; and a significant positive correlation exists with the amount of microalbuminuria, mean blood pressure, and age. Fibrinogen levels were also increased in patients with microalbuminuria and correlated with von Willebrand Factor antigen measurements.[38] The authors speculated that short-term changes in blood pressure contribute, in part, to microalbuminuria and endothelial damage. Since dyslipidemia is also frequently present in these patients, its contributory role to this process needs further exploration. Indeed, an interaction between blood pressure, oxidant stress and oxidized lipids is proposed as an important interaction that could lead to aggressive cardiovascular disease.

Modification of Risk Factors

Strategies to decrease cardiovascular morbidity and mortality in patients with microalbuminuria have focused on blood pressure control particularly with agents that modify the renin angiotensin II system and treatment of lipids. Many of the factors that are important for cardiovascular disease reduction are also independent risk factors for progressive kidney disease. Persistent proteinuria is associated with development of nephrosclerosis and progressive interstitial fibrosis in patients with essential hypertension.[39-41]

In one randomized trial of patients with essential hypertension, the degree of baseline proteinuria was an important determinant of rate of change of glomerular filtration rate. Patients with baseline protein excretion of less than 500 mg per 24 hours had change in GFR of $+2.8\pm0.4$ ml/min/1.73m^2/year, while those with more than 500 mg per 24 hours had a change of -2.1 ± 0.8 ml/min/1.73m^2/year.[42] Ruilope et al followed hypertensive patients with and without microalbuminuria at presentation who were treated with diuretics and beta blockers. After 5 years those with microalbuminuria at presentation had a significant decrease in GFR despite similar diastolic and systolic blood pressure levels before and after treatment.[10] The Afro-American Study of Renal Disease recently stopped the calcium channel blocker arm of that trial; because participants that were receiving the angiotensin converting enzyme inhibitor, ramipril, had greater reduction in proteinuria and better preservation of renal function. This reduction of protein excretion is independent of decreases in blood pressure.[43] Benazepril was shown to be effective in delaying progression of renal disease in The ACE Inhibitor in Progressive Renal Insufficiency (APRI) trial. The patients with the greatest benefit were those with the largest amount of protein excretion at baseline.[44] The Ramipril Efficacy in Nephropathy (REIN) trial evaluated the effect of ramipril versus placebo on decrease in renal function and risk of terminal renal failure in proteinuric patients with non-diabetic nephropathy. Patients given ramipril had a slower rate of decline of glomerular filtration rate and a greater reduction in urinary protein excretion that was independent of level of blood pressure control.[11] This effect was most evident in patients with massive proteinuria. In addition, in the Heart Outcomes Prevention Evaluation Trial (HOPE), ramipril was found to significantly decrease mortality, myocardial infarction and stroke in high–risk patients with evidence of vascular disease or diabetes.[45] In particular, the risk reduction for cardiovascular events was greatest in those patients who had a serum creatinine > 1.4 mg/dl or who had elevated albumin excretion rates.[1]

Angiotensin-converting enzyme inhibitors and angiotensin II receptor antagonists are more effective than diuretics, B-blockers and calcium antagonists in decreasing microalbuminuria.[10] Schiffrin and Deng compared the effects of angiotensin 1-converting enzyme inhibition and beta-blockade on function of small arteries from hypertensive patients and found that ACE-inhibitors improve endothelial function in resistance arterioles in hypertensive patients. Similar positive effects have been described in small arterioles in the coronary and renal vascular beds after therapy with converting enzyme inhibitors and calcium antagonists.[46] Recent studies have demonstrated that angiotensin II receptor antagonists also have an anti-proteinuric effect in normotensive and hypertensive microalbuminuric subjects[13] and patients with type 1 and type 2 diabetic nephropathy.[47-50]

There is clear evidence that the use of angiotensin-converting enzyme inhibitors and good blood pressure and glycemic control can the delay the progression of renal failure in patients with type 1 diabetes.[51] The recently completed trials in patients with type 2 diabetic nephropathy will provide new insights regarding the use of angiotensin II receptor antagonists in patients with advanced diabetic disease. Treatment of the dyslipidemia that is frequently present in the albuminuric/proteinuric patients with diabetes or essential hypertension have not been specifically carried out. However, small subsets of diabetic patients that have been included in some of the larger lipid lowering trial have clearly suggested a potential benefit. Trials of lipid lowering therapy are currently being conducted in end-stage renal disease patients who have the highest cardiovascular risk. These studies should provide new insights into the management of cardiovascular disease in patients with renal disease.[52]

References

1. Mann JFE, Gerstein HC, Pogue J, Bosch J, Yusuf S, for the HOPE Investigators: Renal insufficiency as a predictor of cardiovascular outcomes and the impact of ramipril: The HOPE Randomized Trial. Ann Intern Med 134:629-36, 2001
2. Mogensen CE, Keane WF, Bennett PH, Jerums G, Parving H-H, Passa P, Steffes MW, Striker GE, Viberti GC: Prevention of diabetic renal disease with special reference to microalbuminuria. Lancet 346:1080-4, 1995
3. Remuzzi G, Bertani T: Pathophysiology of progressive nephropathies. N Engl J Med 339:1448-56, 1998
4. Ruggenenti P, Perna A, Gherardi G, Gaspari F, Benini R, Remuzzi G: Renal function and requirement for dialysis in chronic nephropathy patients on long-term ramipril: REIN follow-up trial. Gruppo Italiano di Study Epidemiologici in Nefrologia(GISEN). Lancet 352:1252-6, 1998
5. Ruggenenti P, Perna A, Gherardi G, Garini G, Zoccali C, Salvadori M, Scolari F, Schena FP, Remuzzi G: Renoprotective properties of ACE-inhibition in non-diabetic nephropathies with non-nephrotic proteinuria. Lancet 354:359-64, 1999
6. Rossing P, Hommel E, Smidt UM, Parving H-H: Reduction in albuminuria predicts diminished progression in diabetic nephropathy. Kidney Int Suppl 45:S145-9, 1994
7. Peterson JC, Adler S, Burkart JM, Greene T, Hebert LA, Hunsicker LG, King AJ, Klahr S, Massry SG, Seifter JL, Modification of Diet in Renal Disease (MDRD) Study Group: Blood pressure control, proteinuria and the progression of renal disease. Ann Intern Med 123:754-62, 1995
8. Eddy AA: Molecular insights into renal interstitial fibrosis. J Am Soc Nephrol 7:2495-508, 1996
9. Nomura A, Morita Y, Maruyama S, Hotta N, Nadai M, Wang L, Hasegawa T, Matsuo S: Role of complement in acute tubulo-interstitial injury of rats with aminonucleoside nephrosis. Am J Pathol 151:539-47, 1997
10. Ruilope LM, Campo C, Rodriguez-Artalejo F, Lahera V, Garcia Robles R, Rodicio JL: Blood pressure and renal function: therapeutic implications. J Hypertens 14:1259-63, 1996
11. Gruppo Italiano di Studi Epidemiologici in Nefrologia: Randomised placebo-controlled trial of effect of ramipril on decline in glomerular filtration rate and risk of terminal renal failure in proteinuric, non-diabetic nephropathy. Lancet 349:1857-63, 1997
12. Buter H, Navis G, Dullaart RPF, de Zeeuw D, de Jong PE: Time course of the antiproteinuric and renal haemodynamic responses to losartan in microalbuminuric IDDM. Nephrol Dial Transplant 16:771-5, 2001
13. Russo D, Pisani A, Balletta MM, De Nicola L, Savino FA, Andreucci M, Minutolo R: Additive antiproteinuric effect of converting enzyme inhibitor and losartan in normotensive patients with IgA nephropathy. Am J Kidney Dis 33:851-6, 1999
14. Viberti GC, Hill RD, Jarrett RJ, Argyropoulos A, Mahmud U, Keen H: Microalbuminuria as a predictor of clinical nephropathy in insulin-dependent diabetes mellitus. Lancet i:1430-2, 1982
15. Messent JW, Elliot TG, Hill RG, Jarrett RJ, Keen H, Viberti GC: Prognostic significance of microalbuminuria in insulin-dependent diabetes mellitus: a twenty-three-year follow-up study. Kidney Int 41:836-9, 1992
16. Mogensen CE: Microalbuminuria predicts clinical proteinuria and early mortality in maturity-onset diabetes. N Engl J Med 310(6):356-60, 1984
17. Jarrett RJ, Viberti GC, Argyropoulos A, Hill RD, Mahmud U, Murrels TJ: Microalbuminuria predicts mortality in non-insulin-dependent diabetics. Diabet Med 1:17-9, 1984
18. Schmitz A, Vaeth M: Microalbuminuria: a major risk factor in non-insulin-dependent diabetes. A ten-year follow-up study of 503 patients. Diabet Med 5:126-34, 1988
19. Winocour PH, Harland JO, Millar JP, Laker MF, Alberti KG: Microalbuminuria and associated cardiovascular risk factors in the community. Atherosclerosis 93:71-81, 1992
20. Gerber LM, Shmukler C, Alderman MH: Differences in urinary albumin excretion rate between normotensive and hypertensive white and non white subjects. Arch Intern Med 152:373-7, 1992
21. Bigazzi R, Bianchi S: Microalbuminuria as a marker of cardiovascular and renal disease in essential hypertension. Nephrol Dial Transplant 10:10-4, 1995
22. McFarlane SI, Banerji M, Sowers JR: Insulin resistance and cardiovascular disease. J Clin Endocrinol Metab 86:713-8, 2001
23. Keane WF: Proteinuria: its clinical importance and role in progressive renal disease. Am J Kidney Dis 35:S97-105, 2000
24. Bianchi S, Bigazzi R, Campese VM: Microalbuminuria in essential hypertension: significance, pathophysiology and therapeutic implications. Am J Kidney Dis 34:973-95, 1999

25. Bigazzi R, Bianchi S, Campese VM, Baldari GL: Prevalence of microalbuminuria in a large population of patients with mild to moderate essential hypertension. Nephron 61:94-7, 1992
26. Cerasola G, Cottone S, Mule G, Nardi E, Mangano MT, Andronico G, Contorno A, Li Vecchi M, Gaglione P, Renda F, Piazza G, Volpe V, Lisi A, Ferrara L, Panepinto N, Riccobene R: Microalbuminuria, renal dysfunction and cardiovascular complication in essential hypertension. J Hypertens 14:915-20, 1996
27. Agrawal B, Berger A, Wolf K, Luft FC: Microalbuminuria screening by reagent strip predicts cardiovascular risk in hypertension. J Hypertens 14:223-8, 1996
28. Bigazzi R, Bianchi S, Nenci R, Baldari D, Baldari G, Campese VM: Increased thickness of the carotid artery in patients with essential hyeprtension and microalbuminuria. Journal of Human Hypertension 9:827-33, 2001
29. Grimm RH, Svendsen KH, Kasiske BL, Keane WF, Wahi M: Proteinuria is a risk factor for mortality over 10 years of follow-up. The MRFIT Research Group. Kidney Int Suppl 52:S-10-4, 1997
30. Tuttle KR, Puhlman ME, Cooney SK, Short R: Urinary albumin and insulin as predictors of coronary artery disease: an angiographic study. Am J Kidney Dis 34:918-25, 1999
31. Calvino J, Calvo C, Romero R, Gude F, Sanchez-Guisande D: Atherosclerosis profile and microalbuminuria in essential hypertension. Am J Kidney Dis 34:996-1001, 1999
32. Bianchi S, Bigazzi R, Valtriani C, Chiaponni I, Sgherri G, Baldari G, Natali A, Ferrannini E, Campese VM: Elevated serum insulin levels in patients with essential hypertension and microalbuminuria. Hypertension 23:681-7, 1994
33. Bigazzi R, Bianchi S, Baldari G, Campese VM: Clustering of cardiovascular risk factors in salt-sensitive patients with essential hyeprtension: role of insulin. Am J Hypertens 9:24-32, 1996
34. Bigazzi R, Bianchi S, Baldari D, Sgherri G, Baldari G, Campese VM: Microalbuminuria in salt-sensitive patients. A marker for renal and cardiovascular risk factors. Hypertension 23:195-9, 1994
35. Pyörälä K, Pedersen TR, Kjekshus J, Faergeman O, Olsson AG, Thorgeirsson G: Cholesterol lowering with simvastatin improves prognosis of diabetic patients with coronary heart disease. A subgroup analysis of the Scandinavian Simvastatin Survival Study(4S). Diabetes Care 20:614-20, 1997
36. Plehn JF, Davis BR, Sacks FM, Rouleau JL, Pfeffer MA, Bernstein V, Cuddy TE, Moye LA, Piller LB, Rutherford J, Simpson LM, Braunwald E: Reduction of stroke incidence after myocardial infarction with pravastatin: the Cholesterol and Recurrent Events(CARE) study. The Care Investigators. Circulation 19:216-23, 1999
37. Ravid M, Savin H, Jutrin I, Bantal T, Katz B, Lishner M: Long-term stabilizing effect of angiotensin-converting enzyme inhibition on plasma creatinine and on proteinuria in normotensive type II diabetic patients. Ann Intern Med 118:577-81, 1993
38. Pedrinelli R, Giampietro O, Carmassi F, Melillo E, Dell'Omo G, Catapano G, Matteucci E, Talarico L, Morale M, DeNegri F, DiBello V: Microalbuminuria and endothelial dysfunction in essential hypertension. Lancet 344:14-8, 1994
39. Eddy AA: Interstitial nephritis induced by protein-overload proteinuria. Am J Pathol 135:719-33, 1989
40. Eddy AA, Giachelli CM: Renal expression of genes that promote interstitial inflammation and fibrosis in rats with protein-overload proteinuria. Kidney Int 47:1546-57, 1995
41. Bertani T, Cutillo F, Zoja C, Broggini M, Remuzzi G: Tubulo-interstitial lesions mediate renal damage in adriamycin glomerulopathy. Kidney Int 30:488-96, 1986
42. Toto RD, Mitchell HC, Smith RD, Lee HC, McIntire D, Pettinger WA: "Strict" blood pressure control and progression of renal disease in hypertensive nephrosclerosis. Kidney Int 48:851-9, 1995
43. Keane WF, Eknoyan G: Proteinuria, albuminuria, risk, assessment, detection, elimination(PARADE): a position paper of the National Kidney Foundation. Am J Kidney Dis 33:1004-10, 1999
44. Maschio G, Alberti D, Janin G, Locatelli F, Mann JFE, Motolese M, Ponticelli C, Ritz E, Zucchelli P: Effect of the angiotensin-converting-enzyme inhibitor benazepril on the progression of chronic renal insufficiency. N Engl J Med 334:939-45, 1996
45. Yusuf S, Sleight P, Pogue J, Bosch J, Davies R, Dagenais G: Effects of an angiotensin-converting-enzyme inhibitor, ramipril, on cardiovascular events in high-risk patients. The Heart Outcomes Prevention Evaluation Study Investigators. N Engl J Med 342:145-53, 2000
46. Li JS, Schiffrin EL: Effect of calcium channel blockade or angiotensin-converting enzyme inhibition on structure of coronary, renal, and other small arteries in spontaneously hypertensive rats. J Cardiovasc Pharmacol 28:68-74, 1996
47. Lozano JV, Llisterri JL, Aznar J, Redon J: Losartan reduces microalbuminuria in hypertensive microalbuminuric type 2 diabetics. Nephrol Dial Transplant 16:1-5, 2001
48. Lacourciere Y, Belanger A, Godin C, Halle JP, Ross S, Wright N, Marion J: Long-term comparison of losartan and enalapril on kidney function in hypertensive type 2 diabetics with early nephropathy. Kidney Int 58:762-9, 2000
49. Fernandez-Andrade C, Russo D, Iversen B, Zucchelli P, Aranda P, Guerra L, Casado S: Comparison of losartan and amlodipine in renally impaired hypertensive patients. Kidney Int 54:S-120-4, 1998
50. Fauvel JP, Berra N, Pozet N, Madonna O, Zech P, Laville M: Effects of losartan on renal function in patients with essential hypertension. J Cardiovasc Pharmacol 28:259-63, 1996
51. Lewis EJ, Hunsicker LG, Bain RP, Rohde RD: The effect of angiotensin-converting-enzyme inhibition on diabetic nephropathy. The Collaborative Study Group. N Engl J Med 329:1456-62, 1993
52. Keane WF, Brenner BM, Mazzu A, Agro A, for the CHORUS Steering Committee: The CHORUS (Cerivastatin in Heart Outcomes in Renal Disease: Understanding Survival) protocol: a double-blind, placebo-controlled trial in patients with ESRD. Am J Kidney Dis 37:S48-53, 2001

5 Oxidative Stress and Inflammation in Hemodialysis Patients

MARGARET SPITTLE MD, NICHOLAS A. HOENICH PH.D, GARRY HANDELMAN PH.D, ROHINI ADHIKARLA MD, PETER HOMEL PH.D AND NATHAN W. LEVIN MD.

Abstract

Cardiovascular disease is a major cause of mortality and morbidity in patients receiving hemodialysis for end stage renal disease (ESRD). Several groups of factors have been identified as being responsible. These include the traditional causes such as hypertension, hyperlipidemia, diabetes, smoking and race, and factors arising from the underlying renal disease and the dialysis procedure itself. The relationship between these factors and the development of atherosclerosis is complex; oxidative stress has, however, emerged as an important co-factor for the development of endothelial dysfunction and atherogenesis. Oxidant stress markers include F2 isoprostanes and ethane. Measurements in dialysis patients showed much higher levels of predialysis esterified plasma F2 isoprostanes 1.62 ±0.73 ng/ml compared with control subjects (0.27 ±0.10 ng/ml 0 ($p < 0.001$)). The high levels of F2-iso-prostanes also correlated with high plasma CRP levels ($r=0.48$, $p=0.015$). Breath ethane levels for patients was 6.32 ± 3.16 pMoles/kg-min (n=19) in contrast to control subjects of 3.08 ± 1.50 pMol/kg-min. (n=11) ($p<0.005$).

In keeping with other reported studies in the literature, we demonstrated elevated levels of CRP in patients undergoing regular dialysis therapy. Univariate analysis of data collected in a cohort of 557 patients over a two year period demonstrated a negative correlation of C-reactive protein quartiles with albumin, hematocrit, and creatinine levels, and a positive correlation with age, ferritin, hopitalization, rehospitalization and death. A multiple logistic regression also indicated a highly significant relationship between log CRP and rehospitalization ($p<0.001$) and death ($p<0.025$). In a subgroup of this cohort (n=104), CRP levels also correlated with titers of IgG antibodies to porphymonas gingivalis ($p<0.05$) an indicator of periodontal disease.

Introduction

The benefits of renal replacement therapy by hemodialysis and associated therapies are well recognized. Despite considerable improvements in the technology uremic patients have a higher prevelance of cardiovascular complications than other populations of a comparable age. A recent study by Foley[1] indicated that cardiovascular mortality in dialysis patients is 10-20 times higher than in the general population when stratified for risk factors such as diabetes and age. A number of factors are involved in the etiology of this complication, which result in an acute phase response or systemic reaction to inflammatory stimuli or tissue injury. Such systemic reaction may be characterized by an increased synthesis and release of acute phase proteins, such as C-reactive protein (CRP) and fibrinogen, as well as the suppression of other acute phase proteins, such as albumin and transferrin.

Extracorporeal circulatory procedures only treat the consequences of renal diseases rather than affecting the mechanics involved in their pathogenesis. The regulation of this response involves highly complex mechanisms and includes the initial release of cytokines such as interleukin-1 (IL-1), IL-6, IL-8 and tumor necrosis factor-alpha *(TNF-a)*. The most common clinical tool to detect the presence of inflammation, is CRP; although cytokines, serum amyloid A, alpha 2 macroglobulin and ferritin are other indicators.

Renal disease itself which is not treated by extracorporeal circulatory procedures is associated with a variety of pathogenic mechanisms, including the generation of reactive oxidative species or oxidative stress. The purpose of this paper is to explore the interrelationship between oxidative stress and inflammation and to examine their role in dialysis related pathology.

Oxidant Stress and Inflammation

Oxidant Stress

Oxidant stress is present in both health and disease. Although oxygen is essential to human life, paradoxically it can also cause great harm The dangerous effects of oxygen arise because oxygen atoms have one unpaired electron in their outer valence shell, and

M.M. Avram.(ed.), Improving Prognosis for Kidney Disorders, 45-52.

oxygen in molecular form has two unpaired electrons. Since a radical is defined as any atom or molecule that has one or more unpaired electrons in an outer valence shell, oxygen atoms and molecules are, therefore, free radicals and bi-radicals respectively. As a result of this, oxygen has the potential to be involved in a variety of oxidation/reduction reactions, which may produce several reactive intermediates. Examples of such reactive oxygen species (ROS) include the superoxide anion radical ($O_2^{\bullet -}$), hydrogen peroxide (H_2O_2) and the highly reactive hydroxyl radical ($^{\bullet}OH$). There are many environmental sources of ROS, including products of photochemical smog such as nitric oxide ($NO^{\bullet}$) nitric dioxide ($NO_2^{\bullet}$), and ozone (O_3), another by-product of industrial combustion processes. X-rays and gamma rays also contribute to our exposure to oxygen radicals, due to their indirect effects resulting from radiolysis of body water.[2] Tobacco smoking produces a variety of radical and non-radical oxidant species; and certain drugs, including acetaminophen and doxorubicin, can cause serious toxicity through the generation of ROS[3,4] In addition to environmental sources of ROS, there are a number of biological sources. While over 95% of the oxygen we breathe undergoes an efficient enzymatic reduction in our cells in the mitochondrial electron transport chain that yields simply water, the nature of this process predisposes electron carriers in parts of the chain to involvement in side reactions with molecular oxygen, generally resulting in the generation of $O_2^{\bullet -}$. This system is thought to be the main physiological intracellular source of ROS, utilizing approximately 1-2% of the daily oxygen consumption. Polymorphonuclear leukocytes and other phagocytic cells produce $O_2^{\bullet -}$ as part of their defense against invading microorganisms, with the radicals targeted into the phagolysosome under normal conditions.[5] The third main biological source of ROS is the autoxidation or metal-catalyzed oxidation of lipids, proteins, carbohydrates and nucleic acids, which are all reduced carbon compounds that are readily susceptible to oxidation.

The term oxidative stress generally expresses the outcome of oxidative damage to biologically important molecules and is usually measured by detection of various modified macromolecules that are generated from the ROS in body tissues, plasma, or other body fluids; since the ROS themselves often have half-lives of just a few seconds. In contrast, the marker molecules usually have longer half-lives, of the order of hours to weeks, and include molecules derived from lipid peroxidation such as malonaldehyde, F2-isoprostanes as well as those derived from oxidation of proteins, such as advanced oxidation protein products (AOPPs). Breath ethane (see below) is an exception. Oxidative

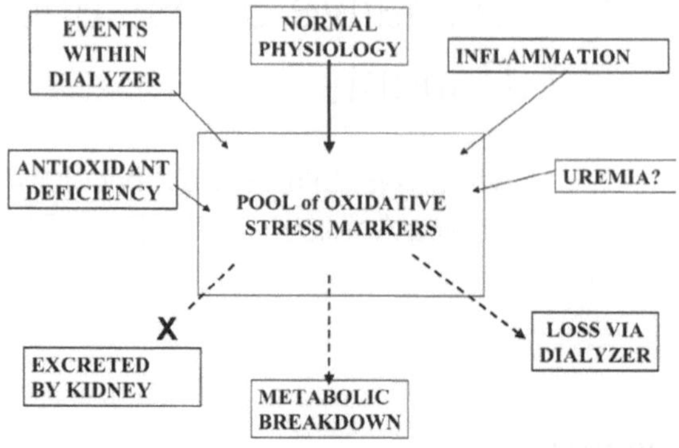

Figure 1. Factors that affect the total pool of oxidative stress markers.

stress occurs at sites of inflammation, during minor injuries and as part of the defense mechanisms of the body in the presence of invading microorganisms. Thus there is a pool of oxidative stress markers within the body resulting from these factors. (**Figure 1**) To deal with the produced oxidative stress markers, the body has a number of different defense mechanisms. Firstly, several antioxidant compounds act as 'scavengers', reacting directly with oxidizing agents. Such antioxidant compounds include water-soluble vitamin C (ascorbic acid), lipid soluble vitamin E (α-tocopherol) and the vitamin A derivative β-carotene. Secondly, a series of antioxidant enzymes exist that catalyze various reactions involving ROS, usually with the help of a transition metal in the enzyme active site. The most well known of these enzymes are superoxide dismutase (SOD) which acts on $O_2^{\bullet -}$ radicals, glutathione peroxidase (GSH-Px) which converts cytoplasmic H_2O_2 to water and oxygen and catalase which is responsible for removing H_2O_2 generated by β-oxidation of long-chain fatty acids. The transition metals most frequently involved in these reactions include selenium, manganese, zinc, copper and iron; and therefore, diets that are deficient in these metals may result in serious problems. A number of damage removal and repair systems are also available to the body to deal with the consequences of oxidative reactions. These systems require the damaged part of the molecule or the entire molecule to be identified, then removed or degraded, before a newly-synthesized replacement of the damaged part is inserted or a completely new molecule is made. Proteases, for example, degrade oxidized proteins to amino acids before a new protein is synthesized. In situations of high degrees of oxidative stress, this proteolytic system may be overwhelmed, at which point damaged proteins cross-link with extensive hydrophobic bonds and aggregate instead of being appropriately degraded. Peroxidation of cell membrane lipids results in more rigid membranes that have reduced selective permeability and often lose integrity. In an attempt to prevent propagation of the oxidation reactions, phospholipase enzymes act on these oxidized lipids to hydrolyze the fatty acids. Fatty acid hydroperoxides can also be detoxified by GSH-Px to produce hydroxy fatty acids. Lysophospholipids that are left in the membrane can serve as substrates for regeneration of new phospholipids. Nucleic acids are also susceptible to oxidative damage with resultant mutations, possible cell death and production of a variety of damage products. It is thought that some direct mechanisms of DNA repair may exist in addition to the more indirect excision-then-repair systems as described above for proteins and lipids. A number of the antioxidant defense and repair systems can be up-regulated in times of increased oxidative stress by alterations in gene expression, but more studies are required to fully characterize adaptive responses in these situations.

Inflammation

As discussed above, the acute phase reaction in mammalians provides protection against invading microorganisms, limits tissue damage and promotes a return to homeostasis. It involves many of the major systems within the body; however, for diagnostic purposes, the major markers of acute phase reactions are C-reactive protein (CRP) and serum amyloid A. (SAA). CRP is a cyclic pentameric protein with five identical 24 kDa subunits, each consisting of 206 amino acids. Its physiological functions include activation of the classical complement pathway and modulation of platelet activation by inhibiting the action of platelet activating factor. CRP also interacts with nuclear components such as chromatin, histones and small ribonuclear proteins. It binds to nuclear antigens released from apoptotic or necrotic cells, reducing their tissue deposition and limiting autoimmune reactivity. In addition, CRP binds to specific receptors on macrophages, monocytes, and neutrophils, enhancing their phagocytic properties. As well as acting as a marker of inflammation, it has recently been implicated as a risk factor for cardiovascular disease.[6] While it is known to be a risk factor in groups identified as high-risk for cardiovascular disease, evidence is now accumulating that in apparently healthy individuals, baseline CRP predicts risk of future cardiovascular morbidity even at the low levels considered to be in the normal range.[7,8] This suggests that classification of results as being in the 'normal' range may be inappropriate, since such a normal range appears not to exist. The mechanisms involved in this association between CRP and cardiovascular disease are unclear. It may involve direct endothelial cell injury and subsequent atherosclerotic plaque formation or the inflammatory response may contribute to cardiovascular disease by modifying plasma protein composition with increases, for example, in fibrinogen levels.[9,10] In addition, it has recently been shown by immunohistochemical staining to be present in necrotic human atherosclerotic lesions in thickened intimas and in early plaques.[11]

What is the Link between Oxidative Stress and Chronic Inflammation?

Under normal conditions, oxidative stress has beneficial effects for the body. The systemic inflammatory response is also primarily a beneficial reaction. This response is generally triggered and amplified by the cytokines IL-1, IL-6 and TNF released into the circulation by mononuclear cells or locally by Kupffer cells in the liver in response to tissue injury, inflammation or infection. These cytokines then promote the synthesis and release, largely by the liver, of several positive acute-phase proteins. These proteins include components of the complement system, coagulation cascade (such as fibrinogen), proteinase inhibitors (such as alpha-antitrypsin) and metal-binding proteins (such as ceruloplasmin). The acute-phase proteins most frequently measured in clinical practice include C-reactive protein (CRP) and serum amyloid A (SAA), since they have relatively short half-lives and concentrations of these reactants may increase more than 1000-fold over normal concentrations. Albumin and transferrin are examples of negative acute phase proteins, since their concentrations fall in response to inflammation. Albumin levels fall due to a combination of reduced synthesis, increased catabolism and loss from the vascular compartment by extravasation. Poor protein intake may compound the problem. The systemic inflammatory response tends to be advantageous provided it is acting in the short-term (in response to acute stimuli), but deleterious effects supervene if the condition becomes chronic or if the insults are repetitive. There also appears to be a synergism between oxidative stress and the systemic inflammatory response. Oxidative metabolites such as hydrogen peroxide can activate the NF-KB pathway, promoting synthesis of pro-inflammatory cytokines, resulting in amplification of the inflammatory cascade. Furthermore, the acute-phase proteins themselves may modulate the production of oxidative agents. For example, CRP has been shown to enhance intracellular generation of ROS by IgG-stimulated phagocytic cells. In these ways, events related to increased oxidative stress may sustain a state of chronic inflammation and a vicious circle may be generated. Thus oxidant stress impinges on inflammatory processes in dialysis patients in a variety of ways, but the relative importance of each of these in stimulation of inflammation has been difficult to quantitate. Indeed, the reciprocal nature of the process in which inflammation promotes further oxidant stress makes this task even more complicated. Nevertheless, a starting point would be measures of oxidant stress examined both in terms of what is oxidized and their relative half lives. Each of these, in turn, contains a large number of other variables.

Quantification of Markers of Oxidant Stress

Four specific groups of factors can be identified as being implicated in the formation of oxidative stress in patients undergoing hemodialysis. Uremia itself and other co-morbid conditions such as diabetes,[12] hemodialysis induced loss of antioxidants such as Vitamin C which is known to be an anti oxidant *in vitro* and which may also act as an *in vivo* antioxidant due to its ability to regenerate vitamin E from the Vitamin E radical.[13,14] In addition, a study by Koenig et al.[15] indicated that selenium concentrations may also be reduced below that of normal controls in dialysis patients. Concurrent with the decreased plasma levels, decreased activity of plasma selenium glutathione peroxidase has also been noted.[16]

As mentioned above, the huge difference in half lives of radicals, such as hypochlorite, hydroxyl, and peroxyl which are measured in seconds, and of modified macromolecules, such as oxidized lipids and proteins measured in days or weeks, may be useful as a guide to understanding inflammatory consequences of oxidant stress. The pathways that lead to markers from lipid peroxidation are illustrated in **Figure 2**.

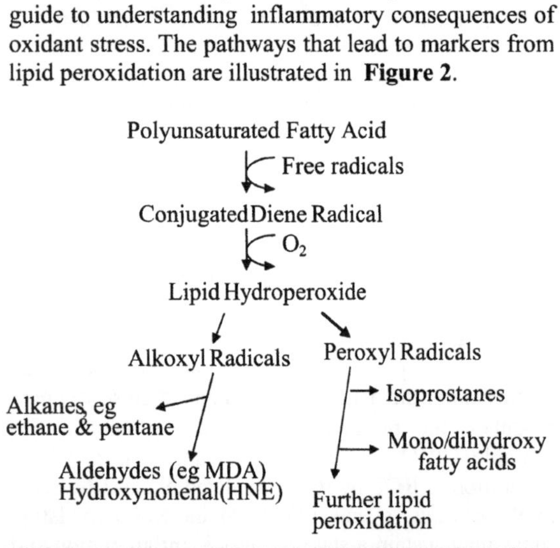

Figure 2. Formation of lipid peroxidation products.

An example of a commonly used indicator of effects of oxidant stress on lipids is malonaldehyde (MDA) which is usually found to be present in increased amounts in dialysis patients. Unfortunately, methods for MDA are not standardized and measure different parts of the MDA pool. Some MDA may be generated by breakdown of lipid peroxides in vitro. Another possibility is the retention of MDA in renal failure. A superior indicator of oxidant stress may be the measurement of isoprostanes which are derived from the effect of free radicals on archidonic acid. These compounds are an end product and are chemically stable. Because of their relatively long half life, they be may represent a longer period of oxidative stress than, for example, breath ethane.

In a comparative study, our group has compared isoprostane levels in patients undergoing hemodialysis with normal controls. Control subjects were screened using fasting blood samples, and were excluded for elevated plasma cholesterol (>250 mg/dL), plasma triglycerides (>200 mg/dL), and blood glucose (>150 mg/dL). Normal renal function in controls was established by lack of urinary protein or casts and by plasma creatinine < 1.5 mg/dL. Blood samples for isoprostanes were drawn with EDTA anticoagulant and centrifuged within 10 minutes of collection. Plasma was snap-frozen in liquid nitrogen in plastic vials with tight-fitting caps and stored at -80°C until measurement of isoprostane content. Samples from ESRD patients were typically collected during the course of the dialysis session. Plasma esterified isoprostanes were measured by gas chromatography-mass spectrometry with negative chemical ionization (GC-MS-NCI) CRP was determined by enzyme-linked immunoassay (ELISA) with a lower detection limit of 0.1 mg CRP/L. Plasma albumin and creatinine were determined by standard clinical methods (Spectra-East Labs, Rutherford, New Jersey).

F2-isoprostanes, CRP and other variables were compared between dialysis patients and controls by using Student's T-test for independent samples. The Pearson correlation coefficient was used to measure the association between plasma F2-isoprostanes and plasma CRP, after logarithmic transformation of each variable. Analyses were carried out with Systat for Windows, version 7.0.1 (SPSS Inc., Chicago, IL). The results obtained are summarized in **Figure 3**. The average value for total esterified plasma F-2 isoprostanes was much higher for ESRD patients (1.62±0.73 ng/ml) than for control subjects (0.27 ±0.10 ng/ml) ($p < 0.001$). There was no overlap between the patient and control groups; the lowest isoprostane value reported for ESRD patients (0.64 ng/ml) was higher than the highest isoprostane value in the control

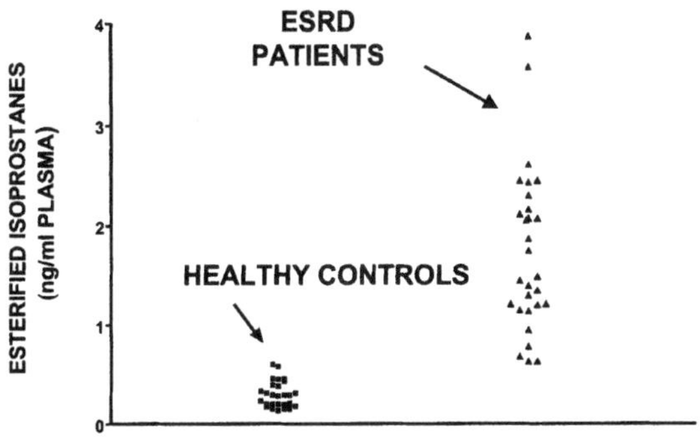

Figure 3. Plasma isoprostane levels for patients on hemodialysis drawn pre dialysis and normal controls

subjects (0.47 ng/ml) Diabetes was responsible for ESRD in 13 patients, and esterified F2-isoprostanes in diabetic patients was 1.53±0.54 ng/ml. In 12 other non diabetic patients, esterified F2-isoprostane levels were 1.71±0.84 ng/ml ($p < 0.001$) for these patients compared to controls. The high levels of F2-isoprostanes in the dialysis patients correlated with high plasma CRP levels ($r = 0.48$, $p = 0.015$), as has been reported in previous investigations.[17]

Ethane arises as a product of oxidative attack on n-3 fatty acids (such as 20:5n3 and 20:6n3), both *in vitro* and *in vivo*. Breath ethane is strikingly increased in experimental animals following injection of iron-complexes into the peritoneum.[18] A portion of the ethane formed during metabolism appears in the breath where it can be measured by gas chromatography. Experimental studies recently competed by our group have indicated that the average breath ethane value for 19 hemodialysis patients was 6.32 ± 3.16 pMoles/kg-min in contrast to the average for the 11 control subjects of 3.08 ± 1.50 pMol/kg-min. ($p<0.005$). The observed overlap between dialysis patients and controls can be interpreted in different ways. On the one hand, it may indicate that only a portion of dialysis patients experience the type of oxidative stress that would elevate breath ethane. Alternatively, it may be that hemodialysis patients fluctuate intermittently between a state of low and high oxidative stress analogous to fluctuations in C-reactive protein but with a much more rapid rate of change for ethane. Isoprostane level might then be thought to provide a more integrated record of oxidative stress, while ethane provides more information about short duration attacks by oxygen radicals.

Quantification of Effects of Markers of Inflammation

In a longitudinal study, we have studied a cohort of 557 patients over a two year period lasting from January 1998 to December 1999. During the study period, measurements of CRP were undertaken using a nephelometric method that had a lower limit of detection of 6.9 mg/l. All patients in the group were receiving high flux dialysis delivered using dialyzers containing polysulfone membranes used in conjunction with bicarbonate buffered dialysis fluid delivered by proportionating systems incorporating volumetric fluid removal control. The data collected was subdivided into quartiles in respect of CRP. The relationship of these quartiles relative to demographic details as well the usual monthly metabolic and hematological parameters is summarized in **Table 1.**

Table 1. Relationship between CRP levels and commonly measured parameters during hemodialysis

	CRP levels(mg/l)[1]				p value
	8.2	**12.8**	**20.9**	**49.5**	
Age (yrs)	54 ±12	54±13	62±12	62±11	<0.0001
Gender (F)	55%	50%	43%	42%	0.103
Diabetes	25%	30%	32%	38%	<0.001
Albumin (g/dl)	3.9±0.6	3.9±0.4	3.9±0.7	3.6±0.5	<0.001
HCT (%)	35.3±3.3	35±3.6	34.5±3.4	33.8±3.4	<0.001
Ferritin (ng/ml)	368±244	450±633	393±252	511±431	0.033
Creatinine (mg/dl)	9.8±3.4	9.9±3.0	9.1±3.1	8.2±2.9	<0.001
PTH (ng/ml)	265±280	285±369	225±238	216±269	NS
Kt/V	1.51±0.3	1.59±0.7	1.48±0.3	2.1±0.6	NS
eNPCR (g/kg/d)	1.1±0.8	1.3±2.2	1.2±1.4	1.2±1.4	NS
Anti HCV +ve	36%	25%	19%	15%	<0.001
Hospitalization	59%	65%	76%	78%	<0.001
Rehospitalization	25%	39%	42%	54%	<0.001
Death	13%	6%	19%	37%	<0.001

[1] Expressed in quartiles

Whilst non-infectious causes may be the most likely cause of the inflammatory response in patients undergoing dialysis, such patients may also be subject to chronic and persistent infections. One of the less recognized clinical associations being periodontal disease. Studies in the general population have shown that destructive periodontal disease is associated with elevated CRP concentrations and raised incidence of atherosclerotic complications.[19] We have studied the relationship between levels of IgG antibodies to porphyromonas gingivalis, the organism most frequently associated with periodontal disease, and CRP levels in a random group of 104 patients drawn from patients receiving dialysis. Blood samples were drawn before dialysis sessions and IgG antibodies were determined using a commercially produced ELISA assay. Positivity to antibodies were noted in 91 patients (87.5%). Data for two patients suspected of suffering from an acute infection and who also had high antibody titres (>3200Eu) were excluded. In the remaining patients, the range of antibody titers were between 0.28-289.9Eu with a mean of 57.3±72.3 Eu. The CRP level in this group was 14.37±20.78 mg/L, and a significant correlation existed between the two parameters ($p<0.05$)

Discussion

Patients treated by renal replacement therapy remain subject to a wide range of biochemical abnormalities some of which may be induced by the dialysis process itself. Our finding that plasma isoprostanes are elevated in patients on hemodialysis is consistent with the hypothesis that these patients are under increased oxidative stress. Diverse mechanisms might account for increased oxidative stress, including antioxidant deficiency, neutrophil activation during dialysis, and chronic inflammation. Degranulation of neutrophils passing through the dialyser may also play a role.[20] The elevated levels of F2-isoprostanes seen in ESRD patients might also derive from impaired clearance of esterified isoprostanes, which may be altered during renal failure. Since the clearance of esterified F2-isoprostanes is not well understood at present, other mechanisms besides oxidative stress may contribute to the elevated levels of F2-isoprostanes. Our control subjects were mostly Caucasian, whereas the dialysis patients were preponderantly Hispanic and African-American. However, a subgroup analysis of the dialysis patients indicated that the 5 Caucasian subjects had the highest plasma isoprostanes among the 25 dialysis patients (1.74±0.63 ng/mL), compared with Hispanic (1.39 ±0.43 ng/mL) and African-American (1.57±0.73 ng/mL) dialysis patients.

The levels of esterified F-2 isoprostanes correlate with plasma CRP ($r=0.48$, $p = 0.015$), following logarithmic transformation of each variable. This correlation needs to be evaluated in a larger group of patients. This relation between CRP and oxidative stress requires further investigation in view of the prominent role that CRP plays in the outcome of patients receiving dialysis treatment.

The mechanisms whereby CRP contributes directly or indirectly to cardiovascular disease are at present incompletely understood. Several mechanisms have, however, been suggested which include the binding of CRP to damaged cells and activation of the complement system promoting atherosclerotic lesions[21]: binding and aggregation of low density lipoproteins[22] and stimulation of tissue factor production by monocytes.[23] Of particular interest among the many effects of oxidant stress is the measurement of oxidized – LDL because of the role it plays in the formation of atheroeschlerotic plaques.[24] Amino acid damage due to oxidants, especially to methionine, may be instrumental in reducing calmodulin activity. In the course of dialysis, exposure to endotoxin in dialysate (as one example) may be followed by monocyte activation and release of oxidant species from leucocytes. The oxidants could amplify inflammatory cascades via activation of the NF-KB pathway which promotes synthesis of inflammatory cytokines and may be responsible for some of the inflammatory components as measured by CRP and other acute phase reactants in dialysis patients.

CRP levels in dialysis are influenced by a number of non-dialysis related factor,s such as age, sex and race; and these factors may also influence the development of atherosclerosis. Women, the young, and African Americans all have relatively lower levels of this indicator of inflammation.[25] Is it relevant that mortality rates follow this same pattern? Because adjusted mortality is inversely proportional to body water volume (measured as V, derived from urea kinetic modeling) one possibility is an inverse relationship between V and CRP; but a recent analysis on the data above shows this not to be the case (Spittle, M., submitted for ASN 2001). It is conceivable that these demographic differences may be explained by more studies in respect of plasma level responses to oxidant stress and acute phase reactants. Elevated CRP levels in dialysis patients as well as in the normal population may be triggered by a number of factors. Our study has demonstrated a relationship between the levels of antibodies to periodontal pathogens and CRP, and it should be recognized that other chronic persistent infections may also contribute to the development of atheroclerotic plaques. A recent hypothesis formulated by Osswarde et al.[26] suggested that atherogenesis may develop as a consequence of chlamydial infection. The significance of inflammation is mysterious in its relation to obesity and particularly in child obesity. Cook et al.[27] measured CRP in 699 children aged 10-11 years. CRP levels were 47% higher in girls than boys, and rose with age by 15%/year. CRP levels were 270% (95% CI, 155-439%) higher in the top fifth than the bottom fifth of Ponderal index (weight/height^3). After adjustment, CRP levels remained 104% (95% CI, 23-236%) higher in the 56 children of South Asian origin. CRP was unrelated to: birth weight, height, social class, Helicobacter pylori infection or passive smoke exposure. CRP was correlated with several cardiovascular risk factors, but only fibrinogen ($r = 0.33$, $P = 0.0001$), HDL-cholesterol ($r = -0.13$, $P = 0.0006$), heart rate ($r = 0.12$, $P = 0.002$) and systolic blood pressure ($r = 0.08$, $P = 0.02$) remained statistically significant after adjustment. These findings indicate that there may be a role for inflammation throughout life in the development of atherosclerosis and cardiovascular disease. The ARIC (Atherosclerosis Risk in Communities Study) studied 13,000 individuals, 45-64 years of age, over a 3 year period. Those in the highest quartile of fibronogen gained more weight than those in the lowest quartile (1.65 95% CL 1.38 – 1.97). There were similar positive ratios for those with high WBC count, Factor VIII, and Von Willebrand factors.[28] These findings suggest that inflammatory processes stimulate weight gain leading to cardiovascular disease and may explain the findings of Cook et al.[27]

In conclusion, our data demonstrates that hemodialysis patients are exposed to both oxidative stress and inflammation. These factors add significant risk of morbidity and mortality. A particular observation is a link between C reactive protein and the titre of IgG antibodies to periodontal pathogens is suggestive that patients may have an increased susceptibility to peridontitis arising from poor dental hygiene or impaired immunity. This finding presents an opportunity for treatment of periodontal disease with a potentially favourable effect on the progression of atherosclerosis.

Much more needs to be learned concerning the reasons for inflammation including the role of genetic influences.

References

1. Foley RN, Parfrey PS, Sarnak MJ. Clinical epidemiology of cardiovascular disease in chronic renal disease. Am J Kidney Dis 132(5 Suppl 3):S112-9, 1998
2. Davies KJA: Oxidative stress: the paradox of aerobic life. Biochem Soc Symp 61:1-31, 1995
3. Dahlin DC, Miwa GT, Lu AY, Nelson SD: N-acetyl-p-benzoquinone imine: a cytochrome P-450-mediated oxidation product of acetaminophen. Proc Natl Acad Sci USA 81:1327-31, 1984
4. Marcillat O, Zhang Y, Davies KJ: Oxidative and non-oxidative mechanisms in the inactivation of cardiac mitochondrial electron transport chain components by doxorubicin. Biochem J 259:181-9, 1989
5. Babior BM: The respiratory burst oxidase. Adv Enzymol Relat Areas Mol Biol 65:49-95, 1992
6. Morrow DA, Ridker PM: C-reactive protein, inflammation, and coronary risk. Med Clin North Am 84:149-61, 2000
7. Ridker PM, Cushman M, Stampfer MJ, Tracy RP, Hennekens CH: Inflammation, aspirin, and the risk of cardiovascular disease in apparently healthy men. N Engl J Med 336:973-9, 1997
8. Ridker PM, Buring JE, Shih J, Matias'M, Hennekens CH: Prospective study of C- reactive protein and the risk of future cardiovascular events among apparently healthy women. Circulation 98:731-3, 1998
9. Tomura S, Nakamura Y, Doi M, Ando R, Ida T, Chida Y, Ootsuka S, Shinoda T, Yanagi H, Tsuchiya S, Marumo F: Fibrinogen, coagulation factor VII, tissue plasminogen activator, plasminogen activator inhibitor-I, and lipid as cardiovascular risk factors in chronic hemodialysis and continuous ambulatory peritoneal dialysis patients. Am J Kidney Dis 27:848-54, 1996
10. Ridker PM, Stampfer MJ, Rifai N: Novel risk factors for systemic atherosclerosis: A comparison of C-reactive protein, fibrinogen, homocysteine, lipoprotein(a), and standard cholesterol screening as predictors of peripheral arterial disease. JAMA 285:2481-2485, 2001.
11. Torzewski M, Rist C, Mortensen RF, Zwaka TP, Bienek M, Waltenberger J, Koenig W, Schmitz G, Hombach V, Torzewski J: C-reactive protein in the arterial intima: role of C-reactive protein receptor-dependent monocyte recruitment in atherogenesis.Arterioscler Thromb Vasc Biol 20:2094-2099, 2000.
12. Keaney JF Jr, Loscalzo J. Diabetes, oxidative stress, and platelet activation. Circulation 99:189-91, 1999
13. Bohm V, Tiroke K, Schneider S, Sperschneider H, Stein G, Bitsch R. Vitamin C status of patients with chronic renal failure, dialysis patients and patients after renal transplantation. Int J Vitam Nutr Res 67:262-6, 1997
14. Halpner AD, Handelman GJ, Harris JM, Belmont CA, Blumberg JB. Protection by vitamin C of loss of vitamin E in cultured rat hepatocytes. Arch Biochem Biophys 359:305-9, 1998
15. Koenig JS, Fischer M, Bulant E, Tiran B, Elmadfa I, Druml W. Antioxidant status in patients on chronic hemodialysis therapy: impact of parenteral selenium supplementation. Wien Klin Wochenschr 109:13-9, 1997
16. Saint-Georges MD, Bonnefont DJ, Bourely BA, Jaudon MC, Cereze P, Chaumeil P, Gard C, D'Auzac CL. Correction of selenium deficiency in hemodialyzed patients. Kidney Int Suppl 27:S274-7, 1998
17. Yeun JY, Kaysen GA: Factors influencing serum albumin in dialysis patients. Am J Kidney Dis 32:s118-25, 1998
18. Dillard CJ, Downer JE, Tappel AL: Effects of antioxidants on lipid peroxidation in iron-loaded rats. Lipids 19:127-33, 1984.
19. Slade GD, Offenbacher S, Beck JD, Heiss G, Pankow JS. Acute-phase inflammatory response to periodontal disease in the US population. J Dent Res 79: 49-57, 2000.

20. Grooteman MP, Bos JC, van Houte AJ, van Limbeek J, Schoorl M, Nube MJ: Mechanisms of intra-dialyser granulocyte activation: a sequential dialyser elution study. Nephrol Dial Transplant 12:492-9, 1997
21. Griselli M, Herbert J, Hutchinson WL, Taylor KM, Sohail M, Krausz T, Pepys MB. C-reactive protein and complement are important mediators of tissue damage in acute myocardial infarction. J Exp Med190:1733-40, 1999
22. Pepys MB, Rowe IF, Baltz ML. C-reactive protein: binding to lipids and lipoproteins. Int Rev Exp Pathol 27:83-111, 1985
23. Cermak J, Key NS, Bach RR, Balla J, Jacob HS, Vercellotti GM. C-reactive protein induces human peripheral blood monocytes to synthesize tissue factor. Blood 82:513-20, 1993
24. Esterbauer H, Gebicki J, Puhl H, Jurgens G. The role of lipid peroxidation and antioxidants in oxidative modification of LDL. Free Radic Biol Med 13: 341-70, 1992
25. Zimmermann J, Herrlinger S, Pruy A, Metzger T, Wanner C. Inflammation enhances cardiovascular risk and mortality in hemodialysis patients. Kidney Int 55:648-58, 1999
26. Ossewaarde JM, Feskens EJ, De Vries A, Vallinga CE, Kromhout D. Chlamydia pneumoniae is a risk factor for coronary heart disease in symptom-free elderly men, but Helicobacter pylori and cytomegalovirus are not. Epidemiol Infect 120:93-9, 1998
27. Cook DG, Mendall MA, Whincup PH, Carey IM, Ballam L, Morris JE, Miller GJ, Strachan DP. C-reactive protein concentration in children: relationship to adiposity and other cardiovascular risk factors. Atherosclerosis 149:139-50, 2000
28. Folsom AR, Aleksic N, Park E, Salomaa V, Juneja H, Wu KK. Prospective study of fibrinolytic factors and incident coronary heart disease : the atherosclerosis risk in communities (aric) study. Arterioscler Thromb Vasc Biol 21:611-7, 2001

6 Prognostic Value of Enrollment Parathyroid Hormone in Hemodialysis and Peritoneal Dialysis Patients for Survival. A 14 years Follow-up

MORRELL MICHAEL AVRAM, MD, NEAL MITTMAN, MD, MAUNG M. MYINT, MD, AND PAUL FEIN, MD

Abstract

Excess parathyroid hormone (PTH) is involved in the pathogenesis of many of the manifestations of the uremic syndrome. We have prospectively examined the relationship of enrollment serum intact PTH, as well as various demographic characteristics and other biochemical parameters, to all-cause mortality in hemodialysis (HD) and peritoneal dialysis (PD) patients. We enrolled 345 HD and 277 PD patients and monitored the patients up to 14 years. Observed survival computed by the Kaplan-Meier method and survival after adjustment for age, race, gender, months on dialysis at enrollment, diabetic status, and nutritional markers were significantly better for patients with enrollment PTH >200 pg/mL than for those with PTH 65–199 pg/mL and those with PTH <65 pg/mL. Enrollment serum PTH was an independent predictor of survival both in HD and PD patients. For HD patients, age and months on HD at enrollment were inversely associated with PTH level; while black race, creatinine and phosphorus were directly associated with PTH. For PD patients, age, diabetes and months on PD at enrollment were inverse predictors; while black race, albumin, creatinine and phosphorus were positively associated with PTH. In summary, lower than expected levels of PTH in dialysis patients is associated with decreased survival. We hypothesize that inadequate protein and/or phosphorus intake result in impaired development of the expected secondary hyperparathyroidism, as well as the excess mortality risk inherent with malnutrition.

Introduction

Hyperparathyroidism and elevated level of PTH are common complications of dialysis patients.[1] The level of parathyroid hormone (PTH) rises in direct proportion to the reduction in glomerular filtration rate (GFR). During progressive renal insufficiency, the fall in residual GFR results in a reduced filtered load of phosphate. If intake remains constant, phosphate retention and mild hyperphosphatemia will occur. This modest phosphate retention is central to the development of secondary hyperparathyroidism.[2] However, the mechanism whereby mild hyperphosphatemia causes secondary hyperparathyroidism is uncertain. Initially, reduced serum calcium due to complexing of calcium phosphate in phosphate excess was thought to stimulate the secretion of PTH. More recently, inhibition of renal production of calcitriol has been proposed, leading to hypocalcemia and increased PTH secretion. Regardless of the exact mechanism, the excess PTH is an appropriate "trade-off" initially: it normalizes both the calcium and the phosphate levels despite the reduction in GFR. Ultimately, this secondary hyperparathyroidism is maladaptive, causing a serious and debilitating bone disease, renal osteodystrophy.[3] In addition, a number of studies have implicated PTH as a multisystem uremic toxin.[4,5] For this reason, clinicians have been trained to aggressively treat secondary hyperparathyroidism by using phosphate binders and intravenous vitamin D supplementation as well as counseling dietary restrictions. Counterintuitively, we have noted and previously reported that higher PTH values at enrollment were associated with significantly better survival in PD as well as HD patients.[6] This controversial finding has been subsequently confirmed by Coco and Rush.[7] We now report on the prognostic importance of single enrollment levels of PTH to predict long-term survival in hemodialysis (HD) and peritoneal dialysis (PD) patients and compare PTH values with demographic characteristics and other biochemical markers to determine overall mortality risk.

Methods

Patients

Beginning in 1987, patients undergoing dialytic therapy (345 HD and 277 PD) at the Avram Center for Kidney Diseases were enrolled. All patient outcomes

M.M. Avram.(ed.), Improving Prognosis for Kidney Disorders, 53-59.

were followed through August 2001. Follow-up was censored on renal transplantation, dialysis modality change, or transfer to another dialysis center. On enrollment, the following demographic and clinical data were collected: age, race, gender, etiology of ESRD, total months on dialysis prior to enrollment, diabetic status, and seropositivity to human immunodeficiency virus (if known).

Biochemical Data

On enrollment, non-fasting baseline predialysis venous blood samples were drawn at a routine visit. Multiphasic biochemistry screening was obtained for each patient using the SMAC autoanalyzer (Technicon, Tarrytown, NY), and included albumin, creatinine, serum urea nitrogen, and total cholesterol. Serum intact PTH was measured by radioimmunoassay (Nichols Institute Diagnostics, San Juan Capistrano, CA). Enrollment value was the first value of a given nutritional marker for the patient obtained at or immediately after enrollment.

Dialysis Prescription

Hemodialysis patients were treated with bicarbonate-based dialysate and volumetric ultrafiltration control. Cellulose-based membranes (predominantly cellulose acetate and cellulose triacetate) were used prior to 1998 for more than 95% of all treatments. Thereafter, all patients were switched to polysulfone membranes. Initially, the hemodialysis prescription was guided by the goal of achieving a urea reduction ratio of >60% on the first treatment of the week (i.e. 68 hours after the preceding dialysis), later increased to >65%. Prior to 1992, most patients treated with continuous ambulatory peritoneal dialysis (PD) received four 2-liter Dianeal solution exchanges per day. After 1992, PD prescription was guided to achieve a target weekly Kt/V of 1.7, later increased to 2.1. Dextrose concentration in the dialysate varied with the need for ultrafiltration.

Statistical Analysis

Continuous variables are presented as mean ± SD. For selected comparisons between two group means, parametric (T-test) or non-parametric (Mann-Whitney test) wherever applicable, were used. Correlations were reported as either the Pearson correlation coefficient or the Spearman rank correlation coefficient. Simple linear regression was used to identify the predictors of PTH. Multiple linear regression was used to produce a predictive model for PTH. Observed survival of HD and PD patients was computed by Kaplan-Meier method. Survival was evaluated by univariate and multivariate Cox proportional hazards model using age, race, gender, diabetes, prior months on dialysis, comorbidity, and nutritional status as independent variables. PTH, which was not normally distributed, was log-transformed before entering the analysis. A two-tailed *P* value <0.05 was considered to be statistically significant. Calculations were performed using SPSS for Windows 9.0.1 (SPSS Inc., Chicago, IL).

Results

Hemodialysis

Demographics

The mean age of the HD patients was 60 ± 15 years; 44% of the HD patients were diabetic and 53% were female. The composition of the population by race was 60% black, 24% white, and 16% Hispanic. The etiology of ESRD was diabetes in 37%, hypertension in 32%, chronic glomerulonephritis in 10%, polycystic kidney disease in 6%, obstruction in 3%, HIV in 2% and other/unknown in 9 mg %. Mean prior months on HD at enrollment was 30.2 ± 42.6 months. At enrollment, the mean PTH level was 362 ± 447 pg/mL, and the median PTH was 208 pg/mL. In addition, the mean enrolment values were: albumin 3.73 ± 0.5 g/dL; serum creatinine 11.9 ± 4.8 /dL; and total cholesterol 182 ± 49 mg/dL. Mean predialysis serum phosphorus was 5.4 ± 1.9 mg/dL. The mean and maximum follow-up times were 3.48 and 13.9 years, respectively.

Survival Analysis by PTH

During the period of observation, 230 (67%) HD patients died. The cumulative observed survival of HD patients with enrollment PTH >200 pg/mL was significantly higher than those with PTH 65–200 pg/mL and those with PTH <65 pg/mL (*P*=0.009). After adjusting for age, race, gender, diabetes, months on HD, and enrollment nutritional indices (albumin, creatinine, and cholesterol), the results were similar—patients with PTH >200 pg/mL at enrollment had significantly better survival (*P*=0.008) **(Figure 1A)**. **Table 1** shows the univariate Cox regression analysis of predictors of mortality in these dialysis patients. Age, female gender and presence of diabetes were associated with higher relative mortality risk in HD patients; while higher levels of serum albumin, serum creatinine, total cholesterol, and log PTH at enrollment were associated with lower mortality risk.

Table 2 shows the multivariate Cox regression analysis for predictors of mortality. In this model, which adjusted for other variables that affected survival in the univariate model, age, enrollment serum albumin, enrollment serum cholesterol, and log PTH were found to be significant independent predictors of mortality.

Table 1. Predictors of Mortality in Dialysis Patients: Univariate Cox Regression Analysis

Variable	HD		PD	
	Relative Risk	*P*	Relative Risk	*P*
Age (years)	1.035	<0.0001	1.031	<0.0001
Gender (female *vs.* male)	1.28	0.05	0.83	NS
Race (black *vs.* other)	0.96	NS	0.57	0.001
Diabetes (yes *vs.* no)	1.88	<0.0001	2.14	<0.0001
Prior months on dialysis	0.998	NS	0.988	NS
Albumin (g/dL)	0.44	<0.0001	0.43	<0.0001
Creatinine (mg/dL)	0.91	<0.0001	0.89	<0.0001
Cholesterol (mg/dL)	0.996	0.003	0.997	0.048
Log PTH (pg/mL)	0.72	0.006	0.43	<0.0001
Phosphorus (mg/dL)	1.018	NS	0.84	0.003

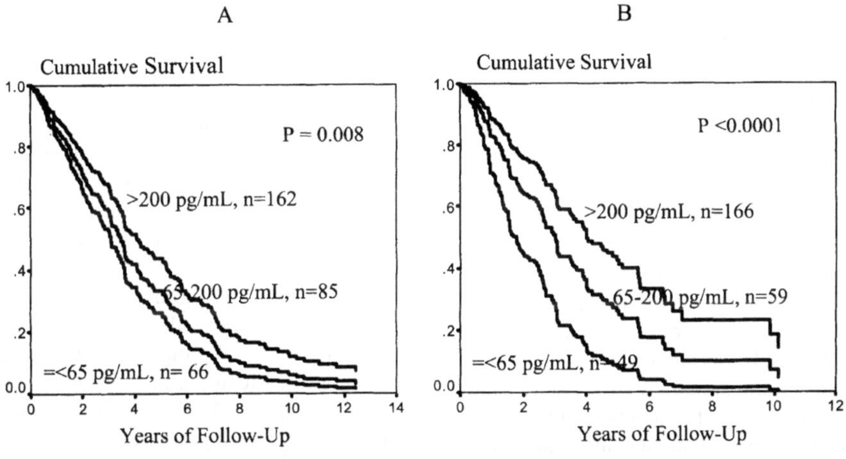

Figure 1. (**A**) Expected patient survival by enrollment level of PTH in 345 hemodialysis patients after adjustments were made for age, race, gender, diabetes, months on HD, albumin, cholesterol and creatinine. (**B**) Expected patient survival by enrollment level of PTH in 277 peritoneal dialysis patients after adjustments were made for age, race, gender, diabetes, months on PD, HIV status, albumin, cholesterol and creatinine.

Table 2. Predictors of Mortality in Dialysis Patients: Multivariate Cox Regression Analysis

Variable	HD		PD	
	Relative Risk	*P*	Relative Risk	*P*
Age (years)	1.028	<0.0001	1.021	0.001
Gender (female *vs.* male)	1.18	NS	0.94	NS
Race (black *vs.* other)	0.99	NS	0.79	NS
Diabetes (yes *vs.* no)	1.32	NS	1.37	NS
Prior months on dialysis	1.002	NS	0.99	NS
Albumin (g/dL)	0.56	0.001	0.53	<0.0001
Creatinine (mg/dL)	0.98	NS	0.976	NS
Cholesterol (mg/dL)	0.995	0.001	0.999	NS
Log PTH (pg/mL)	0.75	0.03	0.49	<0.0001

Table 3. Correlations of PTH with Age and Biochemical Profile in HD and PD

Variable	HD	PD
	Correlation Coefficient	Correlation Coefficient
Age (years)	-0.18**	-0.13*
Albumin (g/dL)	0.08	0.22**
Creatinine (mg/dL)	0.13*	0.20**
Cholesterol (mg/dL)	-0.058	0.04
Calcium (mg/dL)	-0.16**	-0.16*
Phosphorus (mg/dL)	0.23**	0.19**

* $P<0.05$
** $P<0.0001$

For each year of age, there was an associated increase of 2.8% in relative mortality risk. Every increase of 1 g/dL of serum albumin at HD enrollment was associated with a 44% reduction in relative risk, and every 1 mg/dL increase in serum cholesterol was associated with a 0.5% reduction in relative mortality risk. A 10-fold increase in PTH (e.g. from 10 pg/mL to 100 pg/mL) was associated with a 25% lower relative mortality risk.

Predictors of PTH

Table 3 shows correlations of PTH with age, prior months on dialysis, and biochemical profile. PTH correlated directly with serum creatinine and serum phosphorus, and was inversely correlated with age, prior months on HD, and serum calcium. **Table 4** shows the univariate regression analysis for independent predictors of PTH level in dialysis patients. Increasing age and more prior months on dialysis at enrollment were associated with lower levels of PTH. African ancestry, and higher levels of serum creatinine and serum phosphorus were strong predictors of higher PTH level.

Multivariate stepwise regression analysis confirmed that age (β=-0.13, P=0.017), black race (β=0.22, $P<0.0001$), and serum phosphorus (β=0.24, $P<0.0001$) are independent predictors of serum PTH level in HD patients. Enrollment PTH was significantly lower in diabetic patients compared to non-diabetic patients (305 pg/mL *vs.* 409 pg/mL, P=0.034) on HD, and diabetes was a significant predictor of non-transformed mean PTH at enrollment (β=-0.125, P=0.02). Patients of African descent had significantly higher PTH than Caucasian and Hispanic patients (433 pg/mL for black vs. 350 pg/mL for whites and 281 pg/mL for Hispanics, P=0.001).

Peritoneal Dialysis

Demographics

The mean age of the PD patients was 53 ± 15 years; 42% of the PD patients were diabetic and 55% were women. The composition of the population by race was 62% black, 20% white, and 18% Hispanic. The etiology of ESRD in this group was similar to that in the HD group except there were more patients with known HIV infection among PD patients than HD patients (9.4% vs. 2%). Mean prior months on PD at enrollment was 4.75 ± 14.7 months. At enrollment, the mean PTH level was 364 ± 346 pg/mL, and the median PTH was 260 pg/mL. In addition, the mean enrollment values were: albumin 3.45 ± 0.64 g/dL; serum creatinine 11.3 ± 4.6 mg/dL; and total cholesterol 203 ± 63 mg/dL. Mean predialysis serum phosphorus was 5.1 ± 1.8 mg/dL. The mean and maximum follow-up were 2.69 and 14.1 years, respectively.

Survival Analysis by PTH

During this study period, 146 (53%) PD patients died. The cumulative observed survival of patients with

Table 4. Predictors of PTH in Dialysis Patients: Univariate Regression Analysis

Variable	HD		PD	
	Beta Coefficient	*P*	Beta Coefficient	*P*
Age (years)	-0.17	0.001	-0.134	0.026
Male gender	0.019	NS	-0.004	NS
Black race	0.22	<0.0001	0.212	0.001
Diabetes	-0.81	NS	-0.17	0.005
Prior months on dialysis	-0.014	NS	0.042	NS
Albumin (g/dL)	0.084	NS	0.195	0.001
Creatinine (mg/dL)	0.11	0.039	0.22	<0.0001
Cholesterol (mg/dL)	-0.056	NS	0.045	NS
Phosphorus (mg/dL)	0.21	<0.0001	0.156	0.012

enrollment PTH >200 pg/mL was significantly better than patients with enrollment PTH of 65–200 pg/mL and those with PTH <65 pg/mL ($P<0.0001$). Survival adjusted for enrollment age, race, gender, months on PD, HIV status, and for enrollment nutritional markers (albumin, creatinine, cholesterol) also showed similar results ($P<0.0001$) (**Figure 1B**).

Table 1 shows the univariate Cox regression analysis for predictors of mortality in dialysis patients. Age and presence of diabetes were associated with higher mortality risk in PD patients; while African heritage and higher enrollment levels of serum albumin, serum creatinine, serum cholesterol, serum phosphorus and log PTH were associated with lower mortality risk.

Table 2 shows the multivariate Cox regression analysis for predictors of mortality. In this model, which adjusted for other variables that affected survival in the univariate model, age, enrollment serum albumin, and log PTH were found to be significant independent predictors of mortality. In this model, each year of age imparted a 2% increase in relative mortality risk for PD patients; while for every 1 g/dL increase in serum albumin at PD enrollment, there was a 47% reduction in relative risk. For each 10-fold increase in PTH (e.g., from 10 pg/mL to 100 pg/mL), there was a 51% reduction in mortality risk.

Predictors of PTH

Table 3 shows correlations of PTH with age and biochemical profile in dialysis patients. PTH correlated directly with serum albumin, serum creatinine, and serum phosphorus, and was inversely correlated with age and serum calcium.

Table 4 shows the univariate regression analysis for independent predictors of PTH level in dialysis patients. Increasing age and presence of diabetes were associated with lower levels of PTH. African ancestry and higher levels of serum albumin, serum creatinine and serum phosphorus were predictors of higher PTH level. Multivariate stepwise regression analysis confirmed black race (β=0.19, P=0.001), diabetes (β= 0.16, P=0.007), enrollment serum albumin (β=0.15, P= 0.012) and serum phosphorus (β=0.15, P=0.013) as independent predictors of enrollment PTH. Enrollment PTH was significantly lower in diabetic patients compared to non-diabetic patients (280 pg/mL vs. 425 pg/mL, P=0.001), and diabetes was a significant predictor of non-transformed mean PTH at enrollment (β=-0.207, P=0.001). Patients of African descent had significantly higher PTH than Caucasian and Hispanic patients (433 pg/mL for black *vs.* 226 pg/mL for white and 283 pg/mL for Hispanic patients, $P<0.001$).

Discussion

Secondary hyperparathyroidism is a usual consequence of progressive renal failure.[1] The rise in PTH roughly parallels the fall in GFR. Excess parathyroid hormone has long been considered detrimental to the health of patients on renal replacement therapy. In addition to the potentially debilitating bone disease that can occur, many uremic manifestations have been attributed to high PTH levels in this population: neurotoxicity, cardiomyopathy, impaired insulin secretion, abnormal lipid metabolism, impaired immune function, metabolic acidosis, and impaired protein catabolism/anabolism have all been reported.[4,5,8,9] Better understanding of the pathophysiology of secondary hyperparathyroidism and the availability of intravenous vitamin D replacement have substantially improved the clinician's ability to interrupt the toxic cascade of uncontrolled hyperparathyroidism. This study represents a unique group of prevalent and incident dialysis patients who were enrolled prior to the general availability of intravenous vitamin D preparations to effectively manage secondary hyperparathyroidism.

We previously reported an observation that seemed counterintuitive; that is, higher levels of PTH were associated with improved survival in both HD and PD patients. We hypothesized that patients with higher PTH were better nourished than those with lower PTH.[6] The results of this prospective study confirm and extend our previous reports of the prognostic importance of low serum PTH in long-term survival of HD and PD patients.[6] In fact, low levels of PTH at enrollment were associated with increased all-cause mortality in HD and PD patients followed up to 14 years. Single enrollment values of PTH >200 pg/mL were predictors of better raw survival, as well as better survival after adjustment for other variables known to influence mortality, such as age, race, gender, previous months on dialysis, as well as nutritional markers for both HD and PD patients. This degree of secondary hyperparathyroidism would be considered "normal" for a person requiring maintenance renal replacement therapy who has not received intravenous vitamin D therapy. In fact, such a person with a lower PTH, particularly with a PTH < 65 pg/mL, might be considered to have perturbed homeostasis.

In regression analysis, lower PTH as a continuous log function variable was a significant mortality predictor for HD and PD patients, both in the univariate and multivariate analyses. In addition to PTH, we found other demographic and biochemical predictors of increased mortality risk, such as age and serum albumin, which have been well documented by our group and others.[10-13] PTH was inversely correlated with age and directly correlated with serum creatinine (a marker for somatic protein stores) in patients undergoing both dialytic modalities. African heritage was highly predictive of higher levels of PTH, similar to the findings of Gupta et al.[14] Race has previously been reported to be an important predictor of serum creatinine as well as survival in dialysis patients.[15,16] Advanced age has been associated with lower PTH levels and with adynamic bone disease. In addition, diabetic patients on HD and PD had lower levels of PTH, which is consistent with prior reports.[6,17,18] Not surprisingly, PTH was inversely correlated with serum calcium and directly correlated with serum phosphorus.[6]

Retention of phosphate is accepted as crucial to the development of secondary hyperparathyroidism. Low phosphorus diets can prevent or ameliorate the development of secondary hyperparathyroidism in rats [19,20] and in humans[21] with renal insufficiency. Hypophosphatemia has been associated with relative hypoparathyroidism and adynamic bone disease in pre-dialysis patients, which is moderately amenable to phosphate supplementation.[22] In the majority of dialysis patients, phosphorus intake exceeds the amount of phosphate removal, requiring the addition of oral phosphate binders. Dietary phosphorus intake is closely correlated with dietary protein intake.[23] Protein restriction in patients with renal insufficiency results in lower serum phosphorus and lower PTH without changes in serum calcium or calcitriol.[24] Therefore, low protein diet ameliorates secondary hyperparathyroidism by directly inhibiting PTH secretion, probably through phosphorus restriction.[24]

These data support the hypothesis that malnutrition associated with inadequate protein (and phosphorus) intake in our low PTH groups may explain the excess mortality. Recently, other investigators have also reported that lower PTH levels may reflect poor nutritional status and predict the risk of short-term mortality in dialysis patients.[7,25,26] Contrarily, Chertow et al reported that, with adequate adjustment for case mix and nutritional indicators, there was a direct, linear relationship between PTH and one-year mortality in a large group of hemodialysis patients.[27] However, this study reported a group of prevalent HD patients in 1998, well into the intravenous vitamin D era. Therefore, some patients in the low (<150 pg/mL) PTH groups may have had iatrogenic suppression of PTH, independent of protein/phosphorus intake. Our HD patients were enrolled prior to the use of intravenous vitamin D, and we tested the significance of lower than expected PTH, rather than stratifying PTH well above the therapeutic target range.

The association of increased mortality with low levels of PTH in a dialysis population offers a paradox but not a therapeutic dilemma. The need to control excessive degrees of secondary hyperparathyroidism (PTH >300 pg/mL) remains an important goal to minimize the debilitating effects of unchecked renal osteodystrophy in our patients. This study calls attention to the patients on the other end of the spectrum, those who have lower than expected levels of PTH, especially without aggressive PTH management. As recognized by Sherlock Holmes, the culprit's guilt (or in this case, the patient's underlying metabolic abnormality) is noted because the dog didn't bark.

References

1. Llach F, Massry SG: On the mechanism of secondary hyperparathyroidism in moderate renal insufficiency. J Clin Endocrinol Metab 61:601-6, 1985
2. Delmez JA, Slatopolsky E: Hyperphosphatemia: Its consequences and treatment in chronic renal failure. Am J Kidney Dis 19:303-17, 1992
3. Sherrard D, Herez G, Pei Y, Maloney NA, Greenwood C, Manuel A, Saiphoo C, Fenton SS, Segre GV: The spectrum of bone disease in end-stage renal failure–an evolving disorder. Kidney Int 43:436-42, 1993
4. Avram MM, Feinfeld DA, Huatuco AH: Search for the uremic toxin: Decreased motor-nerve conduction velocity and elevated parathyroid hormone in uremia. N Engl J Med 298:1000-3, 1978
5. Avram MM, Iancu M, Morrow P, Feinfeld D, Huatuco A: Uremic syndrome in man: new evidence for parathormone as a multisystem neurotoxin. Clin Nephrol 11:59-62, 1979
6. Avram MM, Sreedhara R, Avram DK, Muchnick RA, Fein P: Enrollment parathyroid hormone level is a new marker of survival in hemodialysis and peritoneal dialysis therapy for uremia. Am J Kidney Dis 28:924-30, 1996
7. Coco M, Rush H: Increased incidence of hip fractures in dialysis patients with low serum parathyroid hormone. Am J Kidney Dis 36:1115-21, 2000
8. Nishizawa Y, Shoji T, Kawagishi T, Mori H: Atherosclerosis in uremia: possible roles of hyperparathyroidism and intermediate density lipoprotein accumulation. Kidney Int 62:S90-2, 1997
9. Tzanno-Martins C, Futata E, Jorgetti V, Duarte AJ: Immune response in hemodialysis patients: is there any difference when low and high iPTH levels are compared? Clin Nephrol 54:22-9, 2000
10. Avram MM, Mittman N, Bonomini L, Chattopadhyay J, Fein PA: Markers for survival in dialysis: A seven year prospective study. Am J Kidney Dis 26:209-19, 1995
11. Lowrie EG, Lew NL: Death risk in hemodialysis: The predictive value of commonly measured variables and an evaluation of death rate differences between facilities. Am J Kidney Dis 15:458-63, 1990
12. Avram MM, Goldwasser P, Erroa M, Fein PA: Predictors of survival in continuous ambulatory peritoneal dialysis patients: the importance of prealbumin and other nutritional and metabolic markers. Am J Kidney Dis 23:91-8, 1994
13. Avram MM, Goldwasser P, Derkatz D, Gusik S-A: Correlates of long-term survival on hemodialysis, in Friedman EA (ed):

Death on Hemodialysis: Preventable or Inevitable? , Dordrecht, The Netherlands, Kluwer Academic Publishers, 1994, pp169-76

14. Gupta A, Kallenbach LR, Zasuwa G, Divine GW: Race is a major determinant of secondary hyperparathyroidism in uremic patients. J Am Soc Nephrol 11:330-4, 2000
15. Lowrie EG, Lew NL, Huang WH: Race and diabetes as death risk predictors in hemodialysis patients. Kidney Int (Suppl.) 42:S22-S31, 1992
16. Abuelo JG, Shemin D, Chazan JA: Serum creatinine concentration at the onset of uremia: Higher levels in black males. Clin Nephrol 37:303-7, 1992
17. Avram MM: Lower parathyroid hormone and creatinine in diabetic uremia, in Avram MM (ed): Parathyroid hormone in kidney failure. New York, Karger, 1980, pp 4-8
18. Martinez I, Saracho R, Moina I, Montenegro J, Llach F: Is there a lesser hyperparathyroidism in diabetic patients with chronic renal failure? Nephrol Dial Transplant 13:S9-S11, 1998
19. Slatopolsky E, Caglar S, Gradowska L, Canterbury J, Reiss E, Bricker NS: On the prevention of secondary hyperparathyroidism in experimental chronic renal disease using "proportional reduction" of dietary phosphorus intake. Kidney Int 2:147-51, 1972
20. Yi H, Fukagawa M, Yamato H, Kumagai M, Watanabe T, Kurokawa K: Prevention of enhanced parathyroid hormone secretion, synthesis and hyperplasia by mild dietary phosphorus restriction in early chronic renal failure in rats: possible direct role of phosphorus. Nephron 70:242-8, 1995
21. Aparicio M, Combe C, Lafage MH, de Precigout V, Potaux L, Bouchet JL: In advanced renal failure, dietary phosphorus restriction reverses hyperparathyroidism independent of changes in the levels of calcitrol. Nephron 63:122-3, 1993
22. Carvalho AB, Lobao RRS, Cuppari L, Draibe SA, Ajzen H: Does hypophosphataemia induce hypoparathyroidism in predialysis patients? Nephrol Dial Transplant 13:S12-4, 1998
23. Ruffino M, de Bonis E, Martin M, Rebollo S, Martin B, Miquel R, Cobo M, Hernandez D, Torres A, Lorenzo V: Is it possible to control hyperphosphatemia with diet, without inducing protein malnutrition? Nephrol Dial Transplant 13:S65-7, 1998
24. Combe C, Aparicio M: Phosphorus and protein restriction and parathyroid function in chronic renal failure. Kidney Int. 46:1381-6, 1994
25. Akizawa T, Kinugasa E, Kurihara S, Tsukamoto Y, Fukagawa M, Kawaguchi Y, Kurokawa K: Parathyroid hormone deficiency is an indicator of poor nutritional state and prognosis in dialysis patients. J Am Soc Nephrol 10:615A, 1999 (Abstract)
26. Heaf JG, Lokkegard H: Parathyroid hormone during maintenance dialysis: influence of low calcium dialysate, plasma albumin and age. J Nephrol 11:203-10, 1998
27. Chertow GM, Lazarus JM, Lew NL, Lowrie EG: Intact parathyroid hormone is directly related to mortality in hemodialysis. J Am Soc Nephrol 11:573A, 2000 (Abstract)

7 Prealbumin As an Important Predictor for Survival and Nutritional Status in Hemodialysis and Peritoneal Dialysis Patients

NEAL MITTMAN, MD, MORRELL MICHAEL AVRAM, MD, KYIN K. OO, MD, AND JYOTI CHATTOPADHYAY, PHD

Abstract

Malnutrition is highly prevalent in dialysis patients and is one of the factors contributing to the high mortality rate in hemodialysis (HD) and peritoneal dialysis (PD) patients. We, and others, have previously reported that single enrollment levels of serum nutritional markers such as albumin, cholesterol, creatinine, and prealbumin are directly correlated with mortality in HD and PD patients. We have prospectively examined the relationship of enrollment prealbumin levels, as well as demographic characteristics and other biochemical markers, to all causes of mortality in 130 hemodialysis and 128 peritoneal dialysis patients who were monitored for up to 10 years. The Kaplan-Meier method was used to compute observed survival, and the Cox proportional hazards model was used to identify independent predictors of mortality risk. For HD patients, enrollment serum prealbumin remained a strong independent predictor of long-term survival after adjusting for age, race, gender, months on dialysis, diabetic status, and other nutritional markers. In PD as well as HD patients, observed and adjusted survival (after adjusting for above confounding variables) of patients with prealbumin greater than 30 mg/dL was significantly higher than those with prealbumin less than 30 mg/dL. For HD and PD patients, age and diabetes were inversely associated with prealbumin concentration; while levels of albumin, creatinine, and total cholesterol were directly associated with prealbumin concentration. In this study, prealbumin was the best single biochemical predictor of mortality for HD patients and a useful tool to assess nutritional risk in both HD and PD.

Introduction

The incidence and prevalence of end-stage renal disease (ESRD) continues to increase worldwide. According to the United States Renal Data System in 2000, 397,971 patients received renal replacement therapy in 1998 compared to 186,819 in 1989.[1] With advances in dialysis technology and therapeutic management, the mortality rate in ESRD patients has declined modestly. In the United States, there has been a 38.5% reduction in first-year adjusted death rate for incident ESRD patients during the period from 1988 to 1997.[2] Nevertheless, the first-year adjusted mortality rate of dialysis patients remains high: 18.5% in 1997.[2] Comorbid factors such as advanced age, malnutrition, infection, cardiovascular disease, and malignancy, as well as technical factors such as adequacy of dialysis, vascular access complications, and peritoneal membrane characteristics may all contribute to this high mortality rate.

Protein energy malnutrition is highly prevalent in HD and PD patients and is a major contributing factor to the high mortality rate in this population.[3] Over the past decade, various nutritional parameters have emerged as powerful predictors of mortality in dialysis patients.[3,4] As early as 1985, we reported the relationship of serum urea nitrogen (BUN) and creatinine to survival of HD patients.[5] Subsequently, we and others reported that, in addition to advanced age and diabetes, serum measures of nutritional markers such as albumin, cholesterol, creatinine, and prealbumin are important predictors of survival in HD and PD patients.[6-10]

Assessment of nutritional status in dialysis patients using laboratory measures is problematic, because there is no "gold standard" measurement. A low serum albumin level has been most commonly used as an indicator of malnutrition in dialysis patients.[7] Serum albumin, however, responds slowly to nutritional intervention because of its long half-life and large body pool.[11] Because of these difficulties with serum albumin, several authors have searched for more sensitive and earlier markers for malnutrition in dialysis patients. Among the newer indices of nutrition, serum prealbumin has received increasing attention. Due to its rapid turnover rate, short half-life, high tryptophan content, and small pool size, prealbumin is a highly sensitive marker of nutritional status.[12] We have previously reported the importance of serum prealbumin

M.M. Avram.(ed.), Improving Prognosis for Kidney Disorders, 61-67.

in predicting nutritional status and mortality in HD and PD patients over 14 months to five years of observation.[8,13-15] Recently, Chertow et al confirmed that prealbumin provides prognostic value in HD patients, independent of albumin and other established predictors of mortality.[16] We now report on the ability of single enrollment levels of prealbumin to predict long-term survival in HD and PD patients and compare serum prealbumin measurements with demographic characteristics and other markers of nutritional status to determine overall mortality risk.

Patients and Methods

Patients

One hundred thirty HD and 128 PD patients undergoing dialytic therapy at the Avram Center for Kidney Diseases were enrolled in the study beginning in January, 1991. All patient outcomes were followed through August, 2001. Patients were excluded from follow-up if they had undergone renal transplantation, changed dialysis modality, or transferred to another dialysis facility. On enrollment, demographic and clinical data collected included age, race, gender, diabetic status, etiology of ESRD, total months on dialysis at enrollment, and seropositivity to human immunodeficiency virus (if known).

Biochemical Data

On enrollment, nonfasting, predialysis, venous blood samples were drawn at a routine visit to establish baselines. Multiphasic biochemistry screening was performed for each patient using the SMAC autoanalyzer (Technicon, Tarrytown, NY), and included albumin, creatinine, serum urea nitrogen, and total cholesterol. Serum prealbumin was measured by rate nephelometry on a Beckman Array Protein System (Beckman Instruments Inc, Brea, CA). "Enrollment" value was the first value of a given nutritional marker for the patient obtained at or immediately after enrollment.

Dialysis Prescription

Hemodialysis patients were treated with bicarbonate-based dialysate and volumetric ultrafiltration control. Cellulose-based membranes (predominantly cellulose acetate and cellulose triacetate) were used prior to 1998 for more than 95% of all treatments. Thereafter, all patients were switched to polysulfone membranes. Initially, the hemodialysis prescription was guided by the goal of achieving a urea reduction ratio of >60% on the first treatment of the week (i.e., 68 hours after the preceding dialysis). This was later increased to >65%. Prior to 1992, most patients treated with continuous ambulatory peritoneal dialysis (PD) received four 2-liter Dianeal solution exchanges per day. After 1992, PD prescription was guided to achieve a target weekly Kt/V of 1.7, later increased to 2.1. Dextrose concentration in the dialysate varied with the need for ultrafiltration.

Statistical Analysis

Continuous variables are reported as mean (± SD). For selected comparisons between two group means, parametric (t-test) or non-parametric (Mann-Whitney test) tests were used. Correlations were reported as either the Pearson correlation coefficient or the Spearman rank correlation coefficient. Simple linear regression was used to identify the predictors of prealbumin. Multiple linear regression was used to produce a predictive model for prealbumin. Observed survival of HD and PD patients was computed by Kaplan-Meier method. Survival was also evaluated using univariate and multivariate Cox proportional hazards model using age, race, gender, diabetes, prior months on dialysis, comorbidity, and nutritional status as independent variables. A two-tailed P value <0.05 was considered to be statistically significant. Calculations were performed using SPSS for Windows 9.0.1 (SPSS Inc., Chicago, IL).

Results

Hemodialysis

Demographics

The mean age of HD patients was 60 years. Forty-three percent of the patients were diabetic and 52% were female. The causes of ESRD were as follows: 38% diabetes, 34% hypertension, 6% glomerulonephritis, 9% polycystic kidney disease, 3% obstruction, 3% HIV, and 7% other/unknown. The ethnic composition of the population was 52% black, 31% white, and 17% Hispanic. The mean time on HD at enrollment was 55 ± 54 months. At enrollment, the mean serum prealbumin level was 26.5 ± 6.5 mg/dL. In addition, the mean enrollment albumin was 3.77 ± 0.35 g/dL, mean serum creatinine 11.8 ± 3.7 mg/dL, mean total cholesterol 172 ± 47 mg/dL, and mean predialysis serum urea nitrogen was 82 ± 22 mg/dL.

Survival Analysis by Prealbumin

During the study period, 94 of the 130 HD patients (72%) died. The cumulative observed survival of HD patients with enrollment prealbumin >30 mg/dL was significantly (P=0.003) better than that of patients with prealbumin ≤30 mg/dL (**Figure 1A**). Similar results were seen when survival for the two groups (prealbumin ≤30 or >30 mg/dL) was adjusted for age, race,

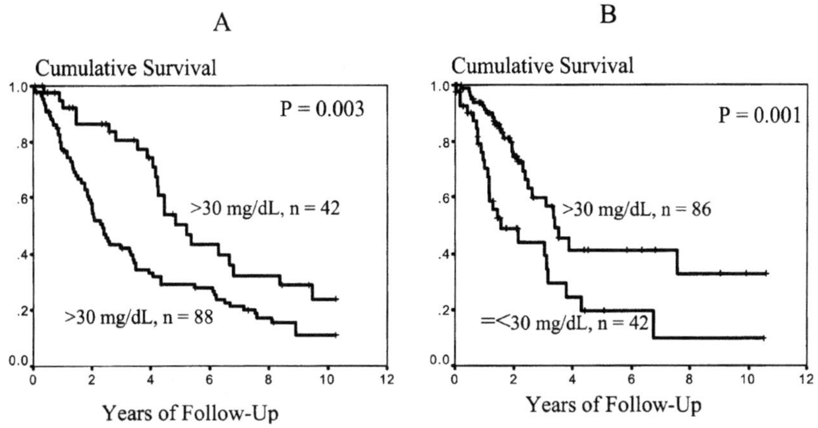

Figure 1. (**A**) Observed survival by enrollment level of prealbumin in 130 hemodialysis patients. (**B**) Observed survival by enrollment level of prealbumin in 128 peritoneal dialysis patients.

gender, diabetic status, prior months on HD, and enrollment serum albumin (P=0.009). By univariate Cox regression analysis (**Table 1**), age, female gender, and presence of diabetes were positive predictors of mortality in HD patients; while prior months on dialysis, serum prealbumin, albumin, and creatinine levels were associated with improved survival. For example, diabetics had a relative risk of 2.45 (P<0.0001), indicating almost a two and half-fold increase in relative risk; while serum prealbumin had a relative risk of 0.91 (P<0.0001). Thus, for each 1 mg/dL increase in serum prealbumin level at enrollment, there was a 9% decrease in the relative risk of death. The independent predictors of patient survival were determined using a multivariate Cox proportional hazard analysis, which adjusts for other variables known to influence survival (**Table 2**). In this model, only age and serum prealbumin were significant independent predictors of mortality risk. For each year of age at enrollment, there was a 3% increase in mortality risk; while for every mg/dL increase in serum prealbumin at enrollment, there was a 5% reduction in mortality risk during the study. The predictors of mortality were further examined using Cox stepwise regression analysis. Serum prealbumin (RR=0.94, P=0.002) was also the single best predictor of survival in this model.

Predictors of Prealbumin

Table 3 shows the correlations of prealbumin with age and other biochemical markers in HD patients. Prealbumin correlated positively with albumin, creatinine, total cholesterol, and predialysis urea nitrogen in HD patients. Therefore, higher levels of these nutritional markers were associated with a higher prealbumin value. By univariate regression analysis, the presence of diabetes (β= -0.28, P=0.001) was associated with lower prealbumin level. Serum prealbumin was higher in men (β =0.19, P=0.035), and in the presence of higher serum albumin (β=0.53, P<0.0001), serum creatinine (β=0.46,

Table 1. Predictors of Mortality in Dialysis Patients: Univariate Cox Regression Analysis

Variable	**HD (N=130)**		**PD (N=128)**	
	Relative Risk	***P***	**Relative Risk**	***P***
Age (years)	1.039	<0.0001	1.057	<0.0001
Race (black *vs.* other)	0.991	NS	0.52	0.02
Gender (female *vs.* male)	1.45	0.05	0.79	NS
Diabetes (yes *vs.* no)	2.45	<0.0001	3.26	<0.0001
Prior months on dialysis	0.995	0.03	0.98	0.013
Prealbumin (mg/dL)	0.91	<0.0001	0.95	0.001
Albumin (g/dL)	0.37	0.002	0.49	0.007
Creatinine (mg/dL)	0.84	<0.0001	0.87	<0.0001

Table 2. Predictors of Mortality in Dialysis Patients: Multivariate Cox Regression Analysis

Variable	HD (N=130)		PD (N=128)	
	Relative Risk	*P*	Relative Risk	*P*
Age (years)	1.028	0.006	1.054	<0.0001
Race (black *vs.* other)	1.18	NS	0.64	NS
Gender (female *vs.* male)	1.17	NS	0.76	NS
Diabetes (yes *vs.* no)	1.59	NS	2.40	0.004
Prior months on dialysis	1.004	NS	0.994	NS
Prealbumin (mg/dL)	0.95	0.016	0.99	NS
Albumin (g/dL)	0.91	NS	0.86	NS
Creatinine (mg/dL)	0.92	NS	0.99	NS

P<0.0001), serum total cholesterol (β=0.47, P<0.0001), and BUN. Multivariate regression analysis confirmed that serum albumin (β=0.29, P<0.0001), serum creatinine (β=0.28, P<0.0001), serum total cholesterol (β=0.39, P<0.0001), and predialysis BUN (β=0.19, P=0.005) independently predict higher serum prealbumin level. Enrollment serum prealbumin in diabetic HD patients (n=56) was lower than that of non-diabetic HD patients (n=74) (24.4 vs. 28.1 mg/dL, P=0.001).

Peritoneal Dialysis

Demographics

The mean age of PD patients was 53 ± 16 years. Thirty-four percent of the patients were diabetic, and 59% were female. The cause of ESRD in PD patients was similar to that of HD patients. The ethnic composition of the population was 58% black, 20% white, and 22% Hispanic. Mean time on PD at enrollment was 21 ± 24 months. The mean enrollment serum prealbumin level was 35.2 ± 11.3 mg/dL, while mean enrollment albumin was 3.6 ± 0.52 g/dL, creatinine was 12.4 ± 4.7 mg/dL, total cholesterol was 217 ± 54 mg/dL, and BUN was 58 ± 20 mg/dL.

Survival Analysis by Prealbumin

Figure 1B shows the observed survival for two groups of patients stratified by serum prealbumin. The cumulative observed survival of PD patients with enrollment prealbumin >30 mg/dL was significantly (P=0.001) higher than that of patients with prealbumin ≤30 mg/dL. Cumulative survival adjusted for race, gender, diabetes, previous months on PD, enrollment serum creatinine and by HIV seroreactivity also showed similar results, i.e., patients with enrollment serum prealbumin >30 mg/dL had better survival (P=0.02). By univariate Cox regression analysis (**Table 1**), age and presence of diabetes were positive predictors of mortality in PD patients; while African ancestry, more months on PD at enrollment, and higher levels of serum prealbumin, serum albumin, and serum creatinine were associated with better survival in PD patients. For example, age had a relative risk of 1.057 (P<0.0001), indicating that for each year of life at enrollment, there was almost a 6% increase in mortality risk. Serum prealbumin had a relative risk of 0.95 (P=0.001). Thus, each 1 mg/dL increase in serum prealbumin level at enrollment was associated with a 5% decrease in relative risk of death. In the multivariate Cox proportional hazards model (**Table 2**), adjusting for factors that influence survival in the univariate model, only age and diabetic status were independent mortality predictors. For each year of life, there was a 5% increase in relative risk. Diabetics had 2.4-fold increase in mortality risk (RR=2.40). In this model, prealbumin and all nutritional parameters ceased to be independent predictors of survival for PD patients.

Predictors of Prealbumin

Table 3 shows the correlations of prealbumin with age and other biochemical markers in PD patients.

Table 3. Correlations of Prealbumin with Age and Biochemical Profile in HD and PD

Variable	HD (N=130)	PD (N=128)
	Correlation Coefficient	Correlation Coefficient
Age (years)	-0.15	-0.3**
Albumin (g/dL)	0.53**	0.62**
Creatinine (mg/dL)	0.46**	0.34**
Cholesterol (mg/dL)	0.47**	0.43**
Predialysis BUN (mg/dL)	0.34**	0.21*

**P<0.0001, *P<0.05

Prealbumin was positively correlated with serum albumin, serum creatinine, total cholesterol and serum urea nitrogen, while it negatively correlated with age. By uni-variate regression analysis, increasing age (β= -3.48, P=0.001) and presence of diabetes (β= -3.69, P=0.001) were associated with lower prealbumin level. Serum prealbumin was higher in the presence of higher serum albumin (β=8.72, P<0.0001), serum creatinine (β=4.1, P<0.0001), serum total cholesterol (β=5.2, P<0.0001), and BUN (β=2.33, P=0.022). Multivariate regression analysis confirmed that higher serum albumin (β=0.51, P<0.0001) and creatinine (β=0.28, P<0.0001) are independent predictors of higher serum prealbumin level, and that the presence of diabetes was associated with lower prealbumin level (β=-0.195, P=0.005). As in HD patients, enrollment serum prealbumin in diabetic PD patients was significantly lower than in non-diabetic patients (30.3 vs. 37.7 mg/dL, P<0.0001). In addition, the serum prealbumin level was significantly higher in PD patients compared to HD patients (35.2 mg/dL vs. 26.5 mg/dL, P<0.05).

Discussion

The results of this ten-year prospective study confirm and highlight the prognostic importance of serum prealbumin measurements in the survival of HD and PD patients. Lower levels of serum prealbumin at enrollment were associated with increased all-cause mortality in both HD and PD patients. In univariate Cox regression analysis, prealbumin was a highly significant independent predictor of mortality in both HD and PD patients; and in multivariate analysis, prealbumin was the single best biochemical predictor of survival for HD patients.

Protein energy malnutrition is prevalent in the dialysis population and is currently accepted as an important factor contributing to high mortality in dialysis patients.[4,17] We and others have previously reported the predictive value of several biochemical indices of nutritional state on mortality in HD and PD patients.[6-8,10,15,16,18-23] Serum albumin remains the most commonly used biochemical index for nutritional state. However, serum prealbumin is a more sensitive marker of nutritional status than albumin and reflects changes more rapidly in nonuremic patients.[12,24] Prealbumin has been shown to increase with protein and calorie intake and to decline with inadequate protein intake;[25] as with serum albumin, prealbumin reflects visceral protein stores. In HD patients, clinically significant changes in albumin can be reliably predicted by earlier changes in serum prealbumin.[26] In this study, serum prealbumin was highly correlated with markers for visceral (albumin and cholesterol) and somatic protein stores (creatinine), as well as a marker of recent protein intake (serum urea nitrogen). Direct correlation of prealbumin with other nutritional markers suggests that prealbumin is a powerful indicator of overall nutritional status in HD and PD patients. Serial measurements of serum prealbumin in HD patients can reliably identify patients in need of nutritional intervention.[21]

By univariate and multivariate analysis, we identified the above nutritional markers as well as several demographic characteristics such as age and diabetes that were significant predictors of prealbumin in dialysis patients. Lower serum prealbumin has been reported in aging rats.[27] In the current study, age was a strong predictor of prealbumin, especially in PD patients. Lower prealbumin levels in diabetic patients compared to nondiabetics has been noted previously and may be an indication of poorer nutritional status in diabetics, leading to higher mortality seen in these patients.[21,28]

Serum prealbumin impacted the relative risk of death in HD patients to a greater degree than in PD patients; e.g., in univariate analysis, the decrease in relative risk for every unit increase in prealbumin was higher and more significant for HD patients than PD patients (RR=0.91 or 9% risk reduction per unit, P<0.0001 for HD vs. RR=0.95 or 5% risk reduction per unit, P=0.001 for PD). The effect of serum albumin on mortality risk also was greater in HD than PD patients. The Cox multivariate regression analysis showed only age and prealbumin as significant independent predictors of all causes of mortality in HD patients. This was confirmed by a Cox stepwise multivariate regression analysis. The 5% reduction in relative risk per 1 mg/dL increase in serum prealbumin in the multivariate analysis is very similar to the findings of Chertow et al.[16] Therefore, serum prealbumin appears to be a better predictor of survival in HD patients than albumin, the most widely used marker of nutritional health in dialysis patients. The high degree of correlation between serum prealbumin and other nutritional markers (albumin, creatinine and cholesterol) explains the multivariate analysis results; i.e., serum prealbumin, when added to the model, already reflects a significant part of the nutritional risk seen with low values of the other markers. Therefore, the other nutritional indices, which are known to influence survival, cease being independent predictors.

The predictive power of prealbumin in PD patients appears to be somewhat different from that of HD patients. Although serum prealbumin is a mortality predictor in PD patients as a continuous and a categorical variable in the univariate model, the addition of age and diabetic status in the multivariate analysis confounds the mortality risk of prealbumin and all nutritional markers in PD patients. Age was highly correlated with prealbumin in PD patients; while diabetic status was associated with lower prealbumin levels (β=-0.195, p=0.005). Therefore, the addition of age and diabetic status to the multivariate model accounted for a substantial portion of the mortality risk associated with prealbumin. Serum prealbumin is known to be higher in HD patients than in the general population, an effect attributed to elevated levels of retinol-binding protein and impaired degradation of prealbumin.[29] However, the serum prealbumin level was significantly higher in PD patients compared to HD patients, a finding also reported by others,[30] and may reflect other pathophysiological mechanisms that are independent of nutritional state. For example, the ongoing peritoneal effluent protein losses may alter hepatic synthesis or affect the degradation of prealbumin. In addition, prealbumin is known to be a negative "acute phase reactant."[31] Therefore, multiple influences in opposing directions may explain differences by dialysis technique. The ideal level of prealbumin required to maintain adequate nutritional status of PD patients may be higher than that of HD patients.

In summary, it is well documented that protein energy malnutrition is a significant contributor to mortality in hemodialysis and peritoneal dialysis patients. We prospectively examined all-cause mortality risk in dialysis patients over ten years, and found that serum prealbumin was a more sensitive predictor of risk than albumin—the most commonly utilized biochemical marker of nutritional state. Serial prealbumin measurements should be incorporated in prospective trials of nutritional assessment and intervention in this high-risk population. Further work will be necessary to elucidate the differences in serum prealbumin by dialysis modality, as well as to define the negative acute phase reactant effect in prealbumin's mortality risk.

Acknowledgements

Supported in part by the National Kidney Foundation of New York/New Jersey and the Nephrology Foundation of Brooklyn.

References

1. United States Renal Data System: USRDS 2000 Annual Data Report. The National Institutes of Health, National Institute of Diabetes and Digestive and Kidney Diseases, Bethesda, MD, 2000
2. United States Renal Data System: USRDS 2000 Annual Data Report: Survival, mortality and causes of death. Am J Kidney Dis 36:S127-42, 2000
3. Hakim RM, Levin N: Malnutrition in hemodialysis patients. Am J Kidney Dis 21:125-37, 1993
4. Acchiardo SR, Moore LW, Latour PA: Malnutrition as the main factor in morbidity and mortality of dialysis patients. Kidney Int (Suppl.) 24:S199-S203, 1983
5. Avram MM, Slater PA, Gan A, Iancu M, Pahilan AN, Okanya D, Rajpal K, Paik SK, Zouabi M, Fein PA: Predialysis BUN and creatinine do not predict adequate dialysis, clinical rehabilitation, or longevity. Kidney Int 28:S100-4, 1985
6. Avram MM, Mittman N, Bonomini L, Chattopadhyay J, Fein PA: Markers for survival in dialysis: A seven year prospective study. Am J Kidney Dis 26:209-19, 1995
7. Lowrie EG, Lew NL: Death risk in hemodialysis: The predictive value of commonly measured variables and an evaluation of death rate differences between facilities. Am J Kidney Dis 15:458-63, 1990
8. Avram MM, Goldwasser P, Erroa M, Fein PA: Predictors of survival in continuous ambulatory peritoneal dialysis patients: the importance of prealbumin and other nutritional and metabolic markers. Am J Kidney Dis 23:91-8, 1994
9. Avram MM, Sreedhara R, Avram DK, Mushnick RA, Fein P: Enrollment parathyroid hormone level is a new marker of survival in hemodialysis and peritoneal dialysis therapy for uremia. Am J Kidney Dis 28:924-30, 1996
10. Avram MM, Goldwasser P, Derkatz D, Gusik S-A: Correlates of long-term survival on hemodialysis, Death on Hemodialysis:Preventable or Inevitable? Edited by Friedman EA. Kluwer Academic Publishers, 1994, pp 169-76.
11. Klein S: The myth of serum albumin as a measure of nutritional status. Gastroenterology 99:1845-6, 1990
12. Mears A: Outcomes of continuous process improvement of a nutritional care program incorporating serum prealbumin measurements. Nutrition 12:479-84, 1996
13. Avram MM, Sreedhara R, Mittman N: Prealbumin is a strong predictor of nutritional risk and five year mortality in dialysis patients. ASAIO 1997(Abstract)
14. Goldwasser P, Michel M-A, Collier J, Mittman N, Fein P, Gusik S-A, Avram MM: Prealbumin and Lipoprotein (a) in Hemodialysis: Relationships With Patient and Vascular Access Survival. Am J Kidney Dis 22:215-25, 1993
15. Sreedhara R, Avram MM, Blanco M, Batish R, Mittman N: Prealbumin is the best nutritional predictor of survival in hemodialysis and peritoneal dialysis. Am J Kidney Dis 28:937-42, 1996
16. Chertow GM, Ackert K, Lew NL, Lazarus JM, Lowrie EG: Prealbumin is as important as albumin in the nutritional assessment of hemodialysis patients. Kidney Int 58:2512-7, 2000
17. Kopple JD: Nutritional status as a predictor of mortality in maintenance dialysis patients. ASAIO J 43:246-50, 1997
18. Avram MM, Bonomini LV, Sreedhara R, Mittman N: Predictive value of nutritional markers (albumin, creatinine, cholesterol, and hematocrit) for patients on dialysis for up to 30 years. Am J Kidney Dis 28:910-7, 1996
19. Goldwasser P, Mittman N, Antignani A, Burrell D, Michel MA, Collier J, Avram MM: Predictors of mortality in hemodialysis patients. J Am Soc Nephrol 3:1613-22, 1993
20. Avram MM, Sreedhara R, Fein PA, Oo KK, Chattopadhyay J, Mittman N: Survival of hemodialysis and peritoneal dialysis over 12 years with emphasis on nutritional parameters. Am J Kidney Dis 37:S77-S80, 2001
21. Duggan A, Huffman FG: Validation of serum transthyretin (prealbumin) as a nutritional parameter in hemodialysis patients. J Ren Nutr 8:142-9, 1998

22. Combe C, Chauveau P, Laville M, Fouque D, Azar R, Cano N, Canaud B, Roth H, Leverve X, Aparicio M: Influence of nutritional factors and hemodialysis adequacy on the survival of 1,610 French patients. Am J Kidney Dis 37:S81-8, 2001
23. Lowrie EG, Lew NL: The predictive value of commonly measured variables and an evaluation of death rate differences between facilities. Am J Kidney Dis 15:458-82, 1990
24. Ingenbleek Y, De Visscher M, De Nayer P: Measurement of prealbumin as index of protein-calorie malnutrition. Lancet 2:106-9, 1972
25. Spiekerman AM: Proteins used in nutritional assessment. Clin Lab Med 13:353-69, 1993
26. Neyra NR, Hakim RM, Shyr Y, Ikizler TA: Serum transferrin and serum prealbumin are early predictors of serum albumin in chronic hemodialysis patients. J Ren Nutr 10:184-90, 2000
27. Chevalier S, Blaner WS, Azais-Braesco V, Tuchweber B: Dietary restriction alters retinol and retinol-binding protein metabolism in aging rats. J Gerontol A Biol Sci Med Sci 54:B384-92, 1999
28. Avram MM: Dialysis in diabetic patients: three decades of experience of, from 1964 to 1997, Diabetic Renal-Retinal Syndrome. 21st Century Management Now. Edited by Friedman EA, L'Esperance JrFA. Kluwer Academic Publishers, 1998, pp 67-78
29. Cano N, Costanzo-Dufetel JD, Calaf R, Durbec JPLP, Pascal S, Stroumza P, Labastie-Coeyrehourcq J: Prealbumin-retinol binding protein-retinol complex in hemodialysis patients. Am J Clin Nutr 47:664-7, 1988
30. Koomen GCM, Krediet RT, Hoek FJ, Arisz L: Different relationships between plasma albumin (pALB) and prealbumin (pPREALB) in CAPD, HEMO and random patients. Perit Dial Int 14:S32, 1994(Abstract)
31. Zazra JJ: Biochemical Markers of Nutrition: Technical aspects. J Ren Nutr 7:65-8, 1997

8 How to Attain Optimal Antiproteinuric Dose of Losartan in Non-Diabetic Patients with Nephrotic Range Proteinuria

GOZEWIJN D. LAVERMAN, MD, ROBERT H. HENNING, MD, PHD, PAUL E. DE JONG, MD, PHD, GERJAN NAVIS, MD, PHD AND DICK DE ZEEUW, MD, PHD

Abstract

Although the antiproteinuric response to antihypertensive treatment is the main predictor of renoprotective efficacy in long-term renal disease, dose finding studies of antihypertensives have only been based on blood pressure so far. The present study aimed to find the optimal antiproteinuric dose of the angiotensin II antagonist losartan. An open-label dose-response study using subsequent six-week treatment periods was performed in ten non-diabetic patients with proteinuria (Uprot) of 5.8 ± 0.8 g/d and a mean arterial pressure (MAP) of 103 ± 3.7 mmHg without antihypertensive medication. All patients had a normal to moderately impaired renal function. After the baseline period, five periods followed with respectively a daily losartan dose of 50 mg, 100 mg, 150 mg, again 50 mg, and a recovery without losartan. At the end of each period, Uprot and MAP were measured. The consecutive doses of losartan had a similar antihypertensive response (-11.3 ± 2.8% at the 100 mg dose). The optimal antiproteinuric response was reached at 100 mg losartan (-30 ± 8%). The 50 mg dose (-13 ± 7%) was less effective and the 150 mg dose (-28 ± 8%) was not more effective. We conclude that 100 mg losartan is the optimal dose for reduction of proteinuria in non-diabetic patients with nephrotic-range proteinuria.

Introduction

One of the major challenges of nephrology is to stop the progressive course of renal function loss in chronic renal disease. Attacking the accompanying hypertension and proteinuria is the cornerstone of renoprotective therapy, since antihypertensive drugs have been demonstrated to result in a more favourable outcome in both diabetic[1,2] and non-diabetic renal disease.[3-7]

The REIN study showed that the amount of proteinuria is the best independent predictor of the rate of progression,[8] and antihypertensive drugs that interfere in the renin-angiotensin system (RAS) have been proven to be superior in reducing proteinuria both in diabetics[9] and non-diabetics[10,11]. In addition, for therapeutic purposes, it is important that the short-term antiproteinuric response to RAS inhibition has been shown to be the strongest predictor of renoprotective efficacy in several studies[12-14].

To obtain optimal reduction of proteinuria, proper dosing is important. The dose-response for antihypertensives with an antiproteinuric action has generally been established from their antihypertensive effect. However, there is evidence to suggest that the dose-response for blood pressure and proteinuria may not be similar.[15] In addition, Rudberg et al found a reduction of proteinuria independent from a lowering of blood pressure.[16] With these considerations in mind, several authors have advocated specific titration of antihypertensive agents for the antiproteinuric response.[17,18]

The angiotensin II antagonist (AIIA) losartan has been shown to effectively reduce proteinuria. A recent abstract reported on the dose-response in diabetic patients with low levels of albuminuria.[19] However, no proper dose-response data are available in non-diabetic patients. In the present study, therefore, we investigated the antiproteinuric response of losartan in a dose-response study in non-diabetic patients with nephrotic range proteinuria, with the purpose of defining the optimal dose for proteinuria reduction.

Methods

Patients and Protocol

Patients on symptomatic antiproteinuric treatment were selected from our renal outpatient department. Inclusion criteria for this study were: stable proteinuria ≥ 2 g/24h and diastolic blood pressure between 80 and 110 mmHg off medication, a creatinine clearance ≥ 30 ml/min/1.73m^2 and age between 18 and 70 years. All antihypertensive drugs had been withdrawn for at least four weeks before inclusion in the study.

M.M. Avram.(ed.), Improving Prognosis for Kidney Disorders, 69-73.

Patients with a history of cardiovascular disease and with diabetes mellitus were excluded, as well as users of NSAID's (>2 doses/ week) and patients with contra-indications for the use of AIIA. The patients were instructed to take the study medication once daily, in the morning, except on the study days: on those days the study drug was not taken before data collection at the hospital (between 8 and 8.30 am), allowing to measure blood pressure at trough. In our out-patient department, all proteinuric patients using RAS blockers are instructed to adhere to a dietary sodium-restriction of 5-7 g/24h.

An open-label dose-response study was performed on an ambulatory basis. The study was designed to prospectively compare the antiproteinuric response of increasing doses of the AIIA losartan with the patients' baseline values as their own control. Baseline values of relevant parameters were obtained after six weeks of complete withdrawal from their antihypertensive drugs. During six-week treatment periods, the patients were treated with increasing doses of losartan, that is, losartan 50 mg, 100 mg, 150 mg, again 50 mg and finally a recovery period without medication. This design, with a period of down-titration from 150 mg to 50 mg allowed to unmask the possible existence of a carry-over phenomenon between the periods. The final six weeks without medication was a control-period for stabilty of the background proteinuria. At the end of each period, patients visited the hospital for data-collection. All subjects gave informed consent. The protocol was approved by the local Medical Ethical Committee.

Clinical and Laboratory Procedures

Blood pressure was measured at trough under standardized conditions by a Dinamap® at 1 min intervals with the patient in supine position. From 15 minutes of measurements, the mean of the last four readings was used for further analysis. Mean arterial pressure was calculated as the sum of one third systolic and two-thirds of the diastolic blood pressure. Urinary protein was determined from two consecutive 24-hour urine samples using the pyrogallol red-molybdate method. Serum and urinary electrolytes, urea and creatinine were determined using an automated multi-analyzer (SMA-C, Technicon®).

Data-Analysis

Results are expressed as mean and SEM. The amount of proteinuria and blood pressure at the end of each period are expressed as percentage change from baseline. Two-sided, paired t-tests were used to show differences between the study-periods. Differences were considered significant if the *P*-value was <0.05. Power-analysis for paired t-test was performed with a desired power of 0.8 and alpha 0.05. In order to detect changes in proteinuria of 0.5 g/day with expected standard deviation of 0.5 g/day, a sample size of n=10 was needed. This sample size provides power of 0.8 to detect changes in blood pressure of 8 mHg with expected standard deviation of 8 mmHg.

Table 1. Patient characteristics during previous treatment.

	Age/ sex	Diagnosis	Creat.Cl (ml/min)	Uprot (g/day)	MAP (mmHg)	previous medication
1	35/F	NPS	45	6.2	84	ena 10/HCT 12.5
2	48/M	FSGS	62	1.8	85	ena 20
3	58/M	MGP	84	2.0 (3.9)[1]	89	lis 10/HCT 12.5
4	38/M	IgA	93	2.9	86	los 50
5	53/F	NCBx	74	2.6	86	ena 20
6	53/M	NCBx	113	1.9 (3.4)[2]	106	ena 10/los 100/HCT 12.5
7	52/F	MGP	74	2.7	76	ena 10/HCT 25
8	45/M	MGP	126	2.0	90	ena 10
9	51/M	FSGS	56	0.7	98	ena 10
10	42/F	MGP	81	1.7 (2.8)[1]	82	los 50/HCT 12.5

NPS=nail-patella syndrome, FSGS=focal segmental glomerulosclerosis, MGP=membranous glomerulopathy, IgA=Ig nephritis, NCBx=non-conclusive renal biopsy ena=enalapril, HCT= hydrochorothiazide, lis=lisinopril, los=losartan [1]without HCT, [2]without losartan

Table 2. Individual characteristics after withdrawal of previous treatment

	Uprot (g/d)	BP (mmHg)	MAP (mmHg)	S-chol (mmol/l)	U-Na (mmol/d)	U-ur (mmol/d)
1	11.2	124/79	94	8.6	160	153
2	6.2	153/89	110	6.6	223	413
3	5.9	146/88	107	5.2	65	284
4	3.4	140/79	99	7.2	134	391
5	3.6	129/74	92	6.4	278	575
6	5.2	164/89	114	7.3	229	422
7	6.4	145/86	105	8.1	65	304
8	2.2	120/75	90	5.7	151	245
9	8.2	175/103	127	6.4	172	414
10	6.2	133/73	93	6.3	147	473
mean	**5.8**	**143/83**	**103**	**6.8**	**162**	**367**

Results

Ten patients were included who were previously on symptomatic renoprotective treatment by RAS-blockade (**Table 1**). The proteinuria during this treatment ranged from 0.7 to 6.2 g/day (mean: 2.5 g/day). After withdrawal of these renoprotective drugs, proteinuria increased to a mean baseline value of 5.8 ± 0.8 g/d (**Table 2**). **Table 2** also demonstrates that at least half of the study-subjects were non-hypertensive. All patients completed the study.

Figure 1 shows the responses of mean arterial pressure and proteinuria, expressed as percentage change from baseline. Mean arterial pressure and proteinuria were significantly reduced by all doses of losartan.

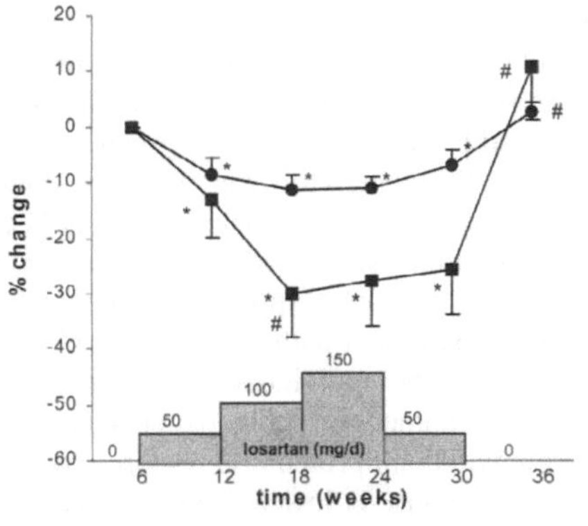

Figure 1. The response of proteinuria (squares) and mean arterial pressure (circles) at the end of six-week treatment periods in ten patients with nephrotic range proteinuria. The values are expressed as mean (SEM) % change from baseline. *p< 0.05 vs. baseline, #p< 0.05 vs. previous dose.

There were no significant differences in antihypertensive efficacy between the doses of losartan. The mean residual proteinuria at the end of the successive treatment periods was 5.0 ± 0.7 g/day (first 50 mg dose), 4.1 ± 0.8 g/day (100 mg dose), 4.3 ± 0.8 g/day (150 mg dose), 4.3 ± 0.8 g/day (second 50 mg dose) and 6.2 ± 0.7 g/day (recovery). The percentual change in proteinuria from baseline between losartan 50 and 100 mg, but not between the 100 and 150 mg dose, was significantly different.

After down-titration from 150 to 50 mg, the mean residual proteinuria remained unchanged. This occurred in eight out of ten patients (individual data not shown).

Individual data on the relative reduction of proteinuria and blood pressure per titration step are shown in **Figure 2**. This figure shows that some patients experienced a preferential reduction of proteinuria, but no change in mean arterial pressure (patients 5, 8 and 10). In five other patients, both proteinuria and mean arterial pressure were reduced substantially. In the two remaining patients an antiproteinuric response was absent despite a clear decrease of blood pressure.

Finally, no significant changes in serum creatinine or potassium levels and no cases of symptomatic hypotension were noticed with increasing doses of losartan.

Discussion

The presented data demonstrate that 100 mg daily is the optimal antiproteinuric dose of the AIIA losartan in normotensive non-diabetic patients with nephrotic range proteinuria.

This study was not designed nor powered to detect small differences in blood pressure since the blood pressure was recorded at the end of the dosing-interval, and

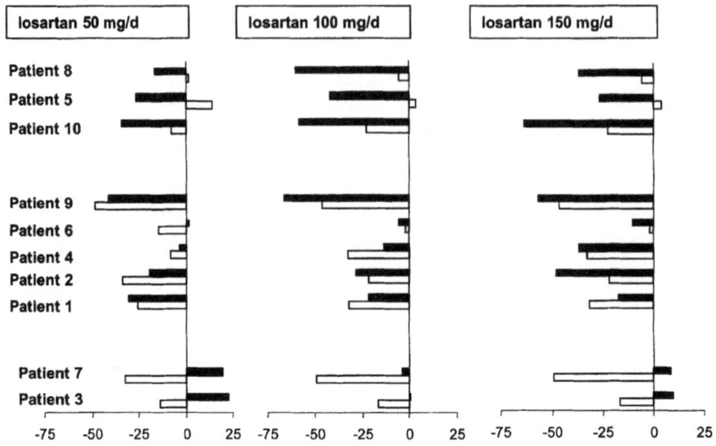

Figure 2. The individual responses (% change from baseline) of proteinuria (black bars) and mean arterial pressure (white bars, *multiplied by two*) at the consecutive uptitration steps. The patients are ranked from top to bottom by a preferential antiproteinuric response (patients 5, 8 and 10), a combined antiproteinuric and blood pressure response (patients 1, 2, 4, 6, 9) and a preferential blood pressure response (patients 3 and 7).

no 24 hour registrations were performed. The mean arterial pressure appeared to be lowest at the 100 mg dose, albeit not significantly lower than at the 50 mg dose. This is in line with the literature in hypertensive patients showing that the dose-response curve of losartan for blood pressure is flat; the antihypertensive efficacy is nearly maximal at starting dose of 50 mg daily.[20]

Our results with respect to proteinuria are in line with the only other documented use of losartan up to 150 mg, which was a recent study on the anti-albuminuric effects of losartan in diabetics.[19] These authors found that albuminuria was maximally reduced by losartan 100 mg. However, those diabetics already had low levels of albuminuria to start with (geometric mean: 1138 mg/day) which might have caused failure to detect further decrease by a higher dose. The present study has additive value in demonstrating that even in patients with a considerable residual proteinuria during 100 mg/day losartan, a higher dose fails to further reduce proteinuria.

A dose-response-study like the present one has the advantage of mimicking the clinical institution of antiproteinuric therapy. Down-titration from 150 mg to 50 mg of losartan per day revealed that proteinuria remained below the level obtained after the first 50 mg period. This phenomenon occurred for proteinuria but not blood pressure and has been demonstrated previously during down-titration of an ACE inhibitor.[21] This finding does not seem to be artefactual as it was seen in nearly all patients. It suggests that there may be sustained beneficial renal effects after shifting from a high to a low dose of losartan.

The antiproteinuric response to losartan reported in the literature ranges from –29% to –59%.[15,19,22] So, the maximal antiproteinuric response of approximately 30% found in the present study is at the lower end of the spectrum. The patients in the present study had lower levels of proteinuria during their regular treatment before entry into the study, which often included a diuretic in addition to ACE inhibition or AIIA. A higher antiproteinuric response could have been induced by adding a diuretic or by a better compliance regarding dietary sodium-intake: the mean sodium excretion amounted 162 mmol/day at baseline (**Table 2**).

It might be argued that enhancement of the antiproteinuric response to the 100 mg dose of losartan is simply caused by longer duration of treatment and not by increasing the dose. However, the time-course of the antiproteinuric response to losartan has been addressed in a previous study with weekly measurements of proteinuria. Proteinuria appeared to be stable after three weeks of treatment with the same dose.[15]

Analysis of the individual responses showed a remarkable phenomenon: some patients appeared to have a preferential antiproteinuric response; whereas in others blood pressure is lowered without reduction of proteinuria. These data seem consistent per individual as they were observed in each step of uptitration. Although our study was not designed for such an analysis, this finding suggests that in individual patients the responses of proteinuria and office blood pressure may be discrepant. To our opinion, this stresses once again the importance of specific attention for the antiproteinuric response, in addition to adequate blood pressure-control.

We conclude that in non-diabetic renal patients with nephrotic range proteinuria and normal to moderately impaired renal function, maximal reduction of proteinuria during monotherapy with losartan is reached at the 100 mg dose. In striving for further reduction, no additional benefit can be expected from uptitration to 150 mg. Instead, we suggest to add a diuretic or to institute sufficient sodium-restriction. Also, the combination with an ACE inhibitor which is currently under investigation, could be considered.

Acknowledgements

This research was supported by the Dutch Kidney Foundation (program grant 5023) and by a medical school grant from Merck Sharp and Dohme BV, Haarlem, the Netherlands.

References

1. Parving HH, Andersen AR, Smidt UM, Svendsen PA: Early aggressive antihypertensive treatment reduces rate of decline in kidney function in diabetic nephropathy. Lancet 1:1175-9, 1983
2. Mogensen CE: Long-term antihypertensive treatment inhibiting progression of diabetic nephropathy. Br Med J (Clin Res Ed) 285:685-8, 1982
3. Peterson JC, Adler S, Burkart JM, Greene T, Hebert LA, Hunsicker LG, King AJ, Klahr S, Massry SG, Seifter JL: Blood pressure control, proteinuria, and the progression of renal disease. The Modification of Diet in Renal Disease Study. Ann Intern Med 123:754-62, 1995
4. Williams PS, Fass G, Bone JM: Renal pathology and proteinuria determine progression in untreated mild/moderate chronic renal failure. Q J Med 67:343-54, 1988
5. Locatelli F, Marcelli D, Comelli M, Alberti D, Graziani G, Buccianti G, Redaelli B, Giangrande A: Proteinuria and blood pressure as causal components of progression to end-stage renal failure. Northern Italian Cooperative Study Group. Nephrol Dial Transplant 11:461-7, 1996
6. Wight JP, Salzano S, Brown CB, El Nahas AM: Natural history of chronic renal failure: a reappraisal. Nephrol Dial Transplant 7:379-83, 1992
7. Ruggenenti P, Perna A, Gherardi G, Benini R, Remuzzi G: Chronic proteinuric nephropathies: outcomes and response to treatment in a prospective cohort of 352 patients with different patterns of renal injury. Am J Kidney Dis 35:1155-65, 2000
8. Ruggenenti P, Perna A, Mosconi L, Pisoni R, Remuzzi G: Urinary protein excretion rate is the best independent predictor of ESRF in non-diabetic proteinuric chronic nephropathies. "Gruppo Italiano di Studi Epidemiologici in Nefrologia" (GISEN). Kidney Int 53:1209-16, 1998
9. Lewis EJ, Hunsicker LG, Bain RP, Rohde RD: The effect of angiotensin-converting-enzyme inhibition on diabetic nephropathy. The Collaborative Study Group [see comments] [published erratum appears in N Engl J Med 1993 Jan 13;330(2):152]. N Engl J Med 329:1456-62, 1993
10. Maschio G, Alberti D, Janin G, Locatelli F, Mann JF, Motolese M, Ponticelli C, Ritz E, Zucchelli P: Effect of the angiotensin-converting-enzyme inhibitor benazepril on the progression of chronic renal insufficiency. The Angiotensin-Converting-Enzyme Inhibition in Progressive Renal Insufficiency Study Group [see comments]. N Engl J Med 334:939-945, 1996
11. Randomised placebo-controlled trial of effect of ramipril on decline in glomerular filtration rate and risk of terminal renal failure in proteinuric, non-diabetic nephropathy. The GISEN Group (Gruppo Italiano di Studi Epidemiologici in Nefrologia) [see comments]. Lancet 349:1857-63, 1997
12. Gansevoort RT, De Zeeuw D, De Jong PE: Long-term benefits of the antiproteinuric effect of angiotensin- converting enzyme inhibition in nondiabetic renal disease. Am J Kidney Dis 22:202-6, 1993
13. Apperloo AJ, De Zeeuw D, De Jong PE: Short-term antiproteinuric response to antihypertensive treatment predicts long-term GFR decline in patients with non-diabetic renal disease. Kidney Int Suppl 45:S174-8, 1994
14. Rossing P, Hommel E, Smidt UM, Parving HH: Reduction in albuminuria predicts diminished progression in diabetic nephropathy. Kidney Int Suppl 45:S145-9, 1994
15. Gansevoort RT, De Zeeuw D, De Jong PE: Is the antiproteinuric effect of ACE inhibition mediated by interference in the renin-angiotensin system? Kidney Int 45:861-7, 1994
16. Rudberg S, Aperia A, Freyschuss U, Persson B: Enalapril reduces microalbuminuria in young normotensive type 1 (insulin-dependent) diabetic patients irrespective of its hypotensive effect. Diabetologia 33:470-6, 1990
17. De Jong PE, Navis G, De Zeeuw D: Renoprotective therapy: titration against urinary protein excretion[comment]. Lancet 354:352-3, 1999
18. Peters H, Ritz E: Dosing angiotensin II blockers--beyond blood pressure [editorial]. Nephrol Dial Transplant 14:2568-70, 1999
19. Andersen, S., Rossing, P., Juhl, T. R., and Parving, H. H. Optimal dose of losartan for renoprotection in diabetic nephropathy [abstract]. J.Am.Soc.Nephrol. 11:112A, 2000.
20. Conlin PR, Spence JD, Williams B, Ribeiro AB, Saito I, Benedict C, Bunt AM: Angiotensin II antagonists for hypertension: are there differences in efficacy? [see comments]. Am J Hypertens 13:418-26, 2000
21. Heeg JE, De Zeeuw D, de Jong P: The effects of lisinopril on renal hemodynamics in patients with renal disease. Current opinion in Cardiology 1989
22. Nielsen S, Dollerup J, Nielsen B, Jensen HA, Mogensen CE: Losartan reduces albuminuria in patients with essential hypertension. An enalapril controlled 3 months study. Nephrol Dial Transplant 12 Suppl 2:19-23, 1997

9 Hypoalbuminemia in the Patient with Renal Disease: Its Causes and Consequences

GEORGE A. KAYSEN, M.D. PH.D.

Introduction

Albumin levels are regulated within well defined limits, although there is some decrease that occurs with normal aging; and albumin levels are slightly lower in women (**Figure 2**).[1] The development of hypoalbuminemia, then, must be traced to the factors that can change the primary variables that regulate its level in health. Virtually all causes of hypoalbuminemia carry with them the potential to cause morbidity. Thus the cause of hypoalbuminemia must be identified, and the effects of the etiology of hypoalbuminemia must be separated from the effect of isolated hypoalbuminemia alone to fully understand the pathophysiology of these processes.

Albumin is synthesized exclusively in the liver at a rate of between 12 and 15 grams per day[7] and is catabolized by the vascular endothelium throughout the body with a half life of approximately 16 days.[2-4] Total albumin mass is approximately 4.5 g/kg body weight.

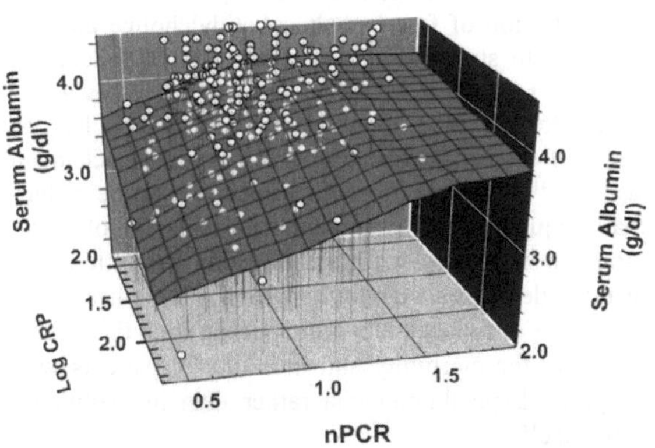

Figure 1. The relationship between serum albumin concentration, serum C reactive protein concentration (CRP) and normalized albumin catabolic rate (nPCR) measured cross sectionally in 287 patients on hemodialysis. C reactive protein levels have been log transformed. The surface is a best fit equation using a negative exponential smoothing function. The open symbols represent values in individual patients. The Vertical line beneath each symbol orients the symbol to the XY plane. Note that there are few patients who simultaneously have a log CRP > 2.0 and an nPCR > 1.0.

Between 40 and 50% of the albumin pool is normally found in the plasma compartment.[5,6] The rest is distributed in interstitial spaces throughout the body, mostly in muscle and skin. Plasma albumin concentration may be decreased because of dilution of the plasma pool during plasma volume expansion, as a result of redistribution of the albumin pool from plasma into interstitial compartments as occurs following burns or during sepsis,[7] as a consequence of a decrease in the rate of albumin synthesis, as a result of increased albumin catabolic rate or as a consequence of the development of external albumin losses; into the urine or gut, or into dialysate, or transcutaneously in the case of trauma or burns. I will review factors that regulate these processes and identify which changes are responsible for hypoalbuminemia in dialysis patients.

Albumin Synthesis

The rate of albumin synthesis is regulated in part by availability of amino acids.[7,8] Because of this relationship, plasma albumin concentration has been used as a clinical marker of nutritional status. However the rate of albumin synthesis responds more to acute changes in dietary protein[9,10] than to general (chronic) nutritional status. When severely malnourished animals or people are re-fed, the rate of albumin synthesis increases promptly, even though total body protein stores are still severely depleted.[11] This very short term regulation appears to be at the post-transcriptional step of initiation of protein synthesis.[12]

In addition to being modulated by dietary protein, albumin[13] is a negative acute phase reactive protein.[13] The acute phase response is initiated by cytokines and signal a cascade of events within hepatocytes.[14,15] Synthesis of positive acute phase reactant proteins, including fibrinogen, C-reactive protein (CRP), α_2 macroglobulin, serum amyloid A (SAA) and lipoprotein (a) (Lp(a)) is stimulated;[16-19] and synthesis of negative acute phase reactive proteins - frequently used as nutritional markers (albumin,[20] prealbumin,[21] apo A-I[22])

M.M. Avram.(ed.), Improving Prognosis for Kidney Disorders. 75-89.

– is suppressed. During the acute phase response, the concentration of positive acute phase reactive proteins is increased in plasma while that of albumin is reduced. The presence of severe protein malnutrition may prevent the increase in synthesis of acute phase proteins even following an appropriate stimulus.[23,24]

Prealbumin (transthyretin, also called thyroid binding globulin) and transferrin are also reduced in response to protein malnutrition and have, like albumin, also been used in nutritional evaluation. Since prealbumin levels, change more rapidly than do albumin levels it has been proposed by some that measurement of this protein replace that of albumin for nutritional surveillance.[25] However, the plasma concentration of none of these proteins is simply a reflection of nutritional status; since these, like albumin, are negative acute phase proteins and subject to the same limitations. Hepatic transferrin gene expression is also subject to iron stores[26] and to oncotic pressure[27] adding a further level of complexity to interpreting plasma levels of this protein.

Albumin Catabolism

Albumin is catabolized through a first order process at sites distributed throughout the vascular endothelium or in a compartment in rapid equilibrium with the plasma compartment.[2,3,28] When plasma albumin concentration is decreased, the **absolute** rate of albumin catabolism would be expected to decrease simply because the concentration of albumin having access to the catabolic sites is decreased. The **fractional** rate of catabolism of a plasma protein is the fraction of the vascular pool catabolized per unit time. In the situation of a protein that is catabolized by a first order process, a change in the fractional catabolic rate is a consequence of a change in the catabolic rate constant and suggests regulation of plasma protein concentration by regulation of protein catabolic rate. In most conditions in which albumin concentration is decreased, malnutrition for example,[10] the fractional rate of albumin catabolism is also reduced. When albumin concentration is increased, the fractional catabolic rate increases, suggesting that regulation of albumin concentration in plasma takes place in part by regulation of albumin fractional catabolic rate. This form of catabolic control dampens the effect of either increases or decreases in the rate of albumin synthesis and protects the albumin pool when the rate of albumin synthesis is decreased.

Hypoalbuminemia in Renal Failure

Hypoalbuminemia is the strongest independent risk factor for death in hemodialysis patients [29,30] or being treated with CAPD[31,32] even when hypoalbuminemia occurs prior to initiation of dialysis.[33]

A change in the concentration of any protein in plasma is a result of a change in its rate of synthesis, in its rate of catabolism, the development of or change in rate of external losses, or a change in the distribution volume of the protein. As will be discussed below, albumin levels are reduced in part by a decrease in the rate of albumin synthesis in dialysis patients and in part because of external losses, either through the hemodialyzer as a consequence of reuse,[34] or through losses across the peritoneal membrane in PD patients. Decreased synthesis may be a consequence of reduced protein intake, the inflammatory response, or a combination of these processes. Any of the processes that tend to reduce albumin levels potentially can produce both morbidity and mortality.

Approximately 50% of plasma protein mass is albumin. Because of its low molecular weight, albumin contributes greatly to supporting plasma colloid osmotic pressure - oncotic pressure (π) and acts as a high capacity binding protein for free fatty acids and divalent cations.[35] Albumin also binds other biologically relevant lipophilic molecules, such as steroid hormones and bilirubin.[8] Despite all of the important functions that albumin serves, hereditary analbuminemia is compatible with life. Rats with hereditary analbuminemia reproduce normally and have normal renal function and blood pressure.[36,37]

Hypoalbuminemia may affect blood viscosity[38] or endothelial cell function as a consequence of increased concentration of free lysophosphatidylcholine altering erythrocyte structure[11] or by inhibiting NO mediated vascular relaxation.[39,40] Since albumin serves as a reservoir for NO, hypoalbuminemia can directly lead to reduced arteriolar relaxation through this mechanism as well.[41] Although hypoalbuminemia may be potentially injurious by the above mechanisms, the observation that hereditary analbuminemia imparts little in the way of decreased viability supports a hypothesis it is the cause of reduced albumin concentration that is responsible for morbidity and mortality in patients with acquired hypoalbuminemia rather than hypoalbuminemia itself.

It has been proposed that the primary cause of hypoalbuminemia is malnutrition,[42-44] which itself is proposed to be a consequence of inadequate dialysis.[45] Hypoalbuminemia from protein malnutrition alone in the absence of renal failure is, however, uncommon in adults. Oral nutritional supplementation has not been strikingly effective in normalizing albumin levels in hypoalbuminemic dialysis patients, although inter dialytic parenteral nutrition (IDPN) has been somewhat

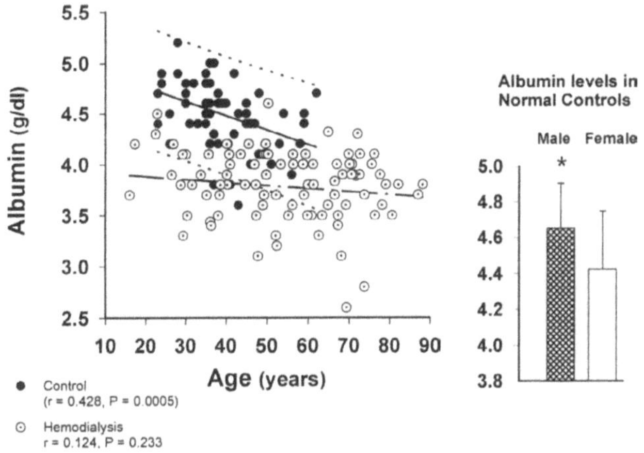

Figure 2. Left panel: Relationship between serum albumin concentration and age in a normal population (solid symbols solid line) and dialysis patients (open symbols broken line) and the 95% confidence limits of these measurements.
Right Panel: Average serum albumin concentration in normal men (cross hatch bar) and women (open bar). All measurements were made using bromcresol green.

more effective in some studies.[46] In contrast, Kwashiorkor responds quite easily when adequate protein is provided.

Recently evidence has accumulated in our laboratory[20,47,48] and elsewhere[28,49-51] suggesting that inflammation, either alone or in combination with malnutrition, plays a significant, and perhaps a controlling, role in causing hypoalbuminemia in hemodialysis patients. Inflammation would be expected either to block the effect of nutritional supplementation on serum albumin concentration or to render dietary protein supplementation less effective. **Figure 1** represents the combined effect of inflammation, measured as the level of C-reactive protein (CRP) in serum and nPCR separately on serum albumin concentration. When analyzed independently, increasing nPCR is associated with an increasing serum albumin concentration over values below 1-1.5g/kg/day. The serum albumin concentration associated with a specific value of nPCR declines with increasing values of CRP; however, one would predict that serum albumin concentration could be increased to nearly normal even in very inflamed patients provided protein intake was sufficient. It is also evident that virtually none of the patients studied in this series consumed that quantity of protein. Whether providing this amount of protein indeed has a salutary effect on serum albumin concentration, however, needs experimental verification. Furthermore, it is also not known whether focusing attention on increasing albumin concentration rather than relieving inflammation will have the desired effect on reducing mortality. CRP levels better predict mortality than by albumin concentration suggesting that hypoalbuminemia may in large part simply serve as a surrogate marker for inflammation.

Albumin Metabolism in End-Stage Renal Disease

Albumin levels are normally greater in men than women (**Figure 2**, right panel) and decrease with advancing age (left panel). While the majority of patients on dialysis have albumin values that fall within the normal range (**Figure 2**), many have albumin levels that fall below normal; and both the sex based and age based variance that normally occurs is effaced.[21] When patients with otherwise normal renal function loose albumin into their urine, they respond by increasing the rate of albumin synthesis;[52] although frequently this response is inadequate to normalize serum albumin concentration. Similarly, patients on PD also increase albumin synthetic rate in response to external losses;[53] and albumin pools are, in fact, preserved to a much greater extent than in nephrotic patients having the same albumin losses. The level of renal function also does not impair the ability of proteinuric rats from also increasing albumin synthesis rate[54] or increasing hepatic albumin mRNA in response to external losses.[55] Thus renal failure per-se does not produce a gross defect in the capacity of patients or animals from having a normal rate of albumin synthesis or from responding to external losses of albumin with an appropriate increase in the rate of albumin synthesis.[52] Hypoalbuminemia, therefore, must be caused by a process other than renal failure.

We found that the proximate cause of hypoalbuminemia ($\leq$ 3.5 g/dl) in hemodialysis patients was a reduced rate of albumin synthesis compared to hemodialysis patients having a normal serum albumin concentration ($\geq$ 4.0 g/dl).[19] Albumin fractional catabolic rate was reduced in the hypoalbuminemic group just as in hypoalbuminemic CAPD patients.[56] Distribution of albumin between the vascular and extravascular pool were the same in hemodialysis,[20] peritoneal dialysis patients[52] and in normal subjects regard-less of serum albumin concentration. Neither plasma volume expansion nor redistribution of albumin out of the plasma compartment played any role at all in contributing to hypoalbuminemia in dialysis patients. We, therefore, must turn our attention to potential processes causing a decrease in the rate of albumin synthesis to establish a mechanism for hypoalbuminemia in this population.

Malnutrition causes decreased albumin synthesis[8-12] and is a potential cause of reduced albumin synthesis, decreased albumin levels, and increased morbidity and mortality in any chronically ill population, including those with ESRD. Malnutrition has been clearly documented in this patient population;[42-44] and it has been generally assumed that hypoalbuminemia in this population is purely nutritionally based, primarily as a consequence of reduced albumin synthesis.

It is proposed that dietary protein intake and calorie intake should be between 1 and 1.2 g/kg and 35 kCal/kg/day respectively in patients on hemodialysis,[57,58] a value greater than the 1 g/kg protein intake recommended for the rest of the population, and generally more protein than most hemodialysis patients consume. Since insufficient dialysis can lead to anorexia,[59] it has been postulated that inadequate dialysis leads to poor nutritional intake followed by the development of hypoalbuminemia. Albumin levels may be increased following increased dialysis dose.[60] It is suggested that optimal dialysis include the use of bio-compatible membranes to deliver Kt/V > 1.4 (urea reduction ratio > 65%).[61]

Were protein malnutrition the only cause of hypoalbuminemia in the dialysis patient population, one would expect to find that nutritional supplementation would be effective in restoring albumin pools as it is in patients with hypoalbuminemia caused by protein malnutrition.[42,44] However, oral nutritional supplementation does not reverse hypoalbuminemia in this patient population.[62-64] Intradialytic parenteral nutrition (IDPN) is also either ineffectual[65,66] or only slowly effective[67] in repair of hypoalbuminemia of hemodialysis patients. The lack of prompt success of nutritional intervention, and especially of enteral nutritional intervention in correcting hypoalbuminemia suggests that non-nutritional factors may contribute to or be responsible for reduced albumin concentration in a fraction of hypoalbuminemic dialysis.

We measured the rate of albumin synthesis in a small group of hypoalbuminemic hemodialysis patients and could find no difference in nutritional factors.[20] We did, however, find that the levels of acute phase proteins were increased, suggesting that inflammation and not malnutrition was the primary cause of reduced albumin synthesis in this small group of patients. Further supporting a hypothesis that the inflammatory response plays a role in establishing albumin levels in hemodialysis patients, presumably by suppressing albumin synthetic rate, Bergström reported in preliminary studies that plasma CRP concentration was the most powerful predictor of serum albumin and was a better predictor of death in 1 year than was albumin concentration.[50] When albumin levels were statistically corrected for CRP, albumin lost its value in predicting death. We found that both CRP and another acute phase protein, serum amyloid A (SAA), predicted albumin concentration in a group of 79 hemodialysis patients by using multiple regression analysis.[47]

Lymphokines, tumor necrosis factor α (TNFα) and interleukin-1 (IL-1),[68] as well as a group of acute phase reactive proteins[51,69] (α^1 acid glycoprotein, ceruloplasmin and C4 complement component), have been found to be increased in hemodialysis patients compared to other patients with chronic renal failure. Cytokine levels were recently reported to also correlate with albumin levels in hemodialysis patients as well as with weight loss,[51] and cytokine levels, like albumin, predicted survival.[49]

External Albumin Losses During Dialysis

Kaplan reported that reuse of specific types of dialyzers (Fresenius 80 A) with bleach causes increased protein losses during dialysis and contributes to hypoalbuminemia.[34] We also found that albumin losses increased with reuse using these dialyzers and this technique to as much as 20 grams in a single dialysis treatment. However, the mechanism of hypoalbuminemia – reduced synthesis – suggests that the relationship between albumin losses and hypoalbuminemia in hemodialysis patients is more complex than simply albumin loss alone in hemodialysis patients. Loss of albumin across the peritoneal dialysis membrane has a statistically significant effect on serum albumin levels in patients maintained on this modality[53,70,71] (**Figure 3**). We found that the response among individual CAPD patients to this external loss was an increase in the rate of albumin synthesis,[53] similar to what occurs in nephrotic patients in response to urinary loss.[52,56,72,73] Unlike the case of patients on hemodialysis however, the transperitoneal losses of albumin are a consequence of a biological event within the dialysis patient that could, at least in part, be a consequence of peritoneal inflammation and not be a separate variable. We found that while both transperitoneal albumin loss and the levels of the acute

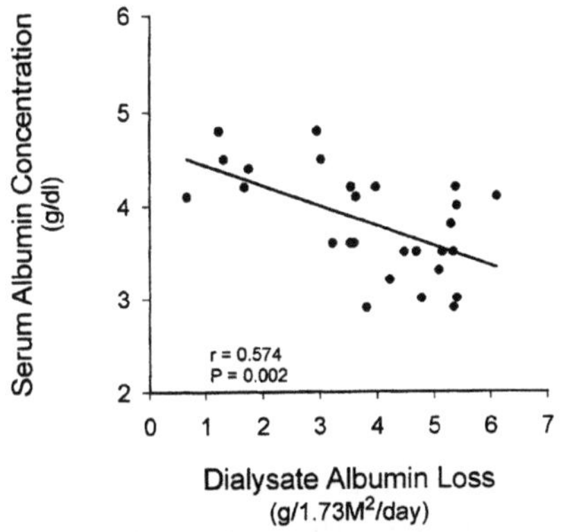

Figure 3. Relationship between serum albumin concentration and 24 hour transperitoneal albumin loss in g/day in 27 peritoneal dialysis patients. Serum albumin concentration was measured by bromcresol green. Peritoneal albumin was measured by rate nephelometry.

phase protein CRP each strongly controlled serum albumin levels in PD patients, that the two variables were statistically independent.[70] Furthermore there was also no relationship between the serum levels of either CRP or SAA and transperitoneal albumin losses, whether expressed either as grams/day or as the peritoneal clearance of albumin (to account for the lower serum albumin levels in patients with high loss rate). These findings are consistent with the observation that albumin synthesis increases in CAPD patients in response to transperitoneal albumin loss,[52] a process that should be suppressed if inflammation were responsible for the peritoneal losses of albumin. This is consistent with observations by Wang et. al. that patients with high tranperitoneal transport rates (high transporters) are not necessarily inflamed.[74]

Han[71] also found that CAPD patients with albumin concentrations $\leq$ 3.5 g/dl had higher dialysate albumin losses and higher CRP levels (17.5 versus 2.5 µg/ml) than those with albumin > 3.5 g/dl. Weekly Kt/V and PCRn did not differ between the two groups, suggesting that differences in dialysis adequacy and in protein catabolic rate were of less importance than albumin losses and a measure of inflammation in predicting albumin levels in CAPD patients and that the two principal variables are external losses and the presence of an inflammatory response. By step-wise regression, they found that multiple risk factors independently correlated with albumin concentration, including C-reactive protein, dialysate albumin as well as nutritional parameters (Lean body mass, BUN, PCRn). These data are quite similar to our own cross sectional study on albumin levels in hemodialysis patients,[20] although the peritoneal losses of albumin were much greater than the transdilayzer albumin losses that we have found during hemodialysis. Thus a body of data are accumulating suggesting that the acute phase response plays an important role in causing hypoalbuminemia in dialysis patients. This would help to explain the relative resistance of these patients to nutritional intervention. The cause of the inflammatory response, however, has not been identified. There is evidence, however, that dialysis with non biocompatible membranes may be one cause of cytokine activation.

Potential Source of Inflammation

Bio-incompatible membranes, such as cuprophane, activate white cells,[75] compliment,[76] and can even exert effects on residual renal function.[77] Activation of cytokines has also been found to occur following dialysis with cuprophane[78] in contrast to biocompatible membranes.[79,80] Reuse technique and numbers of reuse also may contribute to the interaction of blood with dialyzer [20,34] leading to changes in protein loss and possible changes in the acute phase response.

Honkanen also found a very rapid and similar increase in IL-Iβ and serum amyloid A (SAA) during 240 minutes of dialysis with cuprophane, cellulose acetate and polymethylmethachrylate,[81] the latter two being biocompatible membranes. Plasma IL-6[77] and IL-1ß[80] levels may increase during dialysis; and dialysis can also prime blood lymphocytes to release IL-1, IL-2,[82] and TNFα.[83] Indeed, cytokine production occurs even during *in vitro* dialysis of whole blood.[84] Dialysis may even alter blood mononuclear cells in such a manner to make them respond more vigorously to subsequent exposure to endotoxin.[85]

We were unable to find any increase in expression for genes encoding several cytokines in circulating mononuclear cells collected from a small number of hemodialysis patients with high CRP levels, and others also have not been able to identify circulating mononuclear cells as a potential source for stimulating infection in hemodialysis patients.[86]

Another potential way in which dialysis can change albumin levels is by loss of albumin across the dialysis membrane. Clearly this can happen across the peritoneal membrane and contributes to reduced albumin levels in CAPD patients.[53,70,71] Significant amounts of albumin (up to 20 grams per treatment) can be lost across the hemodialysis dialysis membrane after extensive reuse, especially when polysulfone dialyzers were reused with bleach,[20,34] suggesting that dialyzer membrane choice and both reuse number and technique may be in part responsible for deranged albumin homeostasis in hemodialysis patients.[87]

The rate of albumin catabolism decreases both in hypoalbuminemic hemodialysis patients as well as in CAPD patients. In addition, the fractional rate of albumin catabolism also decreases as albumin concentration falls in both hemodialysis and CAPD patients, representing preservation of the normal relationship between fractional catabolic rate and serum albumin concentration. Preservation of this normal relationship will serve to support albumin concentration when other factors (decreased synthesis and loss across the hemodialysis or peritoneal membrane) favor a decreasing level of albumin in blood.

Redistribution of the albumin pool from the vascular to the extravascular space plays no role in the development of hypoalbuminemia in either the hemodialysis or CAPD patient population. If anything, the fraction of albumin found in the extravascular pool decreases slightly in hypoalbuminemic CAPD patients.

Synthesis of acute phase reactive proteins, like that of albumin, is also impeded by protein malnutrition[23,24] even following an appropriate inflammatory stimulus. Thus the absence of an increase in the plasma levels of acute phase reactive proteins does not in and of itself prove that albumin synthesis is not in part inhibited as a component of the inflammatory response. Cytokine release, however, is unimpeded in protein calorie malnourished states.[88] Thus measurement of cytokine levels may provide greater insight into an inflammatory process than direct measurement of acute phase reactant proteins alone.

The cause of inflammation in dialysis patients is unclear. One possibility is that hemodialysis exposes blood and circulating mononuclear cells to membranes that have the potential to cause cytokine release. There is reasonably strong evidence that cuprophane dialyzers cause release of cytokines and promote increased blood levels of acute phase proteins during the course of hemodialysis[78] in contrast to biocompatible membranes.[79,80] Honkanen found a very rapid and similar increase in IL -Iβ and serum amyloid A (SAA) during 240 minutes of dialysis with cuprophane, cellulose acetate and polymethylmethachrylate;[81] although demonstration of this response during dialysis with biocompatible membranes has not been universally replicated, including in our own laboratory.[20] Plasma IL-6 and IL-1ß[81] levels may increase during dialysis; and dialysis can also prime blood lymphocytes to release IL-1, IL-2 and TNFα.[89] Indeed, cytokine production has even been reported during *in vitro* dialysis of whole blood.[82,84] Dialysis may also alter blood mononuclear cells in such a manner to make them respond more vigorously to subsequent exposure to endotoxin.[85] Release of these cytokines result in a prompt increase in the plasma levels of at least some acute phase proteins (CRP,[83] SAA,[81]). Bio-incompatible membranes, such as cuprophane, activate white cells,[75] complement,[76] and can even exert effects on residual renal function.[77] Reuse technique and numbers of reuse also may contribute to the interaction of blood with dialyzer[20,34] leading to changes in protein loss, increased amino acid loss, and possible changes in the acute phase response.

Kaizu[51] reported that pre-dialysis IL-6 levels actually predicted not only albumin levels but also nutritional status measured anthropometrically and serum creatinine. The latter is a surrogate for muscle mass. These findings suggest that inflammation may contribute to malnutrition. This association would not be surprising, since cytokines suppress appetite[90] and also make more severe the loss of tissue mass during periods of reduced nutritional intake.[91] These observations would thus provide a unified mechanism for the cause of hypoalbuminemia in this patient population. They found that dialysis membrane properties was one factor that predicted serum IL-6 level in their patients.

Exposure of blood to dialysis membranes, however, does not explain variability within the dialysis population. The majority of hemodialysis patients have serum CRP and SAA levels within the normal range. Furthermore, the acute phase response also plays an important role in establishing albumin levels in CAPD patients.[71,72] Indeed, in our own patient population we found that CRP and SAA levels were significantly greater in PD patients than in hemodialysis patients (unpublished observations). Exposure of the peri-toneal membrane to plasticizers found in dialysate may be one source of inflammation in this population. Another potential source is the transperitoneal access. Furthermore, the distribution of CRP and SAA values within the hemodialysis patient population is highly skewed, suggesting that patient specific processes, such as type of vascular access, unrecognized infections or variable responses to the dialyzers used, may play a role as well.

Although acute metabolic acidosis induced by feeding of mineral acid causes an immediate decrease in the rate of albumin synthesis in healthy adults,[92] reduced plasma bicarbonate levels do not correlate with hypoalbuminemia in hemodialysis patients;[1,29] and correction of metabolic acidosis with bicarbonate also does not alter albumin levels in dialysis patients.[93]

The Nephrotic Syndrome

The nephrotic syndrome is one clear example of easily identified alteration in normal albumin homeostasis caused by the development of losses not normally present; an alteration in glomerular permselectivity that then leads to urinary albumin losses.[94] Proteinuria, even of very limited extent, is a risk factor for cardiovascular disease[95] and in diabetic patients predicts progression of renal injury.[96] Whether this small level of proteinuria is simply a maker of generalized endothelial dysfunction or, instead, whether even small amounts of proteinuria cause injury to the kidney or atherogenesis by some as yet unidentified process is unknown.[97,98] It is far more certain that greater levels of urinary protein loss are directly injurious to the kidney,[99-101] resulting in interstitial injury,[102,103] likely activating TGF β[104] as well as other chemokines and cytokines,[105] and cause changes in lipoprotein composition that leads to decreased binding to endothelial bound lipoprotein lipase (LpL), which in turn plays an important role in increasing blood lipid levels.[106]

The nephrotic syndrome results from alterations in the permselective characteristics of the glomerular basement membrane (GBM) that allows increased passage of proteins of intermediate size into the urine and consists of the constellation of heavy proteinuria, hypoalbuminemia, hyperlipidemia, increased concentration of several high molecular weight proteins, and edema formation.[107,108] Not all components of this syndrome need be present. It is not known why all manifestations of the nephrotic syndrome are expressed in some patients and not in others.

The nephrotic syndrome results in marked alteration in plasma protein composition. Proteins of intermediate size are reduced in plasma.[109] This includes liver derived proteins such as albumin[110-112] and transferrin,[113-115] as well as proteins synthesized by other tissues, such as immunoglobulin.[116,117] The liver responds to the protein loss or to the decrease in serum albumin concentration or plasma colloid oncotic pressure (π) by increasing the rate of synthesis of a variety of proteins, mostly positive and negative acute phase proteins of specific types. Not all liver derived proteins are affected in this way. The response is independent of which proteins are lost into the urine. For example, hepatic synthesis of transferrin, albumin and fibrinogen are all increased.[109,118] The rates of synthesis of these proteins correlate positively with one another both in the rat[119-121] and human,[109,122,123] and regulation is at the level of transcription.[124] This occurs despite the fact that transferrin and albumin are lost in the urine and their serum concentrations are reduced, while fibrinogen is not lost into the urine and its concentration in plasma is greatly increased.[118,125,126] This alters plasma composition in such a way that the average molecular weight of proteins retained is increased, as is plasma viscosity and the propensity for thrombosis. Synthesis of the large protease inhibitor α2 macroglobulin is also increased in parallel with that of albumin, both in the rat[127] and in humans[122] with the nephrotic syndrome; however, in this case, regulation is post transcriptional.

This change in hepatic gene expression is not a direct result of proteinuria but instead a consequence either of hypoalbuminemia or, more likely, a response to reduced plasma π since essentially the same changes in hepatic gene expression occur in NAR. Both analbuminemia and the nephrotic syndrome are characterized by increased synthesis of fibrinogen, transferrin, α2 macroglobulin, a variety of apolipoproteins, including apo A-I and apo E. In both cases, plasma proteins shift to those of greater molecular weight; although transferrin levels are increased in analbuminemia in contrast to the nephrotic syndrome, since there is no urinary protein losses in hereditary analbuminemia.

Synthesis of many apolipoproteins is also increased and some, like Lp(a) synthesis, again parallels that of albumin;[128] while in the case of others, such as apo B 100 regulation appears to be completely independent of albumin synthesis. Nevertheless the end result is an increased concentration of a variety of highly atherogenic lipoproteins in part as a consequence of increased hepatic synthesis. This is further complicated by a loss of low molecular weight anticoagulant proteins in the urine, such as anti-thrombin III[129,130] and proteins C and S,[131,132] accompanied by an increase in the concentration of large proteins that bind these anticoagulant proteins. These processes lead to a large increase in atherogenic risk. Much of this risk is a consequence of urinary protein loss and the hepatic response by way of increased synthesis of a variety of proteins.

There is little evidence that other organs beside the liver respond by way of increasing protein synthesis in response to urinary protein loss. Although IgG production may be increased *in vivo* in patients with the nephrotic syndrome,[133] the rate of IgG production is depressed[134,135] in lymphocytes isolated from patients with the nephrotic syndrome of various etiologies when they are exposed to mitogens in culture. Urinary IgG losses may cause profound decreases in the immunoglobulin pool, yet synthesis is not increased in experimental models of the nephrotic syndrome.[136]

Hypoalbuminemia and reduced plasma π impart effects that are separate from, but add to the effects of, proteinuria. Hyperlipidemia is a consequence both of increased lipoprotein synthesis and decreased catabolism. Of these, decreased catabolism plays a predominant role, especially with regard to the triglyceride rich lipoproteins, Very Low Density Lipoprotein (VLDL) and chylomicrons (CMs).[106,137] Two processes are necessary for the initial metabolism of these lipoproteins. The first is the binding of the endothelial bound LpL, and the second is lipolysis by LpL. There are at least two defects present in the nephrotic syndrome that impairs this process. One is a defect in binding of these lipoproteins to endothelial bound LpL,[106] and the second is a reduction of endothelial bound LpL on the vascular endothelium. The first of these processes is a direct consequence of proteinuria, not a consequence of reduced serum albumin concentration per se.[106] This can be demonstrated by the observation that VLDL isolated from rats with hereditary analbuminemia, the Nagase Analbuminemic Rat (NAR) actually bind more avidly to LpL than does VLDL isolated from normal animals; while VLDL isolated from nephrotic animals binds considerably more poorly (**Figure 4**).[106] The second defect, the lack of endothelial bound LpL, is a direct consequence of hypoalbuminemia alone. LpL mRNA levels are reduced by about 15% in rats with the nephrotic syndrome; however, secretion and, by inference, synthesis of LpL by perfused hearts isolated from nephrotic rats is essentially normal[106] suggesting that the defect in endothelial bound LpL is a consequence of defective LpL transport from its site of synthesis in mesenchymal tissue (adipose or muscle cells) or defective binding on the vascular endothelium.

LpL is reduced in NAR to an even greater extent than in nephrotic animals[106,138] suggesting that endothelial LpL depletion is a result of reduced albumin concentration or the changed plasma protein composition that is a response to hypoalbuminemia but is not a direct consequence of urinary protein loss. Hyperlipidemia is far more severe in the nephrotic syndrome than in analbuminemia; because, in the former, there is also a defect in the function of lipoproteins; while if anything, analbuminemia, in the absence of proteinuria, is associated with lipoproteins that bind to and are lipolized more readily by LpL than in control.[106] Indeed, catabolism of both VLDL and chylomicrons is essentially normal in analbuminemic rats prior to the onset of proteinuria, despite the absence of albumin from their serum.[138]

Proteinuria and reduced plasma π work together to cause the edema that plays such an important role in the nephrotic syndrome.

Edema Formation: Defenses Against Reduced Plasma π

Capillary hydrostatic pressure serves to force fluid from the vascular compartment into the interstitial space. This hydrostatic force is partially balanced by the difference between plasma π and that exerted by interstitial proteins. Interstitial protein concentration is between 25% and 50% that of plasma protein,[139] and the difference between π exerted by plasma and interstitial proteins ($\Delta\overline{\pi}$) serves to retain salt and water in the vascular space. Fluid not reabsorbed by the time blood has

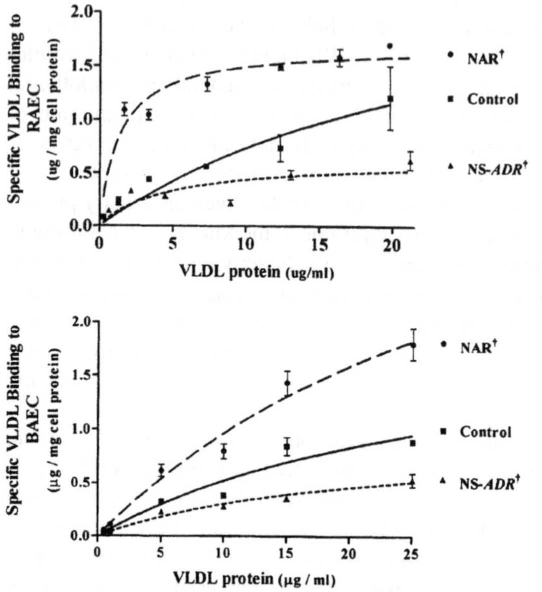

Figure 4. Binding of Very Low Density Lipoprotein (VLDL) from control, Nagase Analbuminemic Rats (NAR) and Nephrotic rats (induced by adriamycin - NS ADR) to aortic endothelial cells. Specific binding of VLDL to aortic endothelial cells was measured after 5 hours measured using ^{125}I labeled VLDL. The upper panel represents binding to rat aortic endothelial cells (*RAEC*) and the lower panel represents binding to bovine aortic endothelial cells (*BAEC*). Error bars represent SEM. † $P < 0.05$ v VLDL from control rats.

reached the venous end of the capillary bed is returned to the vascular space via the lymphatics.

In steady state:

Lymph flow = Kf [(Capillary hydrostatic pressure - tissue hydrostatic pressure) - (plasma π - tissue π)] = $Kf(\Delta\overline{P} - \Delta\overline{\pi})$ (Equation 1).

Where Kf is capillary hydraulic conductivity.[140,141]

When the fall in $\Delta\overline{\pi}$ becomes great enough, the net amount of fluid filtered by the capillaries will exceed maximal lymph flow; and edema will inevitably occur. This increased net transport of fluid into the interstitial space should lead to plasma volume contraction. However, Meltzer et. al.[142] subsequently identified a group of patients with the nephrotic syndrome who had a normal or an expanded plasma volume and reduced plasma renin activity despite a profound reduction in π. These patients represented a subset that had neph-ritic disease as opposed to patients with minimal change nephrotic syndrome. Some patients with minimal change nephrotic syndrome have also been found to have an increase plasma and blood volume.[143,144]

Edema formation in the nephrotic syndrome involves two parallel processes. Reduced plasma π leads to augmented net flux of fluid across the systemic capillary bed, but these alterations may be entirely or largely offset by increased lymphatic return from the periphery and reduction in interstitial π so that $\Delta\pi$ remains unchanged. Edema formation is not generally obligated to occur until total protein concentration is decreased to around 4 g/dl. The second process results from a reduced ability of the nephrotic kidney to excrete a sodium load, either in response to plasma volume expansion[145-147] or in response to atrial natriuretic factor (ANF).[148-150] The inability of the nephrotic kidney to excrete a salt load is intrinsic to the nephrotic kidney itself and is unrelated to systemic volume needs. Studies utilizing unilateral models of proteinuria most clearly demonstrate that impedance to sodium excretion is intrinsic to the nephrotic kidney and not reflective of plasma volume regulation. In one such study, Perico et. al.[56] demonstrated an inability of a proteinuric kidney to excrete fluid or sodium in response to infused ANF even though ANF increased GFR in both the proteinuric kidney and the normal contralateral kidney equally. Clearly both the normal contralateral kidney and the proteinuric kidney were exposed to the same π and the same levels of circulating hormones responsible for plasma volume regulation. The process is a consequence of alteration in a phosphodiesterase that metabolizes cyclic GNP, the effector of ANF.[151]

The proteinuric kidney avidly reabsorbs filtered salt in the distal nephron[152] even in the presence of plasma volume expansion. As a consequence of these combined effects, the systemic capillary bed is faced with increased hydrostatic pressure at the very time that defense mechanisms normally employed to counteract edema formation, increased lymphatic flow and decreased interstitial protein concentration have already been maximized. Edema results from the combined effect of primary renal salt and water retention coupled with reduced defenses against edema formation resulting from the urinary losses of proteins of intermediate weight with the resulting decrease in both and interstitial π. These processes deprive the lymphatic system of the capacity to respond to increased hydrostatic pressure.

Treatment of the Nephrotic Syndrome

Clearly if the nephrotic syndrome is a consequence of a specific treatable disease, treatment should focus on the underlying disease. Minimal change nephrotic syndrome and many cases of focal segmental glomerular sclerosis (FSGS) respond to glucocorticoids.[153] Furthermore, the rate of progression to renal failure in patients with FSGS is slowed in patients who respond to such therapy. Cyclosporin may also be effective in reducing proteinuria caused by several different primary disorders[154,155] including FSGS,[156,157] although the ultimate salutary effect on renal outcome is less well established.

Fortunately urinary protein excretion in the nephrotic syndrome is under the control of a variety of vaso active hormones. Perhaps the easiest of these to manipulate is angiotensin II (Ang II). Both angiotensin II converting enzyme inhibitors (ACEi's)[158] as well as blockers of the type I Ang II receptor (ARBs) are effective in reducing urinary protein and albumin excretion.[159] The proteinuric effect of Ang II may be mediated by interaction with nephrin gene expression.[160] Nephrin is a protein that is important in maintaining the selective nature of the slit diaphragm of the podocyte.[161] Defect in the nephrin gene is responsible for the massive proteinuria that characterizes congenital nephrotic syndrome of the Finnish type.[162] Rats with passive Heymann nephritis exhibit loss of nephrin protein and mRNA in renal podocytes. This reduction in nephrin gene expression is prevented by inhibition of either Ang II generation with and ACEi or by blockade of Ang II receptors.[160] Thus the non-specific but important effect of both ACEi and Ang II receptor blockers may be mediated by their protective effect on nephrin. In patients with very heavy proteinuria, this reduction in urinary protein excretion can be shown to increase renal survival. Reduction in urinary protein excretion also serves to decrease blood lipid levels and to increase serum albumin concentration. Use of these agents forestalls the onset of proteinuria in patients with diabetes and should be considered as a first line therapy for treating proteinuric patients, even in the absence of hypertension, when no specific therapy is available.

Since plasma volume generally tends to be expanded in most patients with the nephrotic syndrome[142] despite reduced plasma π, diuresis is generally of use, in conjunction with dietary sodium restriction, in treating edema. It has also been recognized that dietary protein augmentation increases urinary albumin excretion [52,72] and should play no role in trying to correct the hypoalbuminemia of the nephrotic syndrome. A diet containing between 0.8 g/kg and 1 g of protein per kg body weight should be prescribed. There is also some evidence that soy based proteins may be of greater benefit than animal based proteins,[163] although it is not clear whether this effect is due to the protein composition of soy protein or instead due to other non-protein nutrients such as fat composition.

Since protein is necessary for albumin synthesis and dietary protein augmentation, indeed, leads to increased albumin synthesis, it is unwise to restrict protein much below the values suggested above; and, indeed if protein intake is too restricted this also can contribute to hypoalbuminemia.

It must be realized that while a small decrease in serum albumin into the mid 3 g/dl range may not be of overwhelming clinical importance, patients with massive urinary protein losses who have serum albumin concentrations that are very low are indeed in imminent danger. They have no effective way of maintaining their plasma volume and are subject to acute renal failure. They have massive anasarca and are at risk of infection, and their altered plasma composition renders them susceptive to atheroembolic events, including renal vein thrombosis,[164] sagital sinus thrombosis[165,166] and pulmonary embolism.[167] None of these processes are amenable to albumin infusions if for no other reason than the albumin is promptly lost into the urine. I also suspect that increasing albumin concentration without also decreasing the defect in glomerular perselectivey does little to alter the other adverse effects of nephrotic syndrome and is probably of only limited utility. The primary effort must be directed at reducing proteinuria.

Some investigators have even recommended "medical nephrectomy" using the combination of ACEi's and cyclooxygenase inhibitors to reduce proteinuria, poten-tially sacrificing GFR.

As discussed above, hepatic protein synthesis increases considerably in response to urinary protein loss. Much of this protein is however lost into the urine. Total body protein synthesis however does not increase, and protein catabolism is likewise unchanged.[168] This suggests that protein synthesis must be reduced in extrahepatic compartments. The most likely of these is muscle. Indeed we reported that muscle protein synthesis was reduced in rats with the nephrotic syndrome[169] and this may contribute to the generalized loss of muscle mass seen in severely nephrotic patients. Again, the treatment of this must be directed at reducing urinary protein losses.

Treatment of hypoalbuminemia must always be focused on first identifying the cause of reduced albumin concentration and then directing therapy at that cause. Inflammation or sources of loss of albumin from the body must be identified and if possible reversed. Infection must be treated. At this time it is unknown whether anti inflammatory agents will be of utility in treating patients with no obvious infectious process causing inflammation identified by increased levels of acute phase proteins. Urinary losses of albumin may respond to treatment of the responsible renal disease or respond to manipulations of the angiotensin II system. Tranperitoneal losses may be of such magnitude that patients may require a change in dialysis modality. Bleach should be avoided in reuse techniques depending on the type of dialyzer used.

If protein catabolic rate is less than 1g/kg/day dietary protein supplementation may be useful in restoring albumin pools. Administration of intravenous albumin supplements is expensive, does not correct the underlying problem, has not been shown to have any positive effect on clinical outcome and is to be discouraged. Treat the cause of hypoalbuminemia, not the albumin level.

Acknowledgments

This work was supported in part by the research service of the United States Department of Veterans Affairs, in part by a grant from the National Institutes of Health RO1 DK 50777, and in part by a grant from Dialysis Clinics Incorporated.

References

1. Kaysen GA. Biological basis of hypoalbuminemia in ESRD. J Am Soc Nephrol;9:2368-76, 1998
2. Waldmann, T.A. Albumin Catabolism in: *Albumin Structure, Function and Uses*, edited by Rosemoer, M., Oratz, M., Rothschild, A., pp 255-73, New York, Permagon Press, 1977.
3. Yedgar, S., Carew, T.E., Pittman, R.C., Beltz, W.F. Tissue sites of catabolism of albumin in rabbits. *Am. J. Physiol.* 244 (*Endocrinol. Metab.* 7): E101-E107, 1983.
4. Baynes, J.W., Thorpe, S.R. Identification of sites of albumin catabolism in the rat. *Arch. Biochem Biophys.* 206: 372-9, 1981.
5. Sellers, A.L., Katz, J., Bonorris, G., Okyyama, S Determination of extravascular albumin in the rat. *J. Lab. Clin. Med.* 68: 177-85, 1966.
6. Reeve, E.B., Chen, A.Y. Regulation of interstitial albumin in:Plasma Protein Metabolism, Regulation of synthesis, distribution, and degradation edited by Rothschild, M.A., and Waldmann, T. Academic Press, N.Y., 1970 pp 89-109.
7. Ballmer PE; Ochsenbein AF; Schutz-Hofmann S. Transcapillary escape rate of albumin positively correlates with plasma albumin concentration in acute but not in chronic inflammatory disease. Metabolism: Clinical and Experimental, 43: 697-705, 1994.
8. James. W.P., Hay, A.M. Albumin metabolism: effect of the nutritional state and the dietary protein intake. *J. Clin. Invest.* 47: 1958-72, 1968.
9. Morgan, E.H., Peters, T. Jr. The biosynthesis of rat serum albumin *J. Biol. Chem.* 246: 3500-7, 1971.
10. Kirsch R, Frith L, Black E, Hoffenberg R. Regulation of albumin synthesis and catabolism by alteration of dietary protein *Nature* 217: 578-9, 1968.
11. Hoffenberg, R., Black, E. Brock, J.F. Albumin and gammaglobulin tracer studies in protein depletion states. *J. Clin. Invest.* 45: 143-52 1966.

12. Yap, S.H., Strair, R.K., Shafritz, D.A. Effect of a short term fast on the distribution of cytoplasmic albumin messenger ribonucleic acid in rat liver. *J. Biol. Chem.* 253: 4944-50, 1978.
13. Moshage HJ, Janssen JAM, Franssen JH, Hafkenscheid JCM, Yap SH. Study of the molecular mechanisms of decreased liver synthesis of albumin in inflammation. *J Clin Invest* 79: 1635-41, 1987.
14. Koj A, Gauldie J, Sweeney GD, Regoeczi E, Sauder DN. A simple bioassay for monocyte-derived hepatocyte stimulating factor: Increased synthesis of α2-macroglobulin and reduced synthesis of albumin by cultured rat hepatocytes. *J Immun Meth* 76: 317-27, 1985.
15. Bauer J, Weber W, Tran-Thi T Northoff, G Decker, K Gerok, W Heinrich, PC. Murine interleukin 1 stimulates α_2-macroglobulin synthesis in rat hepatocyte primary cultures. *FEBS letters* 190: 271-4, 1985.
16. Jamieson, JC, Kaplan, HA, Woloski. BMNJ, Hellman, M, Ham, K Glycoprotein biosynthesis during the acute-phase response to inflammation. *Can J Biochem Cell Biol* 61: 1041-8, 1983.
17. Koj, A, Gauldie, J, Regoecsi, E, Sauder, DN, Sweeney, GD. The acute-phase response of cultured rat hepatocytes. *Biochem J* 224: 505-14, 1984.
18. Perlmutter DH, Dinarello CA, Punsal PI, Colten HR. Cachectin/tumor necrosis factor regulates hepatic acute-phase gene expression. *J Clin Invest* 78: 1349-55, 1986.
19. Shiels BR, Northemann W, Gehring MR, Fey GH. Modified nuclear processing of α_1 acid glycoprotein RNA during inflammation. *J Biol Chem* 262: 12826-31, 1987
20. Kaysen GA; Rathore V; Shearer GC; Depner TA. Mechanisms of hypoalbuminemia in hemodialysis patients. *Kidney Int*, 48:510-6, 1995.
21. Rosales FJ; Ritter SJ; Zolfaghari R; Smith JE; Ross AC. Effects of acute inflammation on plasma retinol, retinol-binding protein, and its mRNA in the liver and kidneys of vitamin A-sufficient rats. Journal of Lipid Research, , 37:962-71, 1996.
22. Guo-Fen T, De Jong F, Apostolopoulos J, Nagashima M, Fidge N, Schreiber G, Howlett G. Effect of acute inflammation on rat apolipprotein mRNA levels. *Inflammation* 11:241-51, 1987.
23. Jennings G, Elia M. The acute-phase response to turpentine-induced abscesses in malnourished rats at different environmental temperatures. *Metabolism: Clinical and Experimental*, 41:141-7, 1992.
24. Saito T, Kuwahara A, Shimoda K, Kinoshita T, Sato K, Miyahara M, Kobayashi M. Factors influencing the acute phase protein levels in patients with esophageal cancer. *Japanese Journal of Surgery*, 21:402-11, 1991.
25. Sreedhara, R; Avram, MM; Blanco, M; Batish, R; Avram, MM; Mittman, N. Prealbumin is the best nutritional predictor of survival in hemodialysis and peritoneal dialysis. American Journal of Kidney Diseases, 28:937-42. 1996
26. Idzerda, R.L., H. Huevers, C.A. Finch, and G.S. McKnight. Rat transferrin gene expression: Tissue-specific regulation by iron deficiency. Proc. Natl. Acad. Sci. USA. 83:3723-7, 1986.
27. Kaysen, GA; Sun, X; Jones, H Jr; Martin, VI; Joles, JA; Tsukamoto, H; Couser, WG; al-Bander, H. Non-iron mediated alteration in hepatic transferrin gene expression in the nephrotic rat. Kidney International, 47:1068-77. 1995
28. Docci D, Bilancioni R, Baldrati L, Capponcini C, Turci F, Feletti C. Elevated acute phase reactants in hemodialysis patients. *Clinical Nephrology*, 34:88-91 1990 .
29. Lowrie EG, Lew NL. Death risk in hemodialysis patients: the predictive value of commonly measured variables and an evaluation of death rate differences between facilities. *Am J Kid Dis*, 15:458-82 1990.
30. Lowrie EG, Lew NL, Huang WH. Race and diabetes as death risk predictors in hemodialysis patients. *Kidney Int. Supplement*, 38:S22-31, 1992.
31. Avram MM; Fein PA; Bonomini L; Mittman N; Loutoby R; Avram DK; Chattopadhyay J. Predictors of survival in continuous ambulatory peritoneal dialysis patients: a five-year prospective study. Peritoneal Dialysis International, 16 Suppl 1:S190-4, 1996.
32. Kang SW, Kwon KH, Noh HJ, Park HC, Lee IH, Choi KH, Lee HY, Han DS: Serum albumin as a predictor of morbidity and mortality in continuous ambulatory peritoneal dialysis patients: single center experiences over 700 patients. *J Am Soc Nephrol* 7:1450 (Abst), 1996
33. Avram MM, Goldwasser P, Erroa M, Fein PA. Predictors of survival in continuous ambulatory peritoneal dialysis patients: the importance of prealbumin and other nutritional and metabolic markers. *Am J Kid Dis*, 23:91-8, 1994.
34. Kaplan AA; Halley SE; Lapkin RA; Graeber CW. Dialysate protein losses with bleach processed polysulphone dialyzers. *Kidney Int* 47:573-8 1995.
35. Rothschild MA, Oratz M, Evans CD, Schreiber SS: Albumin Synthesis. In: Albumin Structure, Function and Uses, edited by Rosemoer M, Oratz M, Rothschild A., pp 227-55, New York, Permagon Press, 1977.
36. Fujihara CK; Limongi DM; De Oliveira HC; Zatz R. Absence of focal glomerulosclerosis in aging analbuminemic rats. *Am J Physiol*, 262:R947-54, 1992.
37. Fujihara CK; Limongi DM; Falzone R; Graudenz MS; Zatz R. Pathogenesis of glomerular sclerosis in subtotally nephrectomized analbuminemic rats. *Am J Physiol*, 261:F256-64, 1991.
38. Joles, JA; Willekes-Koolschijn, N; Koomans, HA. Hypoalbuminemia causes high blood viscosity by increasing red cell lysophosphatidylcholine *Kidney Int.* 52:761-70, 1997
39. Cowan CL; Steffen RP. Lysophosphatidylcholine inhibits relaxation of rabbit abdominal aorta mediated by endothelium-derived nitric oxide and endothelium-derived hyperpolarizing factor independent of protein kinase C activation. Arteriosclerosis, Thrombosis, and Vascular Biology, 12:2290-7,1995.
40. Eizawa H; Yui Y; Inoue R; Kosuga K; Hattori R; Aoyama T; Sasayama S. Lysophosphatidylcholine inhibits endothelium-dependent hyperpolarization and N omega-nitro-L-arginine/indomethacin-resistant endothelium-dependent relaxation in the porcine coronary artery. Circulation, 92:3520-6, 1995.
41. Minamiyama Y; Takemura S; Inoue M. Albumin is an important vascular tonus regulator as a reservoir of nitric oxide. Biochemical and Biophysical Research Communications, 225:112-115, 1996.
42. Blumenkrantz MJ, Kopple JD, Gutman RA, Chan YK, Barbour GL, Roberts C, Schen GH, Gandi VC, Tucker CT, Curtis FK, Coburn JW. Methods for assessing nutritional status of patients with renal failure. *Am J Clin Nutr* 33:1567-85, 1980.
43. Schoenfeld PY, Henry RR, Laird NM, Roxe DM. Assessment of nutritional status of the national cooperative dialysis study population. *Kidney Int*; 23 (Suppl 13):80-8, 1983.
44. Acchiardo SR, Moore LW, Latour AP. Malnutrition as the main factor in morbidity and mortality of hemodialysis patients. *Kidney Int.* 24:*Suppl.*16:S-199-S-203, 1983.
45. Owen, WF Jr; Lew, NL; Liu, Y; Lowrie, EG; Lazarus, JM. The urea reduction ratio and serum albumin concentration as predictors of mortality in patients undergoing hemodialysis New England Journal of Medicine, 329:1001-6, 1993.
46. Smolle KH; Kaufmann P; Holzer H; Druml W. Intradialytic parenteral nutrition in malnourished patients on chronic haemodialysis therapy. Nephrology, Dialysis, Transplantation, 10:1411-6, 1995
47. Kaysen, GA; Stevenson, FT; Depner, TA. Determinants of albumin concentration in hemodialysis patients. American Journal of Kidney Diseases, 29:658-68. 1997

48. Kaysen, GA; Yeun, J; Depner, T. Albumin synthesis, catabolism and distribution in dialysis patients. *Mineral and Electrolyte Metabolism*, 23:218-24, 1997.
49. Bologa RM, Levine DM, Parker TS, Serur D, Stenzel KH, Rubin A, Cheigh JS. High cytokine levels may mediate the high mortality of hemodialysis (HD) patients with low albumin and/or cholesterol (TC). . *J Am. Soc. Neph.* 6:573 (Abst) 1995.
50. Bergström J, Heimbürger O, Lindholm B, Qureshi AR. Elevated Serum CRP is a strong predictor of increased mortality and low serum albumin in hemodialysis (HD) patients. *J Am. Soc. Neph.* 6:573 (Abst) 1995.
51. Kaizu, Y; Kimura, M; Yoneyama, T; Miyaji, K; Hibi, I; Kumagai, H. Interleukin-6 may mediate malnutrition in chronic hemodialysis patients. American Journal of Kidney Diseases, 31:93-100. 1998
52. Kaysen GA, Gambertoglio. J, Jiminez I, Jones H, Hutchison FN Effect of dietary protein intake on albumin homeostasis in nephrotic patients. *Kidney Int* 29: 572-577 1986.
53. Kaysen GA, Schoenfeld PY. Albumin homeostasis in patients undergoing continuous ambulatory peritoneal dialysis. *Kidney Int.* 25:107-14, 1984.
54. Kaysen GA, Watson JB. Mechanism of hypoalbuminemia in the 7/8 nephrectomized rat with chronic renal failure. *Am J Physiol* 243:*Renal fluid Electrolyte Physiol.* 12):F372-8, 1982.
55. Zern MA, Yap SH, Strair RK, Kaysen GA, Shafritz DA. The effects of chronic renal failure on protein synthesis and albumin mRNA in rat liver. *J Clin Invest* 73:1167-1174, 1984.
56. Kaysen, GA. Albumin turnover in renal disease. Mineral and Electrolyte Metabolism, 24:55-63. 1998.
57. Kopple J, Shinaberger J, Coburn J, Sorensen M, Rubini M. Optimal dietary protein treatment during chronic hemodialysis. *ASAIO Trans* 15:302-8, 1989.
58. Bergström J. Why are dialysis patients malnourished? American Journal of Kidney Diseases,:26,229-41, 1995
59. Bergström J. Anorexia in dialysis patients. Seminars in Nephrology, 16:222-9,1996
60. Yang C-S; Chen S-W; Chiang C-H; Wang M; Peng S-J; Kan Y-T. Effects of increasing dialysis dose on serum albumin and mortality in hemodialysis patients. American Journal of Kidney Diseases, 27:380-86. 1996
61. Ikizler TA; Wingard RL; Hakim RM. Interventions to treat malnutrition in dialysis patients: the role of the dose of dialysis, intradialytic parenteral nutrition, and growth hormone. American Journal of Kidney Diseases, 26:256-65, 1995
62. Phillips ME, Havard J, Howard JP. Oral essential amino supplementation in patients in maintenance hemodialysis. *Clin Nephrol* 9:241-8 1978.
63. Hecking E, Kohler H, Zobel R Lamellel E-M, Mader H, Opferkuch W, Prellwitz W, Keim HF, Muller D. Treatment with essential amino acids in patients on chronic hemodialysis: A double blind crossover study. *Am J Clin Nutr* 31:1821-6 1987.
64. Compher C, Mullen J, Barker C. Nutritional support in renal failure. *Surg Clin North Am* 71:597-608, 1991.
65. Wolfson, M. Use of nutritional supplements in dialysis patients. *Semin Dial.* 1992;5:285-90.
66. Wolfson M; Foulks CJ. Intradialytic parenteral nutrition: a useful therapy? Nutrition in Clinical Practice, 11:5-11, 1996
67. Capelli JP, Kushner H, Camiscioli TC, Chen S-M, Tores MA. Effect of intradialytic parenteral nutrition on mortality rates in end-stage renal disease care. *Am J Kid Dis* 23:808-16 1994.
68. Herbelin A, Nguyen AT, Zingraff J, Urena P, Descamps-Latscha B. Influence of uremia and hemodialysis on circulating interleukin-1 and tumor necrosis factor alpha. *Kidney Int*, 37:116-25, 1990.
69. Trznadel K, Luciak M, Paradowski M, Kubasiewicz-Ujma B. Hemodialysis and the acute-phase response in chronic uremic patients. *International Journal of Artificial Organs*, 12:762-5 1989.
70. Yeun JY; Kaysen GA. Acute phase proteins & peritoneal dialysate albumin loss are the main determinants of serum albu-min in peritoneal dialysis patients. *Am J Kid Dis*, 30:923-7. 1997
71. Han DS, Lee SW, Kang SW, Choi KH, Lee HY, Cho EY, Lee JH: Factors affecting low values of serum albumin in CAPD patients. Advances in Peritoneal Dialysis 12:288-92, 1996
72. Kaysen, GA; Kirkpatrick, WG; Couser, WG.Albumin homeostasis in the nephrotic rat: nutritional considerations. Am J Physiol, 247:F192-202, 1984.
73. Ballmer, PE; Weber, BK; Roy-Chaudhury, P; McNurlan, MA; Watson, H; Power, DA; Garlick, PJ. Elevation of albumin synthesis rates in nephrotic patients measured with [1-13C]leucine. Kidney International, 41:13213-8,1992.
74. Wang T, Heimburger O, Cheng HH, Bergstrom J, Lindholm B. Does a high peritoneal transport rate reflect a state of chronic inflammation? Perit Dial Int 19:17-22, 1999.
75. Canivet E; Lavaud S; Wong T; Guenounou M; Willemin JC; Potron G; Chanard J. Cuprophane but not synthetic membrane induces increases in serum tumor necrosis factor-alpha levels during hemodialysis. *Am J Kidney Diseases* 23:41-6. 1994
76. Pertosa G; Tarantino EA; Gesualdo L; Montinaro V; Schena FP. C5b-9 generation and cytokine production in hemodialyzed patients. *Kidney Int.* 41:S221-5. 1993
77. Hakim RM; Wingard RL; Parker RA. Effect of the dialysis membrane in the treatment of patients with acute renal failure *New Eng J Med*, 17, 331:1338-42 1994.
78. Memoli B, Libetta C, Rampino T, De Simone W, Meccariello S, Stangherlin P, Dal Canton A, Andreucci VE. Interleukin-6 production of uraemic haemodialysed patients: effects of different membranes. *Nephrology, Dialysis, Transplantation*,6 Suppl 2:96-8 1991.
79. Zaoui P; Hakim RM. The effects of the dialysis membrane on cytokine release. *J Am Soc Neph*, 4:1711-8. 1994
80. Chollet-Martin S; Stamatakis G; Bailly S; Mery JP; Gougerot-Pocidalo MA. Induction of tumour necrosis factor-alpha during haemodialysis. Influence of the membrane type. *Clinical and Experimental Immunology*, 83(2):329-32, 1991
81. Honkanen E, Gronhagen-Riska C, Teppo AM, Maury CP, Meri S. Acute-phase proteins during hemodialysis: correlations with serum interleukin-1 beta levels and different dialysis membranes. *Nephron*, 57:283-7, 1991.
82. Donati D, Degiannis D, Combates N, Raskova J, Raska K Jr. Effects of hemodialysis on activation of lymphocytes: analysis by an in vitro dialysis model. *Journal of the American Society of Nephrology*, 2:1490-7, 1992.
83. Macdonald C; Rush DN; Bernstein KN; McKenna RM. Production of tumor necrosis factor alpha and hemodialysis. *Nephron*, 65:273-7, 1993.
84. Pereira BJ; Snodgrass B; Barber G; Perella C; Chopra S; King AJ. Cytokine production during in vitro hemodialysis with new and formaldehyde- or renalin-reprocessed cellulose dialy-zers. Journal of the American Society of Nephrology 6:1304-8. 1995
84a. Haubitz M, Schulze M, Koch KM. Increase of CRP serum values following haemodialysis. Nephrology, Dialysis, Transplantation, 5:500-3, 1990.
85. Pomianek MJ, Colton CK, Dinarello CA Miller LC Synthesis of tumor necrosis factor α and interleukin-1 receptor antagonist, but not interleukin-1 by human mononuclear cells in enhanced by exposure of whole blood to shear stress. *ASAIO Journal* 42:52-9, 1996.
86. Grooteman, MP; Nubé, MJ; Daha, MR; Van Limbeek, J; van Deuren, M; Schoorl, M; Bet, PM; Van Houte, AJ. Cytokine profiles during clinical high-flux dialysis: no evidence for cytokine generation by circulating monocytes.Journal of the American Society of Nephrology, 8:1745-54. 1997

87. Ikizler TA, Flakoll PJ, Parker RA & Hakim RM. Amino acid & albumin losses during hemodialysis. *Kidney Int.* 46:830-7, 1994.
88. Bradley SF, Vibhagool A, Fabrick S, Terpenning MS, Kauffman CA. Monokine production by malnourished nursing home patients. *Gerontology*, 36:165-70, 1990.
89. Macdonald C; Rush DN; Bernstein KN; McKenna RM. Production of tumor necrosis factor alpha and hemodialysis. *Nephron*, 65:273-277, 1993.
90. Xu, B; Dube, MG; Kalra, PS; Farmerie, WG; Kaibara, A; Moldawer, LL; Martin, D; Kalra, SP. Anorectic effects of the cytokine, ciliary neurotropic factor, are mediated by hypothalamic neuropeptide Y: comparison with leptin. Endocrinology, 39:466-73. 1998
91. Hasselgren, PO; Fischer, JE. Sepsis: stimulation of energy-dependent protein breakdown resulting in protein loss in skeletal muscle. World Journal of Surgery, 22:203-8. 1998
92. Ballmer PE, McNurlan MA, Hulter HN, Anderson SE, Garlick PJ, Krapf R. Chronic metabolic acidosis decreases albumin synthesis and induces negative nitrogen balance in humans. J. Clin. Invest. 95:39-45, 1995.
93. Brady JP, Hasbargen JA. Correction of metabolic acidosis and its effect on albumin in chronc hemodialysis patients. Am. J. Kidney Dis 31:35-40, 1998.
94. Deen, W.M., C.R. Bridges, B.M. Brenner, and B.D. Myers. 1985. Heteroporous model of glomerular size selectivity: application to normal and nephrotic humans. Am. J. Physiol. 249:F374-89.
95. Janssen WM, Hillege H, Pinto-Sietsma SJ, Bak AA, De Zeeuw D, de Jong PE; PREVEND Study Group. Prevention of Renal and Vascular End-stage Disease. Low levels of urinary albumin excretion are associated with cardiovascular risk factors in the general population. Clin Chem Lab Med 2000 Nov;38(11):1107-10
96. Mogensen CE, Christiansen CE. Predicting diabetic nephropathy in insulin-dependent patients. *N. Engl. J. Med.* 311:89-93, 1984.
97. Samuelsson O, Wilhelmsen L, Elmfeldt D, Pennert K, Wedel H, Wikstrand J, Berglund G: Predictors of cardiovascular morbidity in treated hypertension: Results from the primary prevention trial in Goteborg, Sweden. J Hypertens 3:167-76, 1985
98. Keane WF, Eknoyan G. Proteinuria, albuminuria, risk, assessment, detection, elimination (PARADE): a position paper of the National Kidney Foundation. Am J Kidney Dis 1999 May;33(5):1004-10
99. Hunsicker LG, Adler S, Caggiula A, England BK, Greene T, Kusek JW, Rogers NL, Teschan PE: Predictors of the progression of renal disease in the Modification of Diet in Renal Disease Study. Kidney Int 51:1908-19, 1997
100. The GISEN Group (Gruppo Italiano de Studi Epidemiologici in Nefrologia): Randomised placebo-controlled trial of effect of ramipril on decline in glomerular filtration rate and risk of terminal renal failure in proteinuric, non-diabetic nephropathy. Lancet 349:1857-63, 1997
101. P. Ruggenenti, A. Perna, L. Mosconi, R. Pisoni and G. Remuzzi, Urinary protein excretion rate is the best independent predictor of ESRF in non-diabetic proteinuric chronic nephropathies. Kidney Int 53 (1998), pp. 1209-16
102. M. Abbate, C. Zoja, D. Corna, M. Capitanio, T. Bertani and G. Remuzzi, In progressive nephropathies, overload of tubular cells with filtered proteins translates glomerular permeability dysfunction into cellular signals of interstitial inflammation. J Am Soc Nephrol 9 (1998), pp. 1213-24.
103. Y. Wang, J. Chen, L. Chen, Y.C. Tay, G.K. Rangan and D.C. Harris, Induction of monocyte chemoattractant protein-1 in proximal tubule cells by urinary protein. J Am Soc Nephrol 8 (1997), pp. 1537-45
104. Taal MW, Chertow GM, Rennke HG, Gurnani A, Jiang T, Shahsafaei A, Troy JL, Brenner BM, Mackenzie HS. Mechanisms underlying renoprotection during renin-angiotensin system blockade. Am J Physiol Renal Physiol 2001 Feb;280(2):F343-55
105. C. Zoja, R. Donadelli, S. Colleoni et al., Protein overload stimulates RANTES production by proximal tubular cells depending on NF-kappa B activation. Kidney Int 53 (1998), pp. 1608-15
106. Shearer GC, Stevenson FT, Atkinson DN, Jones H, Staprans I, Kaysen GA. Hypoalbuminemia and proteinuria contribute separately to reduced lipoprotein catabolism in the nephrotic syndrome. Kidney Int;59:179-89, 2001
107. Earley LE, Farland M. Nephrotic syndrome Ed 3. In :Diseases of the Kidney, edited by Strauss M.B., Welt, L.G., pp 765-813 Boston, Little Brown Co., 1979.
108. Earley LE, Havel RJ, Hopper J, Graus H. Nephrotic Syndrome. *Calif. Med.* 115:23-41, 1971.
109. Prinsen BH, de Sain-van der Velden MG, Kaysen GA, Straver HW, van Rijn HJ, Stellaard F, Berger R, Rabelink TJ. Transferrin synthesis is increased in nephrotic patients insufficiently to replace urinary losses. J Am Soc Nephrol;12:1017-25, 2001
110. Kaysen GA, Myers BD, Couser WG, Rabkin R, Felts JM. Mechanisms and consequences of proteinuria. *Lab. Invest.* 54:479-98, 1986.
111. Deen WM, Bridges CR, Brenner BM, Myers BD. Heteroporous model of glomerular size selectivity: application to normal and nephrotic humans. *Am. J. Physiol.* 249:F374-89, 1985.
112. Baldamus CA, Galaske R, Eisenbach GM, Krause HP, Stolte H. Glomerular protein filtration in normal and nephrotic rats: A micropuncture study. *Contr. Nephrol.* 1:37-49. 1975.
113. Jensen H, Bro-Jorgensen K, Jarnum S, Olesen H, Yssing M. Transferrin metabolism in the nephrotic syndrome and in protein-losing gastroenteropathy. *Scandinavian J. Clin. Lab. Invest.* 21:293-304, 1968.
114. Hancock, D.E., Onstad, J.W., Wolf, P.L. Transferrin loss into the urine with hypochromic, microcytic anemia. Am. J. Clin. Pathol. 65:72-8, 1976.
115. Prinsen BH, Velden MG, Kaysen GA, Straver HW, Rijn HJ, Stellaard F, Berger R, Rabelink TJ. Transferrin Synthesis Is Increased in Nephrotic Patients Insufficiently to Replace Urinary Losses. J Am Soc Nephrol;12:1017-25, 2001.
116. Giangiacomo J, Cleary TG, Cole BR, Hoffsten P, Robson AM. Serum immunoglobulins in the nephrotic syndrome. A possible cause of minimal-change nephrotic syndrome. *N. Engl. J. Med.* 293:8-12, 1975.
117. Al-Bander, H., Martin, V.I., and G.A. Kaysen. Plasma IgG levels are not defended when urinary protein loss occurs. *Am J Physiol* 262:F333-7, 1992.
118. de Sain-van der Velden MG, Kaysen GA, de Meer K, Stellaard F, Voorbij HA, Reijngoud DJ, Rabelink TJ, Koomans HA. Proportionate increase of fibrinogen and albumin synthesis in nephrotic patients: measurements with stable isotopes. Kidney Int;53:181-8, 1998
119. Sun X, Martin V, Weiss RH, Kaysen GA. Selective transcriptional augmentation of hepatic gene expression in the rat with Heymann nephritis. American Journal of Physiology 264 :F441-7, 1993
120. Sun X, Jones Jr. H, Joles JA, Van Tol A, Kaysen GA. Apolipoprotein gene expression in analbuminemic rats and in rats with Heymann nephritis. *Am. J. Physiol.* 262 (*Renal Fluid Electrolyte Physiol.* 31):F755-61, 1992
121. Kaysen GA, Sun X, Jones Jr. H, Martin VI, Joles JA, Tsukamoto H, Couser WG Al-Bander H. Non-Iron mediated alteration in hepatic transferrin gene expression in the nephrotic rat. *Kidney Int*, 47:1068-77, 1995

122. de Sain-van der Velden MG, Rabelink TJ, Reijngoud DJ, Gadellaa MM, Voorbij HA, Stellaard F, Kaysen GA. Plasma alpha 2 macroglobulin is increased in nephrotic patients as a result of increased synthesis alone. Kidney Int;54:530-5, 1998
123. Prinsen BH, Velden MG, Kaysen GA, Straver HW, Rijn HJ, Stellaard F, Berger R, Rabelink TJ. Transferrin Synthesis Is Increased in Nephrotic Patients Insufficiently to Replace Urinary Losses. J Am Soc Nephrol;12:1017-25, 2001.
124. Kang J, Holland M, Jones H, Kaysen GA. Coordinate augmentation in expression of genes encoding transcription factors and liver secretory proteins in hypo-oncotic states. Kidney Int Aug;56:452-60, 1999
125. Joven J, Cliville X, Camps J, Espinel E, Simo J, Vilella E, Oliver A. Plasma protein abnormalities in nephrotic syndrome: effect on plasma colloid osmotic pressure and viscosity. Clin Chem;43:1223-31,1997
126. Canaan-Kuhl S, Venkatraman ES, Ernst SI, Olshen RA, Myers BD. Relationships among protein and albumin concentrations and oncotic pressure in nephrotic plasma. Am J Physiol;264(6 Pt 2):F1052-9, 1993
127. Stevenson FT, Greene S, Kaysen GA. Serum alpha 2-macroglobulin and alpha 1-inhibitor 3 concentrations are increased in hypoalbuminemia by post-transcriptional mechanisms. Kidney Int;53(1):67-75, 1998.
128. De Sain-Van Der Velden MG, Reijngoud DJ, Kaysen GA, Gadellaa MM, Voorbij H, Stellaard F, Koomans HA, Rabelink TJ. Evidence for increased synthesis of lipoprotein(a) in the nephrotic syndrome. J Am Soc Nephrol; 9:1474-81, 1998.
129. Kauffmann RH, Veltkamp JJ, Van Tilburg NH, Van Es LA. Acquired antithrombin III deficiency and thrombosis in the nephrotic syndrome. *Am. J. Med.* 65:607-13, 1978.
130. Rydzewski A, Myslieiec M, Soszka J. Concentration of three thrombin inhibitors in the nephrotic syndrome in adults. *Nephron* 42:200-3, 1986.
131. D'Angelo S, D'Angelo A, Kaufman CE Jr., Sholer C., Esmon CT, Comp PC. Protein S deficiency occurs in the nephrotic syndrome. *Ann Intern. Med.* 107:42-7, 1987.
132. Cosio FG, Harker C, Batard MA, Brandt JT, Griffin JH. Plasma concentrations of the natural anticoagulants protein C and protein S in patients with proteinuria *J. Lab. Clin. Med.* 106:218-22,1985.
133. Perheentupa *J. Ann. Paediat. Fenn.* 12:189-233, 1966.
134. Heslan JM, Lautie JP, Intrator L, Blanc C, Lagrue G, Sobel AT. *Clinic. Nephrol.* 18:144-7, 1982.
135. Ooi BS, Ooi YM, Hsu A. Hurtsubise, P.E. Diminished synthesis of immunoglobulin by peripheral lymphocytes of patients with idiopathic membranous glomerulonephropathy. *J. Clin. Invest.* 65:789-97, 1980.
136. Al-Bander, H., Martin, V.I., and G.A. Kaysen. Plasma IgG levels are not defended when urinary protein loss occurs. *Am J Physiol* 262:F333-7, 1992.
137. de Sain-van der Velden MG, Kaysen GA, Barrett HA, Stellaard F, Gadellaa MM, Voorbij HA, Reijngoud DJ, Rabelink TJ. Increased VLDL in nephrotic patients results from a decreased catabolism while increased LDL results from increased synthesis. Kidney Int;53:994-1001, 1998.
138. Davies RW, Staprans I, Hutchison FN, and Kaysen GA. Proteinuria, not altered albumin metabolism, affects hyperlipidemia in the nephrotic rat. J Clin Invest 86:600-5. 1990.
139. Aukland K, Nicolaysen G: Interstitial fluid volume: local regulatory mechanisms. *Phys. Rev.* 61:556-643, 1981.
140. Guyton AC, Taylor AE, Granger HJ: (editors) Circulatory Physiology II: Dynamics and Control of Body Fluids pp 149-65. Philadelphia, WB Saunders Co, 1975.
141. Taylor AE: Capillary fluid filtration starling forces and lymph flow. *Circ. Res.* 49:557-75, 1981.
142. Meltzer JI, Keim HJ, Laragh J.H, Sealey JE, Jan KM, Chien S: Nephrotic syndrome: Vasoconstriction & hypervolemia types indicated by renin-sodium profiling *Ann. Int. Med.* 67:387-4, 1979.
143. Dorhout Mees EJ, Roos JC, Boer P, Yoe OH, Simatupang TA: Observations on edema formation in the nephrotic syndrome in adults with minimal lesions. *Am. J. Med.* 67:378-84, 1979.
144. Geers AB, Koomans HA, Roos JC, Boer P, Dorhout Mees EJ: Functional relationships in the nephrotic syndrome. *Kidney Int.* 26:324-30, 1984.
145. Koomans HA, Geers A B, Meiracker AHVD, Roos JC, Boer P, Dorhout Mees EJ: Effects of plasma volume expansion on renal salt handling in patients with the nephrotic syndrome. *Am J Nephrol.* 4:227-34, 1984.
146. Keeler R, Feuchuk D, Wilson N: Atrial peptides and the renal response to hypervolemia in nephrotic rats. *Can J Physiol Pharmacol* 65:2017-75, 1987.
147. Peterson C, Madsen B, Perlman A, Chan AY, Myers BD: Atrial natriuretic peptide and the renal response to hypervolemia in nephrotic humans. *Kidney Int* 34:825-31, 1988.
148. Rabelink AJ, Koomans HA, Gaillard CA, Dorhout Mees EJ: Renal response to atrial natriuretic peptide in nephrotic syndrome. *Nephrol Dial Transplant* 510-4, 1987.
149. Perico N, Delaini F, Lupini C, Benigni A, Galbusera M, Boccardo P, Remuzzi G: Blunted excretory response to atrial natriuretic peptide in experimental nephrosis *Kidney Int* 36:57-64, 1989.
150. Hildebrandt DA, Banks RO: Effect of atrial natriuretic factor on renal function in rats with nephrotic syndrome. *Am J Physiol* 254:(*Renal Fluid Electrolyte Physiol* 23:) F210-6, 1988.
151. Lee EY, Humphreys MH. Phosphodiesterase activity as a mediator of renal resistance to ANP in pathological salt retention. Am J Physiol;271:F3-6, 1996
152. Ichikawa I, Rennke HG, Hoyer JR, Badr KF, Schol N, Troy JL, Lechene CP, Brenner BM: Role for intrarenal mechanisms in the impaired salt excretion of experimental nephrotic syndrome. *J Clin Invest* 71:91-104, 1983.
153. Alexopoulos E, Stangou M, Papagianni A, Pantzaki A, Papadimitriou M. Factors influencing the course and the response to treatment in primary focal segmental glomerulosclerosis. Nephrol Dial Transplant;15:1348-56, 2000
154. Hino S, Takemura T, Okada M, Murakami K, Yagi K, Fukushima K, Yoshioka K. Follow-up study of children with nephrotic syndrome treated with a long-term moderate dose of cyclosporine. Am J Kidney Dis;31:932-9, 1998
155. Hallegua D, Wallace DJ, Metzger AL, Rinaldi RZ, Klinenberg JR. Cyclosporine for lupus membranous nephritis: experience with ten patients and review of the literature. Lupus;9:241-51,2000.
156. Hayashi T, Saito N, Shoji T, Togawa M, Okada N, Tsubakihara Y. Cyclosporin A mono-therapy in nephrotic syndrome with contra-indication of steroid therapy. Intern Med Mar;38:272-5, 1999
157. Klein M, Radhakrishnan J, Appel G. Cyclosporine treatment of glomerular diseases. Annu Rev Med;50:1-15, 1999
158. Heeg JE, de Jong PE, van der Hem GK, de Zeeuw D. Angiotensin II does not acutely reverse the reduction of proteinuria by long-term ACE inhibition. Kidney Int;40:734-41, 1991.
159. Ruilope LM, Aldigier JC, Ponticelli C, Oddou-Stock P, Botteri F, Mann JF. Safety of the combination of valsartan and benazepril in patients with chronic renal disease. European Group for the Investigation of Valsartan in Chronic Renal Disease. J Hypertens;18:89-95, 2000
160. Benigni A, Tomasoni S, Gagliardini E, Zoja C, Grunkemeyer JA, Kalluri R, Remuzzi G. Blocking angiotensin II synthesis/activity preserves glomerular nephrin in rats with severe nephrosis. J Am Soc Nephrol;12:941-8, 2001

161. Ruotsalainen V, Ljungberg P, Wartiovaara J, Lenkkeri U, Kestila M, Jalanko H, Holmberg C, Tryggvason K. Nephrin is specifically located at the slit diaphragm of glomerular podocytes. Proc Natl Acad Sci U S A 96:7962-7, 1999
162. Aya K, Tanaka H, Seino Y Novel mutation in the nephrin gene of a Japanese patient with congenital nephrotic syndrome of the Finnish type. Kidney Int;57:401-4, 2000
163. Gentile MG, Fellin G, Cofano F, Delle Fave A, Manna G, Ciceri R, Petrini C, Lavarda F, Pozzi F, D'Amico G. Treatment of proteinuric patients with a vegetarian soy diet and fish oil. Clin Nephrol;40:315-20, 1993
164. Pasquariello A, Camerini E. Unilateral renal vein thrombosis and pulmonary embolism complicating membranous nephropathy. Am J Nephrol;12:134-6, 1992
165. Urch C, Pusey CD. Sagittal sinus thrombosis in adult minimal change nephrotic syndrome. Clin Nephrol;45:131-2, 1996.
166. Hirata M, Kuroda M, Koni I. Cerebral venous thrombosis in minimal change nephrotic syndrome Nippon Jinzo Gakkai Shi Jun;41:464-8, 1999
167. Zimmerman RL, Novek S, Chen JT, Roggli V. Pulmonary thrombosis in a 10-year-old child with minimal change disease and nephrotic syndrome. A clinical, radiologic, and pathologic correlation with literature review. Am J Clin Pathol;101:230-6,1994
168. de Sain-Van Der Velden MG, de Meer K, Kulik W, Melissant CF, Rabelink TJ, Berger R, Kaysen GA. Nephrotic proteinuria has No net effect on total body protein synthesis: measurements with (13)C valine. Am J Kidney Dis;35:1149-54, 2000.
169. Kaysen GA, Carstensen A, Martin VI. Muscle protein synthesis is impaired in nephrotic rats. Miner Electrolyte Metab;18:228-32, 1992

10 Kidney Disease and Mechanisms that Cause Loss of Muscle Mass

William E. Mitch, M.D., S. Russ Price, Ph. D.

Abstract

The daily turnover of cellular proteins is very large, in the range of the protein contained in 1-1.5 kg of muscle. Consequently, even a small, persistent increase in the rate of protein degradation or decrease in protein synthesis will result in substantial loss of muscle mass and increased morbidity and mortality. Activation of protein degradation in the ubiquitin-proteasome system is the mechanism contributing to loss of muscle mass in kidney disease. Since other catabolic conditions also stimulate this system to cause loss of muscle mass, identification of activating signals is of intense interest. A complication of kidney disease, metabolic acidosis, activates the system in muscle by a process that requires glucocorticoids. The influence of inflammatory cytokines on this system in muscle is more complicated, as evidence indicates that cytokines suppress the system; but again, glucocorticoids block the effect of cytokines to slow protein breakdown in the system. New information identifying mechanisms that activate protein breakdown and the rebuilding of muscle fibers will lead to therapies that successfully prevent the loss of muscle mass in kidney and other catabolic illnesses.

Introduction

In normal adults, the rates of protein synthesis and degradation are very large, amounting to 3.5-4.5 g protein per kg each day.[1] This amount of protein is equivalent to that contained in 1 to 1.5 kg of muscle! The biological reasons for such a high rate of protein turnover are obscure, but a major fraction of daily protein turnover occurs in order to replace proteins that contain transcriptional or translational errors that occur during synthesis.[2] Another major reason is to remove and replace normal proteins that become damaged or undergo modification. In both cases, the proteins are rapidly removed by the ubiquitin-proteasome proteolytic system (see below). Because the rate of protein turnover is so high, it is easy to understand why a small, persistent suppression of protein synthesis or stimulation of protein degradation will lead to substantial loss of muscle protein.

These considerations lead to critical questions about muscle loss and its repair: a) can the loss of muscle mass be prevented; and b) can we initiate or accelerate the process of restoring muscle mass in patients who have lost it? Answers to these questions are emerging from investigations of the mechanisms that accelerate muscle protein breakdown and those stimulating muscle protein growth.

What mechanisms associated with kidney disease cause loss of muscle protein? There is evidence that renal insufficiency per se does not stimulate excessive catabolism and that the compensatory mechanisms that regulate protein turnover function normally in patients with chronic renal failure as long as there is no complicating disease or metabolic acidosis.[3-5] Even in patients with the nephrotic syndrome, nutritional mechanisms are intact so these patients can adapt successfully to a low-protein diet without loss of muscle mass as long as there is no complicating illness.[6] When kidney failure is complicated by other illnesses or metabolic disorders, however, the metabolic mechanisms that should act to maintain muscle mass become impaired. We identified metabolic acidosis as an important factor that stimulates the degradation of essential amino acids and protein in the muscles of rats.[7-12] Others have shown that acidosis exerts the same adverse responses in normal adults and patients with renal insufficiency, including patients being treated by hemodialysis or CAPD (**Table 1**). On the contrary, if acidosis is only partially corrected, there may be no detectable improvement in nutritional parameters.[23]

Recently, there has been intense interest in inflammation as a cause of muscle wasting and arteriosclerosis in patients with kidney disease.[24] There is experimental evidence that inflammation can suppress protein synthesis or stimulate protein degradation, and patients with kidney failure frequently have high serum levels of cytokines and acute phase reactant proteins.[1;25-30] There is also the well-known association between a low level of serum albumin and excessive mortality.[31] This type of indirect evidence has led some to propose that inflammation

M.M. Avram.(ed.), Improving Prognosis for Kidney Disorders, 91-96.

Table 1. Publications illustrating the adverse effects of metabolic acidosis in normal subjects and patients with kidney disease.

Subjects & Reference	Measurements of Effectiveness	Outcome of Trial
Normal adults [13]	Induced acidosis, amino acid and protein metabolism	Acidosis raised amino acid and protein degradation
Normal adults [14]	Induced acidosis, nitrogen balance and albumin synthesis	Acidosis induced negative nitrogen balance and suppressed albumin synthesis
Chronic renal failure [15]	Nitrogen balance before and after treatment of acidosis	$NaHCO_3$ improved nitrogen balance
Chronic renal failure [16]	Essential amino acid and protein degradation before and after treatment of acidosis	$NaHCO_3$ suppressed amino acid and protein degradation
Chronic renal failure [17]	Muscle protein degradation and acidosis	Proteolysis was proportional to acidosis and blood cortisol
Chronic renal failure [18]	Nitrogen balance before and after treatment of acidosis	$NaHCO_3$ reduced urea production and nitrogen balance
Hemodialysis [19]	Protein degradation before and after treatment of acidosis	$NaHCO_3$ decreased protein degradation
Hemodialysis [20]	Serum albumin before and after treatment of acidosis	$NaHCO_3$ increased serum albumin
CAPD [21]	Protein degradation before and after treatment of acidosis	$NaHCO_3$ decreased protein degradation
CAPD [22]	Weight and muscle gain before and after treatment of acidosis	Raising dialysis buffer increased weight and muscle mass

is a major factor causing cardiovascular disease and excessive mortality in chronically uremic patients.[24;32]

Clearly, clinical associations do not identify how inflammation causes a change in protein synthesis or degradation that ultimately cause a loss of lean body mass. This issue is of intense interest because cachexia (defined as an illness-induced loss of skeletal muscle mass) is a major clinical problem in many disorders besides kidney disease and is associated with a high risk of morbidity and mortality. Unfortunately, there are no effective therapies that will prevent the loss of muscle mass in such disorders; the only option for preventing loss of lean body mass is to treat the underlying disease. To devise methods directed at preventing loss of muscle mass, understanding the mechanisms that cause cachexia and those that replenish protein stores is needed. Progress has been made in these areas, but the results are not sufficiently definitive to recommend therapies.

There have been important developments in the search for mechanisms that accelerate protein degradation. It is now clear that the bulk of protein in normal cells is degraded by the ubiquitin-proteasome proteolytic system and that muscle protein breakdown by this system is accelerated in cachexia-producing conditions (e.g., sepsis, cancer, burn injury, etc.).[1;33;34] This system degrades many other proteins besides myofibrils, however, including proteins involved in the regulation of transcription (e.g., the degradation of IκB to activate NF-κB[35]), membrane ion transport proteins (e.g., CFTR[36] and the sodium channel[37]), regulatory proteins[1] and proteins that become antigens on cell surfaces.[38] Consequently, strategies directed at interfering with the ubiquitin-proteasome system throughout the body might have unexpected (and unwanted) consequences for a number of cell functions.

Because the ubiquitin-proteasome system plays a central role in the regulation of muscle mass, it is important to understand how it functions. The initial steps identify and specify which proteins will be degraded by multiple steps that are mediated by enzymes that conjugate ubiquitin to a substrate protein.[1] Ubiquitin is a small protein that is present in all cells and is a member of the heat-shock complex of proteins. The ubiquitin conjugation process is initiated by an E1 enzyme that activates ubiquitin by forming a thiol-ester bond with ubiquitin by an ATP-requiring reaction. The activated ubiquitin is then transferred to one of several E2 enzymes to form an ubiquitin-E2 intermediate complex. The next step confers substrate specificity, because the ubiquitin-E2 complex is brought into contact with the substrate protein by a E3 enzyme that recognizes the substitute as a defective or abnormal protein that should be degraded. The result of these reactions is conjugation of ubiquitin to the substrate protein. The same processes sequentially attach other ubiquitin molecules to the initial ubiquitin until there is a chain of 5 or more ubiquitin molecules attached to the substrate protein. This chain functions as a recognition site for the 26S proteasome complex where the substrate protein is rapidly degraded to small peptides.

Left unchecked, this process would quickly cause a major loss of cell proteins; but several features of the

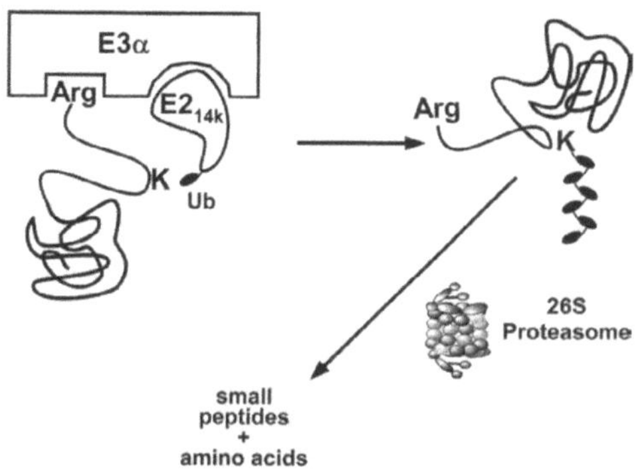

Figure 1. "N-End Rule"Protolysis. Schematic representation of the N-end rule for degradation of proteins by the ubiquitin-proteasome system. Proteins with specific N-terminal amino acids (e.g., arginine) are recognized by E3 enzymes and brought into contact with specific E2 enzymes so that activated ubiquitin molecules can be conjugated to lysines (designated as K) in the protein.

pathway result in specificity of the protocolytic process. Firstly, the enzymes involved in the ubiquitin conjugation reaction confer specificity. Even when muscle cells are stimulated by a cachexia-producing condition, only the $E2_{14K}$ enzyme is activated (this activation response includes an increase in the level of mRNA encoding $E2_{14K}$).[39] Secondly, a specific E3 enzyme in muscle, E3α, appears to be specifically activated in catabolic conditions. The E3α enzyme also exerts specificity by the N-end rule. [40-42] The N-end rule leads to preferential degradation of proteins based on their N- or amino terminal amino acid (see **Figure 1**). [40]Using inhibitors of the E3α enzyme, Solomon and colleagues showed that the E3α enzyme and the N-end rule pathway account for the bulk of protein degraded in muscle and that E3α is specifically activated in rat models of starvation- or sepsis-induced muscle catabolism.[41;42]

An important issue is whether the rate of ubiquitin conjugation to the substrate protein is the rate-limiting step in protein degradation. The conjugation reaction is certainly critical because the chain of ubiquitin molecules must be recognized by the proteasome before the protein is degraded. Even though resting muscle cells contain ubiquitin, in catabolic conditions, there is invariably an increase in the levels of mRNAs that encode ubiquitin and other components of the system.[1] Presumably, the ubiquitin that is present in the resting cell is used to degrade proteins that are turned over each day; but in catabolic conditions, the basal amount of ubiquitin is insufficient, and muscle cells synthesize more ubiquitin to increase the capacity of the system. In support of this proposal, Haas et al reported that cells stimulated to degrade protein had a sharp increase in the pool of ubiquitin, including the free ubiquitin and proteins conjugated to ubiquitin; while Davies and colleagues reported that inhibition of expression of the proteasome C2 subunit led to a block in the ability of hepatic or hemopoetic cells to degrade proteins in response to oxidative stress.[43-46] Secondly, we found that in response to acute diabetes, ubiquitin and ubiquitin-protein conjugates accumulate in muscle related to a sharp increase in the rate of ubiquitin conjugation to muscle protein.[39] These results suggest that the synthesis of new ubiquitin and components of the ubiquitin-proteasome system is required to prevent their levels from becoming rate-limiting. In uremia and diabetes, we found that the increase in mRNAs encoding components of the system is due to stimulation of gene transcription.[12;47;48] Thus, mechanisms that increase proteolysis by the system also stimulate transcriptions of specific genes encoding components of the ubiquitin-proteasome system.

After ubiquitin chains are conjugated to the substrate protein, they can be recognized by the 26S proteasome, a large complex composed of 4 rings of protein subunits (2 outer α rings and 2 inner β rings) with another complex of subunit proteins (the "cap") on each end. These caps not only recognize the ubiquitin-conjugated substrate protein but also remove the ubiquitin molecules which can then be recycled. In another ATP-dependent reaction, the caps unwind the substrate protein so it can be inserted into the central chamber of the proteasome. As the protein descends through the inner chamber, it is degraded into small peptides that are released into the cytoplasm where they are degraded to amino acids by cytoplasmic peptidases. Alternatively, the peptides become attached to the Class 1 MHC complex forming cellular antigens. Another unique feature of protein degradation by the proteasome is that the nucleophilic attack on the peptide bond is catalyzed by threonine hydroxyls (rather than serine hydroxyls or -SH groups) located on the inner face of the hollow core of the proteasome. This leads to a sequential cutting of the substrate protein into peptides of defined lengths.

An important question is what factors activate or control the activity of the ubiquitin-proteasome system? Glucocorticoids are important: removal of the adrenal glands prevented activation of muscle protein degradation by stimuli namely metabolic acidosis, acute diabetes or starvation that activate the system in intact rats.[48-51] In this same model, giving the rats a physiologic dose of glucocorticoids but in the absence of another stimulus, there is no activation of muscle proteolysis. Similar conclusions were reached after studies of cultured muscle cells.[52] Thus, glucocorticoids have a permissive effect on stimulating the ubiquitin-proteasome system; stimuli (e.g., acidosis or diabetes) along with glucocorticoids activate the system to degrade protein and stimulate transcription of genes encoding components of the system.

Treating acidosis is obviously necessary; (**Table 1**) but it has also been suggested that cachexia-induced loss of muscle mass could be prevented if inflammatory mechanisms were effectively blocked because many catabolic conditions (e.g., sepsis, cancer, etc.) are associated with a rise in cytokine production. This is a complicated area, however. As recent reports suggest, cytokines also act to stimulate the formation of new myofibrils by a mechanism that depends on the transcription factor, NF-κB. NF-κB is activated by several cytokines (e.g., tumor necrosis factor (TNF)) by a process that involves its disassociation from a cytosolic inhibitor protein, IκB. IκB, in turn, is degraded by the ubiquitin-proteasome system; and its removal allows NF-κB to translocate to the nucleus where it influences the transcription of genes. In lymphocytes, the genes stimulated by NF-κB participate in inflammatory reactions; but the responses are different in muscle cells. NF-κB expression in cultured muscle cells appears to be involved in regulating the synthesis and degradation of new myofibrils rather than stimulating the loss of muscle protein.[53-55] For example, Guttridge et al reported that treating immature myoblasts with TNF blocked their differentiation into mature myotubes (the stage in muscle cell development that is characterized by myosin synthesis and the accumulation of more myofibrils).[54] It was concluded that TNF-induced activation of NF-κB leads to suppression of a mRNA that encodes another transcription factor, MyoD. MyoD expression mediates the recovery of lost muscle protein, because it is necessary for increasing the formation of myofibrils. In short, MyoD suppression might prevent the accumulation of new muscle protein. The same effects may be active *in vivo,* because Guttridge et al also reported that mice injected with TNF plus IFN-γ experienced a down-regulation of MyoD mRNA in muscle. They speculated that blocking the action of NF-κB would stimulate the growth of muscle mass in patients recovering from catabolic conditions.[54] However, other reports suggest that if NF-κB action were blocked, the cell could not survive catabolic insults with an end result that is deleterious.[53;56;57] Bertrand et al reported that insulin prevents programmed cell death by a mechanism that is mediated through NF-κB.[57] Kaliman et al reported that insulin-like growth factor (IGF) also activates NF-κB even though it is generally perceived to promote the accumulation of muscle protein.[55] In short, conflicting observations about the responses of cultured muscle cells to NF-κB make it unclear how NF-κB influences the regulation of muscle protein turnover nor do they provide insight into whether blocking NF-κB would increase muscle mass in the intact animal (or patient).[58]

What about cytokines in skeletal muscle? We studied the responses of L6 muscle cells to inflammatory cytokines (i.e., TNFα plus IFNγ and LPS) and found that NF-κB interacted with the promoter region of a proteasome subunit.[53] Unexpectedly, however, NF-κB suppressed transcription of the gene. Based on this report and the reasons outlined earlier, it would appear that blocking the production of or effects of NF-κB would have an undesirable effect on muscle proteolysis.[54]

Another complicating issue is that the ubiquitin-proteasome system can degrade free actin or myosin; but by itself, it does not disassemble myofibrils nor degrade proteins contained in an actin-myosin complex.[59] Thus, an initial step in muscle protein loss must involve other proteases that breakdown myofibrils and the actin-myosin complexes. When the mechanisms accounting for the disassembly process are known, potential therapeutic targets might be identified to block the initial stages of muscle protein loss.

In summary, the mechanisms underlying the maintenance of muscle mass are poorly understood but a critical factor is the stimulation of muscle protein degradation by the ubiquitin-proteasome system. Not only is this system responsible for the loss of protein that occurs in catabolic conditions, but it also degrades proteins that are critical for normal function of cells. Consequently, therapeutic methods directed at reducing the loss of muscle protein should avoid interfering with this proteolytic system or must exhibit selectivity in blocking the degradation of specific types of proteins. At the molecular level, factors affecting the biology of muscle protein turnover have been discovered; but new information is needed to develop safe and effective means of preventing the loss of muscle protein and of accelerating muscle protein repair in humans. Despite these hurdles, we are in an exciting time as a more complete understanding of the cellular mechanisms that control muscle mass develops. Surely, these developments will lead to therapeutic breakthroughs.

References

1. Mitch WE, Goldberg AL: Mechanisms of muscle wasting: The role of the ubiquitin-proteasome system. N Engl J Med 335:1897-905, 1996
2. Schild H, Rammensee H-G: Perfect use of imperfection. Nature 404:709-10, 2000
3. Goodship THJ, Mitch WE, Hoerr RA, Wagner DA, Steinman TI, Young VR: Adaptation to low-protein diets in renal failure: Leucine turnover and nitrogen balance. J Am Soc Nephrol 1:66-75, 1990
4. Masud T, Young VR, Chapman T, Maroni BJ: Adaptive responses to very low protein diets: The first comparison of ketoacids to essential amino acids. Kidney Int 45:1182-92, 1994

5. Tom K, Young VR, Chapman T, Masud T, Akpele L, Maroni BJ: Long-term adaptive responses to dietary protein restriction in chronic renal failure. Am J Physiol 268:E668-77, 1995
6. Maroni BJ, Staffeld C, Young VR, Manatunga A, Tom K: Mechanisms permitting nephrotic patients to achieve nitrogen equilibrium with a protein-restricted diet. J Clin Invest 99:2479-87, 1997
7. May RC, Hara Y, Kelly RA, Block KP, Buse MG, Mitch WE: Branched-chain amino acid metabolism in rat muscle: Abnormal regulation in acidosis. Am J Physiol 252:E712-8, 1987
8. May RC, Kelly RA, Mitch WE: Metabolic acidosis stimulates pro-tein degradation in rat muscle by a glucocorticoid-dependent mech-anism. J Clin Invest 77:614-21, 1986
9. May RC, Kelly RA, Mitch WE: Mechanisms for defects in muscle protein metabolism in rats with chronic uremia: The influence of metabolic acidosis. J Clin Invest 79:1099-103, 1987
10. England BK, Greiber S, Mitch WE, Bowers BA, Herring WJ, McKean MJ, Ebb RG, Price SR, Danner DJ: Rat muscle branched-chain ketoacid dehydrogenase activity and mRNAs increase with extracellular acidemia. Am J Physiol 268:C1395-400, 1995
11. Mitch WE, Medina R, Greiber S, May RC, England BK, Price SR, Bailey JL, Goldberg AL: Metabolic acidosis stimulates muscle pro-tein degradation by activating the ATP-dependent pathway invol-ving ubiquitin and proteasomes. J Clin Invest 93:2127-33, 1994
12. Bailey JL, Wang X, England BK, Price SR, Ding X, Mitch WE: The acidosis of chronic renal failure activates muscle proteolysis in rats by augmenting transcription of genes encoding proteins of the ATP-dependent, ubiquitin-proteasome pathway. J Clin Invest 97:1447-53, 1996
13. Reaich D, Channon SM, Scrimgeour CM, Goodship THJ: Ammon-ium chloride-induced acidosis increases protein breakdown and amino acid oxidation in humans. Am J Physiol 263:E735-9, 1992
14. Ballmer PE, McNurlan MA, Hulter HN, Anderson SE, Garlick PJ, Krapf R: Chronic metabolic acidosis decreases albumin synthesis and induces negative nitrogen balance in humans. J Clin Invest 95:39-45, 1995
15. Papadoyannakis NJ, Stefanides CJ, McGeown M: The effect of the correction of metabolic acidosis on nitrogen and protein balance of patients with chronic renal failure. Am J Clin Nutr 40:623-7, 1984
16. Reaich D, Channon SM, Scrimgeour CM, Daley SE, Wilkinson R, Goodship THJ: Correction of acidosis in humans with CRF decreases protein degradation and amino acid oxidation. Am J Physiol 265:E230-5, 1993
17. Garibotto G, Russo R, Sofia A, Sala MR, Robaudo C, Moscatelli P, DeFerrari G, Tizianello A: Skeletal muscle protein synthesis and degradation in patients with chronic renal failure. Kidney Int 45:1432-39, 1994
18. Williams B, Hattersley J, Layward E, Walls J: Metabolic acidosis and skeletal muscle adaptation to low protein diets in chronic uremia. Kidney Int 40:779-86, 1991
19. Graham KA, Reaich D, Channon SM, Downie S, Goodship THJ: Correction of acidosis in hemodialysis decreases whole-body protein degradation. J Am Soc Nephrol 8:632-7, 1997
20. Movilli E, Zani R, Carli O, Sangalli L, Pola A, Camerini C, Cancarini GC, Scolari F, Feller P, Maiorca R: Correction of metabolic acidosis increases serum albumin concentration and decreases kinetically evaluated protein intake in hemodialysis patients: A prospective study. Nephrol Dial Transpl 13:1719-22, 1998
21. Graham KA, Reaich D, Channon SM, Downie S, Gilmour E, Pass-lick-Deetjen J, Goodship THJ: Correction of acidosis in CAPD de-creases whole body protein degradation. Kidney Int 49:1396-400, 1996
22. Stein A, Moorhouse J, Iles-Smith H, Baker R, Johnstone J, James G, Troughton J, Bircher G, Walls J: Role of an improvement in acid-base status and nutrition in CAPD patients. Kidney Int 52:1089-95, 1997
23. Brady JP, Hasbargen JA: Correction of metabolic acidosis and its effect on albumin in chronic hemodialysis patients. Am J Kid Dis 31:35-40, 1998
24. Bergstrom J, Lacson E, Owen WF, Lowrie EG, Glassock RJ, Ikizler TA, Wessels FJ, Moldawer LL, Wanner C, Zimmermann J: What are the causes and consequences of the chronic inflammatory in chronic hemodialysis patients? Sem Dialysis 13:163-76, 2000
25. Lecker SH, Solomon V, Mitch WE, Goldberg AL: Muscle protein breakdown and the critical role of the ubiquitin-proteasome pathway in normal and disease states. J Nutr 129:227S-37S, 1999
26. Dinarello CA: Cytokines: Agents provocateurs in hemodialysis. Kidney Int 41:683-94, 1992
27. Herbelin A, Urena P, Nguyen AT, Zingraff J, Descamps-Latscha B: Elevated circulating levels of Interleukin-6 in patients with chronic renal failure. Kidney Int 39:954-60, 1991
28. Pereira BJ, Shapiro L, King AJ, Falagas ME, Strom JA, Dinarello CA: Plasma levels of IL-1B, TNF-a and their specific inhibitors in undialyzed chonic renal failure, CAPD, and hemodialysis patients. Kidney Int 45:890-6, 1994
29. Herbelin A, Nguyen AT, Zingraff J, Urena P, Descamps-Latscha B: Influence of uremia and hemodialysis on circulating interleukin-1 and tumor necrosis factor a. Kidney Int 37:116-27, 1990
30. Nakanishi I, Moutabarrik A, Okada N, Kitamura E, Kayashi A, Syouji T, Namiki M, Ishibashi M, Zaid D, Tsubakihara Y: Interleukin-8 in chronic renal failure and dialysis patients. Nephrol Dial Transpl 9:1435-42, 1994
31. Kaysen GA: Biological basis of hypoalbuminemia in ESRD. J Am Soc Nephrol 9:2368-76, 1998
32. Qureshi AR, Alvestrand A, Danielsson A, Divino-Filho JC, Gutierrez A, Lindholm B, Bergstrom J: Factors predicting malnutrition in hemodialysis patients: A cross-sectional study. Kidney Int 53:773-82, 1998
33. Mansoor O, Beaufrere Y, Boirie Y, Ralliere C, Taillandier D, Aurousseau E, Schoeffler P, Arnal M, Attaix D: Increased mRNA levels for components of the lysosomal, Ca++-activated and ATP-ubiquitin-dependent proteolytic pathways in skeletal muscle from head trauma patients. Proc Natl Acad Sci USA 93:2714-8, 1996
34. Tiao G, Hobler S, Wang JJ, Meyer TA, Luchette FA, Fischer JE, Hasselgren P-O: Sepsis is associated with increased mRNAs of the ubiquitin-proteasome proteolytic pathway in human skeletal muscle. J Clin Invest 99:163-8, 1997
35. Palombella VJ, Rando OJ, Goldberg AL, Maniatis T: The ubiquitin-proteasome pathway is required for processing the NF-kB1 precur-sor protein and the activation of NF-kB. Cell 78:773-85, 1994
36. Jensen TJ, Loo MA, Pind S, Williams DB, Goldberg AL, Riordan JR: Multiple proteolytic systems, including the proteasome contribute CFTR processing. Cell 83:129-35, 1995
37. Malik B, Schlanger L, Al-Khalili O, Bao H-F, Yue G, Price SR, Mitch WE, Eaton DC: ENaC degradation in A6 cells by the ubiqui-tin-proteasome proteolytic pathway. J Biol Chem 276:12903-10, 2001
38. Rock KL, Gramm C, Rothstein L, Clark K, Stein R, Dick L, Hwang D, Goldberg AL: Inhibitors of the proteasome block the degradation of most cell proteins and the generation of peptides presented on MHC class 1 molecules. Cell 78:761-71, 1994
39. Lecker SH, Solomon V, Price SR, Kwon YT, Mitch WE, Goldberg AL: Ubiquitin conjugation by the N-end rule pathway and mRNAs for its components increase in muscles of diabetic rats. J Clin Invest 104:1411-20, 1999
40. Varshavsky A: The N-end rule: Functions, mysteries, uses. Proc Natl Acad Sci USA 93:12142-9, 1996

41. Solomon V, Lecker SH, Goldberg AL: The N-end rule pathway catalyzes a major fraction of the protein degradation in skeletal muscle. J Biol Chem 273:25216-22, 1998
42. Solomon V, Baracos V, Sarraf P, Goldberg AL: Rates of ubiquitin conjugation increase when muscles atrophy, largely through activation of the N-end rule pathway. Proc Natl Acad Sci 95:12602-7, 1998
43. Grune T, Reinheckel R, Joshi M, Davies KJA: Proteolysis in cultured liver epithelial cells during oxidative stress: Role of the multi-catalytic proteinase complex, proteasome. J Biol Chem 270:2344-51, 1995
44. Grune T, Reinheckel T, Davies KJA: Degradation of oxidized pro-pteins in K562 human hematopoietic cells by proteasome. J Biol Chem 271:15504-9, 1998
45. Grune T, Blasig IE, Sitte N, Roloff B, Haseloff R, Davies KJA: Peroxynitrite increases the degradation of aconitase and other cellular proteins by proteasome. J Biol Chem 273:10857-62, 1998
46. Haas AL, Bright PM: The dynamics of ubiquitin pools within cultured human lung fibroblasts. J Biol Chem 262:345-351, 1987
47. Price SR, Bailey JL, Wang X, Jurkovitz C, England BK, Ding X, Phillips LS, Mitch WE: Muscle wasting in insulinopenic rats results from activation of the ATP-dependent, ubiquitin-proteasome path-way by a mechanism including gene transcription. J Clin Invest 98:1703-8, 1996
48. Mitch WE, Bailey JL, Wang X, Jurkovitz C, Newby D, Price SR: Evaluation of signals activating ubiquitin-proteasome proteolysis in a model of muscle wasting. Amer J Physiol 276:C1132-8, 1999
49. Price SR, England BK, Bailey JL, Van Vreede K, Mitch WE: Acidosis and glucocorticoids concomitantly increase ubiquitin and proteasome subunit mRNAs in rat muscle. Am J Physiol 267:C955-60, 1994
50. May RC, Masud T, Logue B, Bailey JL, England BK: Chronic metabolic acidosis accelerates whole body proteolysis and leucine oxidation in awake rats. Kidney Int 41:1535-42, 1992
51. Wing SS, Goldberg AL: Glucocorticoids activate the ATP-ubiquitin-dependent proteolytic system in skeletal muscle during fasting. Am J Physiol 264:E668-76, 1993
52. Isozaki Y, Mitch WE, England BK, Price SR: Interaction between glucocorticoids and acidification results in stimulation of proteolysis and mRNAs of proteins encoding the ubiquitin-proteasome pathway in BC3H-1 myocytes. Proc Natl Acad Sci USA 93:1967-71, 1996
53. Du J, Mitch WE, Wang X, Price SR: Glucocorticoids induce proteasome C3 subunit expression in L6 muscle cells by opposing the suppression of its transcription by NF-kB. J Biol Chem 275:19661-6, 2000
54. Guttridge DC, Mayo MW, Madrid LV, Wang C-Y, Baldwin AS: NF-kB-Induced loss of MyoD messenger RNA: Possible role in muscle decay and cachexia. Science 289:2363-6, 2000
55. Kaliman P, Canicio J, Testar X, Palacin M, Zorzano A: Insulin-like growth factor-II, phosphatidylinositol 3-kinase, nuclear factor-kB and inducible nitric-oxide synthase define a common myogenic signaling pathway. J Biol Chem 274:17437-44, 1999
56. Baghdiguian S, Martin M, Richard I, Pons F, Astier C, Bourg N, Hay RT, Chemaly R, Halaby G, Loiselet J, Anderson LV, Lopez de Munain A, Fardeau M, Mangeat P, Beckmann JS, Lefranc G: Cal-pain 3 deficiency is associated with myonuclear apoptosis and pro-found perturbation of the I kappa B alpha/NF-kappaB pathway in limb-girdle muscular dystrophy type 2A. Nature, Med 5:503-11, 1999
57. Bertrand F, Desbois-Mouthon C, Cadoret A, Prunier C, Robin H, Capeau J, Atfi A, Cherqui G: Insulin antiapoptotic signaling involves insulin activation of the nuclear factor kappaB-dependent survival genes encoding tumor necrosis factor receptor-associated factor 2 and manganese-superoxide dismutase. J Biol Chem 274:30596-602, 1999
58. Mitch WE, Price SR: Transcription factors and muscle cachexia: have we defined a therapeutic target? Lancet 357:734-5, 2001
59. Solomon V, Goldberg AL: Importance of the ATP-ubiquitin-proteasome pathway in degradation of soluble and myofibrillar proteins in rabbit muscle extracts. J Biol Chem 271:26690-7, 1996

11 Role of Plasma Homocysteine and Plasminogen Activator Inhibitor-1 in the Progression of Diabetic Nephropathy

PETER HOVIND, MD, LISE TARNOW, MD, PETER ROSSING DMSC, COEN D.A. STEHOUWER, MD, JEF J. EMEIS, MD, AND HANS-HENRIK PARVING, PROFESSOR, DMSC.

Abstract

Diabetic nephropathy is a progressive disease and a leading cause of end stage renal disease. However, the decline in glomerular filtration rate (GFR) varies substantially between patients, ranging from 2 to 20 ml/min/year. Thus, identification of predictors of progression in diabetic nephropathy is of importance. Plasma total homocysteine (tHcy) rises with urinary albumin rate in diabetes, and plasminogen activator inhibitor-1 (PAI-1) has been correlated to increased matrix accumulation in various glomerulopathies. The aim of the present prospective observational cohort study was to evaluate the importance of baseline tHcy and PAI-1 as predictors of the rate of decline in GFR. At baseline tHcy and PAI-1 were measured in 157 type 1 diabetic patients with diabetic nephropathy (92 males, age 41 ± 10 years, diabetes duration 28 ± 8 years, GFR (median (range)) 80 (23-143) ml/min/1.73 m^2). Hereafter, GFR was measured yearly with a plasma clearance technique for at least 3 years, median 7 (range 3.0 to 8.3) years. The mean rate of decline in GFR was 3.7 (0.3) ml/min/year. A linear regression analysis revealed a borderline significant relation between rate of decline in GFR and tHcy (p=0.069) and PAI-1 (p=0.087), respectively. Analyzing rate of decline in GFR and tertiles of tHcy and PAI-1, increasing levels of tHcy was correlated with a faster decline in GFR, p=0.025, whereas PAI-1 was not. However, after adjustment for other risk factors for progression of nephropathy, i.e. progression promoters, in a multiple linear regression analysis, neither tHcy nor PAI-1 was independent predictors of rate of decline in GFR. Our study demonstrates a relation between plasma tHcy and the rate of decline in GFR. Plasma tHcy and PAI-1 were, however, not found to be independent predictors of progression in diabetic nephropathy after adjustment for other well established progression promoters.

Introduction

Diabetic nephropathy is a leading cause of end stage renal disease and develops in approximately 35% of type 1 diabetic patients.[1;2] The disease is progressive and characterized by persistent albuminuria, arterial blood pressure elevation and a relentless decline in glomerular filtration rate (GFR).[3] However, the decline in GFR varies substantially between patients, ranging from 2 to 20 ml/min/year.[4-6] In order to improve intervention in patients with accelerated progression of renal disease, the identification of new predictors of progression is of particular importance. Several prospective studies support a relationship between hyperhomocysteinemia and cardiovascular disease,[7-9] and a rise in plasma total homocysteine (tHcy) with increasing urinary albumin excretion rate has been demonstrated in diabetes.[10,11] Plasminogen activator inhibitor-1 (PAI-1) has been associated with coronary heart disease[12] and with matrix accumulation in various glomerulopathies.[13-15] Hence, it is possible that circulating elevated tHcy and PAI-1 may contribute to progression in diabetic kidney disease. The aim of the present prospective observational cohort study was to evaluate the importance of circulating tHcy and PAI-1 at baseline as predictors of the rate of decline in GFR in type 1 diabetic patients with diabetic nephropathy. All patients (n=157) had serial measurements of GFR performed yearly during at least 3 years follow up.

Methods

Patients

In 1993, all type 1 diabetic patients with diabetic nephropathy, who had their GFR measured at Steno Diabetes Center during this year (n=242), were identified for a case-control study.[16,17] Blood samples were

M.M. Avram (ed.), Improving Prognosis for Kidney Disorders, 97-101.

obtained from 199 adult Caucasian patients (122 men, 77 women) with diabetic nephropathy, diagnosed clinically as: Persistent albuminuria >300 mg/24h in at least 2 out of 3 consecutive 24 hours urine collections, presence of diabetic retinopathy and no evidence of renal disease other than diabetic glomerulosclerosis.[18,19] In order to make a valid determination of the rate of decline in GFR, the patients were followed for at least 3 years with yearly GFR measurements until 2001. Of the 199 nephropathic patients, 15 patients had died, 13 patients had progressed to end stage renal failure, 14 patients had moved away from Copenhagen, and 157 patients remained in the study. The local ethical committee approved the experimental design, and all patients gave their informed consent.

Procedures

All investigations were performed in the morning after an overnight fast, in an attempt to avoid diurnal variation. Venous blood was drawn with minimal stasis from an antecubital vein in EDTA tubes. Centrifugation was performed at 1500 g for 10 minutes within an hour and plasma stored at -80 °C. Total (free plus protein bound) homocysteine levels were measured in duplicate as previously described in detail.[20] The intra-assay and inter-assay coefficients of variation were 2.1 % and 5.1 % respectively. Plasma PAI-1 antigen was determined in all samples in a single assay run, using the Thrombonostika PAI-1 ELISA kit (Organon Teknika, Turnhout, Belgium). In parallel assays (n=11) using pooled normal plasma, the intra assay coefficient of variation was 6.8 %. Glomerular filtration rate was measured after a single intravenous injection of 3.7 $MBq^{51}Cr$-EDTA by determining the radioactivity in venous blood samples taken 180, 200, 220 and 240 minutes after the injection,[21] and the results were standardized for 1.73 m^2 body surface area. Hemoglobin A_{1C} (HbA_{1C}) was determined from venous blood samples by high performance liquid chromatography (DIAMAT Analyzer, BIO-RAD, California, USA). Normal range of HbA_{1C} in our laboratory is 4.1-6.4 %. Serum creatinine concentration was assessed by a kinetic Jaffe' method. Urinary albumin concentration was determined by $ELISA_{22}$ from 24 hours urine collections. Arterial blood pressure was measured twice with a Hawksley random zero sphygmomanometer (Hawksley & Sons Ltd, Lancing, Sussex, UK) and appropriate cuff size after at least 10 minutes rest in the supine position. Diastolic blood pressure was recorded at the disappearance of Korotkoff sounds (phase V). Retinopathy was assessed by fundus photography after pupillary dilatation and graded: nil, simplex or proliferative diabetic retinopathy.

Statistical Analysis

Plasma tHcy, PAI-1, serum creatinine and urinary albumin excretion rate were non-normally distributed; and values are given as medians (range) and logarithmically transformed before analysis. All other values are given as means ± SD. In normally or log normally distributed variables, comparison between groups was performed by an unpaired Students-*t*-test or analysis of variance (ANOVA). A linear regression analysis was performed for each patient, and the slope was used to determine the rate of decline in GFR. Multiple regression analysis was performed with rate of decline in GFR as dependent variable and backwards selection including all variables with $p<0.10$ in univariate analysis. A p-value < 0.05 (two sided) was considered statistically significant. All calculations were performed with a commercially available program, SPSS 10.0 (SPSS Inc., Chicago, Illinois, USA).

Results

The characteristics of the 157 patients at baseline are shown in **Table 1**.

During the follow up period of investigation period of 7 (range 3.0 to 8.3) years, the mean rate of decline in GFR rate was 3.7 (0.3) ml/min/year. No relationship between rate of decline in GFR and baseline GFR was detected, NS.

A borderline significant correlation between rate of decline in GFR and plasma tHcy and plasma PAI-1

Table 1. Baseline clinical characteristics and laboratory results of 157 type 1 diabetic patients with diabetic nephropathy.

Sex (men/women)	92 / 65
Age (years)	41 ± 10
Duration of diabetes (years)	27 ± 8
Glomerular filtration rate (ml/min/1.73 m^2)	80 (23 - 143)
Serum creatinine (µmol/l)	92 (54 - 337)
Blood pressure (mm Hg)	148 ± 21 / 85 ± 12
Antihypertensive treatment	76 %
Albuminuria (mg/24hours)*	761 (16 – 8824)
Hemoglobin A_{1c} (%)	9.5 ± 1.5
Serum cholesterol (mmol/l)	5.6 ± 1.2
Retinopathy (simplex/proliferative)	51 / 106
Plasma total homocysteine (µmol/l)	10.8 (5.0 – 37.9)
Plasma PAI-1 (ng/ml)	64 (19-200)

Data are n, means ± SD or medians (range).

*) Some patients with previously persistent albuminuria receiving antihypertensive medication had urinary albumin excretion rate <300 mg/24 hours, at the time of the investigation.

were found. In a univariate linear regression analysis, a ten-fold increase in plasma tHcy (μmol/l) was equivalent to an increase in the decline of GFR of 3.3 ml/min/year (p=0.069); and a ten-fold increase in plasma PAI-1 (ng/ml) corresponded to an increased decline in GFR of 1.7 ml/min/year (p=0.087).

The relationship between the rate of decline in GFR and the potential progression promoters tHcy and PAI-1 separated in tertiles is shown in **Figure 1**.

When analyzing rate of decline in GFR and tertiles of tHcy, it was demonstrated that patients with the lowest levels of tHcy had a slower decline in GFR, ANOVA: p=0.025. No significant relation between rate of decline in GFR and tertiles of PAI-1 was found, ANOVA: p=0.12.

In a multiple linear regression analysis with rate of decline in GFR as dependent variable, including all variables with p<0.10 in univariate analysis (tHcy, PAI-1, blood pressure, albuminuria, hemoglobin A1c, serum cholesterol and gender), tHcy and PAI-1 were not included in the final model and were not independent predictors of decline in GFR.

Discussion

The significance of different progression promoters as predictors of progression is important for the identification of the subset of patients in need of more intensive interventions. Baseline progression promoters have been evaluated in the Captopril Collaborative study with a median follow up time of three years including 409 type 1 diabetic patients with diabetic nephropathy. Though the interrelationship between many risk factors often confounds the assessment of the relative significance of individual risk factors, elevated mean arterial blood pressure, high blood glucose, increased serum creatinine, enhanced proteinuria and presence of edema were found to predict doubling of serum creatinine.[23] In the present study, new additional predictors of progression were evaluated; and a tendency towards increase in the rate of decline in GFR with increasing plasma levels of tHcy and PAI-1 were demonstrated as seen in **Figure 1**. Plasma tHcy and PAI-1 were, however, not found to be independent predictors of progression in diabetic nephropathy after adjustment for other progression promoters.

Plasma tHcy has been identified as a risk factor for vascular disease affecting heart, brain and extremities,[7-9] and has been demonstrated to be a significant predictor of mortality in type 2 diabetes.[24] There is growing evidence that homocysteine induces endothelial dysfunction by promoting oxidative damage.[25] Studies have demonstrated elevated tHcy in type 1 diabetes,[11;26] but results have been conflicting.[10;27] Nevertheless, plasma tHcy has consistently been positively correlated to the level of albuminuria in both type 1 and type 2 diabetes,[10;11;28] and increased tHcy has been related to the severity of diabetic and non-diabetic kidney disease.[10;28;29] The presence of elevated tHcy concentrations may partially explain the observed acceleration of atherosclerosis in end-stage kidney disease, but it remains unclear whether the elevated tHcy is due to impaired metabolism or to reduced excretion in these patients.[25] In our prospective observational cohort study, we did not find acceleration in the rate of decline in GFR in patients with reduced GFR. We demonstrate a borderline significant correlation between tHcy and the rate of decline in GFR, although tHcy was not found to be an independent predictor of the rate of decline in GFR.

PAI-1 plays a critical inhibitory role in the regulation of intravascular fibrinolysis in addition to involvement in tissue repair and remodeling directly or by activation of latent matrix metalloproteinases. PAI-1 is directly induced by angiotensin II and exerts its

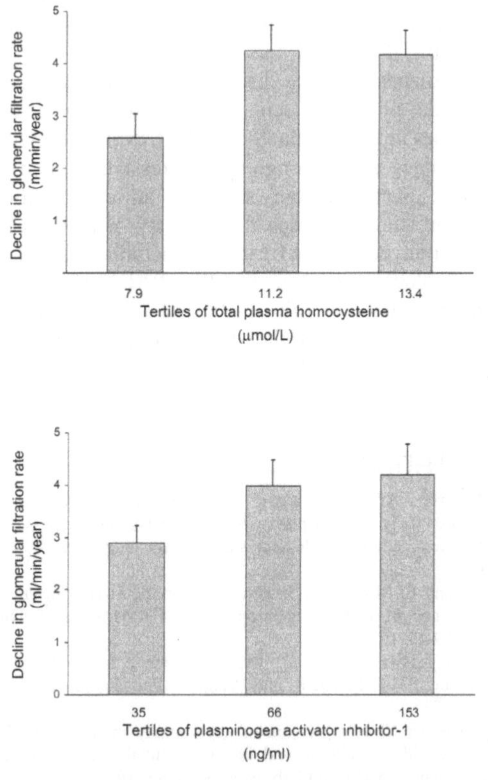

Figure 1.
Impact on decline in glomerular filtration rate of plasma total homocysteine (ANOVA, p=0.025) and plasminogen activator inhibitor-1 (ANOVA, p=0.12) separated in tertiles.

action through inhibition of tissue plasminogen activator (t-PA) and urokinase-like plasminogen activator (u-PA).[30] PAI-1 has been associated with coronary heart disease[12] and with matrix accumulation in glomerular disease.[13-15] In type 1 diabetes, PAI-1 levels did not differ from non-diabetic controls in patients without late diabetic complications,[31;32] whereas elevated PAI-1 has been related to increased urinary albumin excretion rate.[31;33] We have previously demonstrated that plasma PAI-1 is elevated in men with diabetic nephropathy as compared with normo-albuminuric diabetic men.[34] In the present study of progression of diabetic nephropathy, we were unable to detect a relationship between plasma PAI-1 concentration and the decline in kidney function. In an animal study by Fogo et al, the mRNA overexpression of PAI-1 was localized to injured mesangial and endothelial areas; whereas minimal PAI-1 expression was seen in intact glomeruli. Furthermore, levels of PAI-1 were increased in sclerotic glomeruli; and treatment with angiotensin converting enzyme inhibitors (ACE-I) or angiotensin II receptor antagonists (AIIA) significantly inhibited the upregulation of PAI-1.[35] These observations imply several explanations for the findings that plasma PAI-1 concentration did not predict progression of diabetic kidney disease in the present study. Firstly, the possibility remains that circulating PAI-1 levels does not reflect the local PAI-1 expression within the kidney and the ongoing progressive glomerulosclerosis. Secondly, our study is an observational follow up study in which the majority of patients received antihypertensive treatment, including ACE-I, to control blood pressure. Finally, PAI-1 expression might play a major role in the initiation of diabetic nephropathy, whereas the effect on progression of overt diabetic kidney disease could be more modest.

The rate of decline in GFR in diabetic nephropathy can vary widely between patients, from 2 to 20 ml/min/year.[4-6] So-called progression promoters can partly explain the inter-individual variability in the rate of decline in GFR.[36] The knowledge of progression promoters during the course of the disease is essential in every day treatment of the patients in order to postpone, or even prevent, the development of end stage renal disease. In a previous study, we evaluated the course of diabetic kidney disease in 301 type 1 diabetic patients with diabetic nephropathy followed for a median of 7 years with yearly GFR determinations.[37] Arterial hypertension, albuminuria, glycemic control, and dyslipidemia were identified as independent progression promoters. Furthermore, smoking and the ACE insertion/deletion polymorphism have been suggested to be of importance for the decline in renal function in diabetic nephropathy as reviewed by Rossing.[36]

In summary, our study demonstrates a relation between plasma tHcy and the rate of decline in GFR. However, tHcy and PAI-1 were not found to be independent predictors of progression in diabetic nephropathy after adjustment for other progression promoters.

Acknowledgments

The Paul and Erna Sehested Hansen Foundation, The Per S. Henriksen Foundation, and the Danish Diabetes Association are gratefully thanked for financial support. J.J. Emeis is a recipient of grant 28-2623 from the Praeventiefonds.

We acknowledge the excellent technical assistance of Ms C.M. van den Hoogen, and the assistance of B.V. Hansen, Ms B.R. Jensen and Ms U.M. Smidt in conducting this study.

References

1. Andersen AR, Christiansen JS, Andersen JK, Kreiner S, Deckert T: Diabetic nephropathy in Type 1 (insulin-dependent) diabetes: an epidemiological study. Diabetologia 25:496-501, 1983
2. Rossing P, Rossing K, Jacobsen P, Parving H-H: Unchanged incidence of diabetic nephropathy in IDDM patients. Diab 44:739-43, 1995
3. Parving H-H, Østerby R, Ritz E: Diabetic nephropathy, in Brenner BM (ed): The Kidney, Chap 39. Philadelphia, 2000, pp 1731-73.
4. Mogensen CE: Progression of nephropathy in long-term diabetics with proteinuria and effect of initial antihypertensive treatment. Scand J Clin Lab Invest 36:383-8, 1976
5. Parving H-H, Smidt UM, Friisberg B, Bonnevie-Nielsen V, Andersen AR: A prospective study of glomerular filtration rate and arterial blood pressure in insulin-dependent diabetics with diabetic nephropathy. Diabetologia 20:457-61, 1981
6. Viberti GC, Bilous RW, Mackintosh D, Keen H: Monitoring glomerular function in diabetic nephropathy. Am J Med 74:256-64, 1983
7. Boushey CJ, Beresford SA, Omenn GS, Motulsky AG: A quantitative assessment of plasma homocysteine as a risk factor for vascular disease. Probable benefits of increasing folic acid intakes. JAMA 274:1049-1057, 1995
8. Perry IJ, Refsum H, Morris RW, Ebrahim SB, Ueland PM, Shaper AG: Prospective study of serum total homocysteine concentration and risk of stroke in middle-aged British men. Lancet 346:1395-8, 1995
9. Arnesen E, Refsum H, Bonaa KH, Ueland PM, Forde OH, Nordrehaug JE: Serum total homocysteine and coronary heart disease. Int J Epidemiol 24:704-9, 1995
10. Chico A, Perez A, Cordoba A, Arcelus R, Carreras G, de Leiva A, Gonzalez-Sastre F, Blanco-Vaca F: Plasma homocysteine is related to albumin excretion rate in patients with diabetes

mellitus: a new link between diabetic nephropathy and cardiovascular disease? Diabetologia 41:684-93, 1998
11. Hofmann MA, Kohl B, Zumbach MS, Borcea V, Bierhaus A, Henkels M, Amiral J, Schmidt AM, Fiehn W, Ziegler R, Wahl P, Nawroth PP: Hyperhomocyst(e)inemia and endothelial dysfunction in IDDM. Diabetes Care 21:841-8, 1998
12. Hamsten A, Eriksson P: Fibrinolysis and atherosclerosis. Bailliers Clinical Haematology 8:345-63, 1995
13. Nakamura T, Tanaka N, Higuma N, Kazama T, Kobayashi I, Yokota S: The localization of plasminogen activator inhibitor-1 in glomerular subepithelial deposits in membranous nephropathy. J Am Soc Nephrol 7:2434-44, 1996
14. Brown NJ, Nakamura S, Ma L, Nakamura I, Donnert E, Freeman M, Vaughan DE, Fogo AB: Aldosterone modulates plasminogen activator inhibitor-1 and glomerulosclerosis in vivo. Kidney Int 58:1219-27, 2000
15. Fogo AB: Progression and potential regression of glomerulosclerosis. Kidney Int 59:804-19, 2001
16. Tarnow L, Cambien F, Rossing P, Nielsen FS, Hansen BV, Lecerf L, Poirier O, Danilov S, Parving H-H: Lack of relationship between an insertion/deletion polymorphism in the angiotensin-I-converting enzyme gene and diabetic nephropathy and proliferative retinopathy in IDDM patients. Diab 44:489-94, 1995
17. Tarnow L, Cambien F, Rossing P, Nielsen FS, Hansen BV, Lecerf L, Poirier O, Danilov S, Boelskifte S, Borch-Johnsen K, Parving H-H: Insertion/deletion polymorphism in the angiotensin-I-converting enzyme gene is associated with coronary heart disease in IDDM patients with diabetic nephropathy. Diabetologia 38:798-803, 1995
18. Parving H-H, Andersen AR, Smidt UM, Svendsen PAa: Early aggressive antihypertensive treatment reduces rate of decline in kidney function in diabetic nephropathy. Lancet i:1175-9, 1983
19. Mogensen CE, Chachati A, Christensen CK, Close CF, Deckert T, Hommel E, Kastrup J, Lefevre P, Mathiesen ER, Feldt-Rasmussen B, Schmitz A, Viberti GC: Microalbuminuria: an early marker of renal involvement in diabetes. Uremia Invest 9:85-95, 1985
20. te Poele-Pothoff MT, van den BM, Franken DG, Boers GH, Jakobs C, de Kroon IF, Eskes TK, Trijbels JM, Blom HJ: Three different methods for the determination of total homocysteine in plasma. Ann Clin Biochem 32 (Pt 2):218-20, 1995
21. Bröchner-Mortensen J, Rödbro P: Selection of routine method for determination of glomerular filtration rate in adult patients. Scand J Clin Lab Invest 36:35-45, 1976
22. Feldt-Rasmussen B, Dinesen B, Deckert M: Enzyme immunoassay: an improved determination of urinary albumin in diabetics with incipient nephropathy. Scand J Clin Lab Invest 45:539-44, 1985
23. Breyer JA, Bain P, Evans JK, Nahman NS, Lewis E, Cooper ME, McGill JB, Berl T, The Collaborative Study Group: Predictors of the progression of renal insufficiency in patients with insulin-dependent diabetes and overt diabetic nephropathy. Kidney Int 50:1651-8, 1996
24. Stehouwer CD, Gall MA, Hougaard P, Jakobs C, Parving HH: Plasma homocysteine concentration predicts mortality in non-insulin- dependent diabetic patients with and without albuminuria. Kidney Int 55:308-14, 1999
25. Welch GN, Loscalzo J: Homocysteine and atherothrombosis. N Engl J Med 338:1042-50, 1998
26. Targher G, Bertolini L, Zenari L, Cacciatori V, Muggeo M, Faccini G, Zoppini G: Cigarette smoking and plasma total homocysteine levels in young adults with type 1 diabetes. Diabetes Care 23:524-8, 2000
27. Pavia C, Ferrer I, Valls C, Artuch R, Colome C, Vilaseca MA: Total homocysteine in patients with type 1 diabetes. Diabetes Care 23:84-7, 2000
28. Stabler SP, Estacio R, Jeffers BW, Cohen JA, Allen RH, Schrier RW: Total homocysteine is associated with nephropathy in non-insulin- dependent diabetes mellitus. Metabolism 48:1096-101, 1999
29. Bostom AG, Lathrop L: Hyperhomocysteinemia in end-stage renal disease: prevalence, etiology, and potential relationship to arteriosclerotic outcomes. Kidney Int 52:10-20, 1997
30. Fogo A: The role of angiotensin II and plasminogen activator inhibitor-1 in progressive glomerulosclerosis. American Journal of Kidney disease 35:179-88, 2000
31. Jensen T, Feldt-Rasmussen B, Bjerre-Knudsen J, Deckert T: Features of endothelial dysfunction in early diabetic nephropathy. Lancet i:461-3, 1989
32. Auwerx J, Bouillon R, Collen D, Geboers J: Tissue-type plasminogen activator antigen and plasminogen activator inhibitor in diabetes mellitus. Arteriosclerosis 8:68-72, 1998
33. Gruden G, Cavallo-Perin P, Bazzan M, Stalla S, Vuolo A, Pagano G: PAI-1 and factor VII activity are higher in IDDM patients with microalbuminuria. Diab 43:426-9, 1994
34. Tarnow, L., Stehouwer, C. D. A., Emeis, J. J., Poirier, O., Cambien, F., Hansen, B. V., and Parving, H.-H. Plasminogen activator inhibitor-1 and apolipoprotein E gene polymorphisms and diabetic nephropathy. Nephrol Dial Transplant 15:625-30, 2000
35. Oikawa T, Freeman M, Lo W, Vaughan DE, Fogo A: Modulation of plasminogen-activator inhibitor-1 in-vivo - a new mechanism for the anti-fibrotic effect of renin- angiotensin inhibition. Kidney Int 51:164-72, 1997
36. Rossing P: Promotion, prediction, and prevention of progression in diabetic nephropathy. Diabetic Med 15:900-19, 1998
37. Hovind, P., Rossing, P., Tarnow, L., Smidt, U. M., and Parving, H.-H. Progression of diabetic nephropathy. Kidney Int 51: 702-9, 2001

12 Effects of Erythropoietin(EPO)and Aminoguanidine (AG) on Deformability (df) in Diabetic Azotemic and Uremic Patients

CLINTON D. BROWN, ZHONG H. ZHAO, LORRAINE L.THOMAS, R. DEGROOF, ELI A. FRIEDMAN, MD

Abstract

Impaired RBC-deformability (RBC-df) is noted in diabetes and may play a role in the pathogenesis of micrrovasculopathy and nephropathy. We now report the effects of EPO alone and combined EPO and AG (Alteon, Ramsey, NJ) treatment for one year on RBC-df in pre-dialysis patients with renal insufficiency (P-DPs) and patients with end stage renal diseases (ESRD) on maintenance hemodialysis (DPs).

The RBC-df (filterability) is defined as the ability of washed RBCs suspension to filter through polycarbonate membranes of 3μm pores. A qualitative measurement of RBC-df was expressed as a deformability index (DI), defined as the filtration rate of RBCs suspension through the filter divided by filtration rate of the buffer solution, and is inversely related to RBC-df. DI was measured at 0, 6 and 12 months of study. Nine P-DPs (mean serum creatinine 4.1 ± 0.1 mg/dl), who received EPO 50u/kg by subcutaneous injection thrice weekly, are compared to five P-DPs (mean serum creatinine 4.2 ± 0.6) treated without EPO. Twelve DPs (kt/v = 1.5 ± 0.1) were studied. Six DPs received AG 200mg/every other day by mouth and EPO 50u/kg by IV injection, and six received EPO (50u/kg) and placebo served as control.

After 12 months of study: significantly improved RBC-df was noted in nine P-DPs treated with EPO at 6 months (from 2.7 ± 0.1 to 1.6 ± 0.2, p = 0.005) and this positive effect was sustained at 12 months (p =0.005); there was no change in RBC-df in P-DPs receiving usual care without EPO. There was significant and progressive improvement in RBC-df at 6 and 12 months (from 2.2 ± 0.2 to 1.8 ± 0.2, p = 0.01, 1.2 ± 0.1, p = 0.001, respectively) in DPs treated with EPO and AG; there was limited improvement in RBC-df in DPs treated with EPO and placebo.

We conclude that treatment with EPO significantly improved RBC-df in diabetic P-DPs, but EPO alone has no significant effect on RBC-df after 12 months of treatment in diabetic DPs. The combination of EPO and AG restores RBC-df to near normal in diabetic DPs. We speculate that the effect of EPO on RBC-df seen in P-DPs and DPs may be related to the increased synthesis and influx of new and younger RBCs. Ag may confer protection of RBCs in DPs by blocking AGE formation.

M.M. Avram.(ed.), Improving Prognosis for Kidney Disorders, 103-108.

Introduction

Impaired RBC-deformability (RBC-df), a hemorrheologic perturbation induced by diabetes mellitus, may be implicated in the pathogenesis of diabetic microvasculopathy and nephropathy.[1-5] While searching for targets for possible therapeutic intervention in diabetes, we previously demonstrated that the effectiveness of aminoguanidine (Ag), a potent inhibitor of advanced glycosylated end-products (AGEs), improved or reversed the impaired RBC-df, not only in an animal model of diabetes,[6] but in diabetic patients as well.[7] Recombinant human erythropoietin (EPO), administrated for the correction of the anemia in chronic azotemic and uremic patients, have also been shown to improve impaired RBC-df. We assessed the effects of EPO alone and combined EPO plus AG on RBC-df by comparing area under the curve obtained throughout 12 months observation in both diabetic azotemic and uremic patients.

Research Design and Methods

Patients

A total of twenty six diabetic azotemic and uremic patients were studied. Patient demographics and clinical features are shown in **Table 1**. Informed consent was obtained from all subjects.

The pre-dialysis group comprised 14 azotemic patients (mean serum creatinine 4.2 ± 0.2mg/dl), who have renal insufficiency but do not as yet require

Table 1. Patient Demographics and Clinical Features. All parameters were not significantly different between subgroups.

	Predialysis (N=14)			Hemodialysis (N-12)		
	EOP[9]	No EPO[5]	Total	EPO + AG[6]	EPO + Placebo[6]	Total
Age	59.4 ± 4.7	53.4 ± 4.9		56.8 ± 9.1	56.8 ± 5.4	
Gender (M/F)	1/8	4/1		2/4	2/4	
Fasting glucose	125.9 ± 12.6	118.8 ± 3.2		175.2 ± 3.6	207.6 ± 6.2	
SCr. (mg/dl)	4.1 ± 0.4	4.2 ± 0.6	4.2 ± 0.2	8.6 ± 3.5	8.9 ± 1.2	8.8 ± 1.8
MCV (FL)	89.2 ± 1.8	90.6 ± 1.3		90.4 ± 1.3	91.2 ± 2.5	
HCT (%)	27.2 ± 0.9	29.2 ± 0.6	27.9 ± 0.6	33.2 ± 0.9	31.3 ± 1.5	32.3 ± 0.9*
Alb. (g/L)	3.8 ± 0.1	3.8 ± 0.33		3.7 ± 0.5	3.6 ± 0.4	
DI	2.7 ± 0.1	2.5 ± 0.1	2.6 ± 0.1**	2.2 ± 0.2	1.8 ± 0.1	2.1 ± 0.1

*Two to Four months after EPO treatment, hematocrit measured at beginning study, compared with pre-EPO treatment mean hematocrit values, (23.9 ± 0.7)(p = 0.0005)

** Mean DI at baseline is higher in pre-dialysis group (2.6 ± 0.1) than in hemodialysis group (2.1 ± 0.1, p = 0.005), meaning more deformable RBC seen in uremic patients.

dialysis; of these, nine patients (mean creatinine concentration 4.1 ± 0.4mg/dl) treated with EPO 50u/kg by subcutaneous injection thrice weekly were compared to five patients (mean serum creatinine 4.2 ± 0.6mg/dl) treated without EPO.* The hemodialysis group included twelve diabetic patients with ESRD (mean serum creatinine 8.8 ± 1.8mg/dl); six patients (mean serum creatinine 8.6 ± 3.5mg/dl) received Ag (200 mg every other day by mouth) and EPO (50u/kg by subcutaneous injection) thrice weekly, and six (mean serum creatinine 8.9 ± 1.2mg/dl) received EPO (50u/kg) thrice weekly and placebo.

All patients with ESRD initiated hemodialysis (three times per week, each session for four hours, mean kt/v = 1.5 ± 0.1) two to four months prior to study enrollment. EPO was administered to each uremic patient during hemodialysis because of severe anemia (mean hematocrit 23.9 ± 0.7%, measured prior to EPO treatment). RBC-df was measured at baseline, 6 and 12 months of study.

Measuring Erythrocyte Deformability

The RBC-df, measured by filtration technique, is defined by the rate of filtration of a dilute (4% of hematocrit values) suspensions of washed erythrocytes in phosphate buffered saline (PBS) solution through polycarbonate membranes with straight channels of 3μm diameter pore (Nucleopore, Corning, Acton, MA) under a constant negative pressure (-20 cm H2O). The filtration technique is a modification of the technique evolved by Reid et al.[8] and has been fully described in previous publications.[4,6] This technique is generally accepted as providing a relative indication of the ability of a erythrocyte to deform through the microcirculation,[1,3,5,9,13] but the problem most filtration systems have is a substantial change of filter area and decrement in flow rate due to pore blockage[11,14] and its relationship to mean cell volume (MCV).[12] To reduce confounding factors, the technique used was designed to achieve an accurate and reproducible measure by following principles: using suspensions of washed erythrocytes in PBS to eliminate hyperglycemia and hyperviscous plasma; polycarbonate membranes with pore size 3μm chosen because it is more sensitive to small changes in erythrocyte rheology compared to the 5μm pore filter;[9] Imugard ® IG 500 cotton wool (Terumo, Tokyo, Japan) pre-filtration method was used to exclude filter plugging by leukocytes and platelets and to prevent various cell-protein interactions.[10, 11]

To avoid the influence of buffer on MCV, we paid strict attention to buffer pH and osmolality (PBS of pH 7.4 and osmolality 295-300 mmol/kg). pH and osmolality remain constant from batch to batch.[12] This system, that has been used in our laboratory for nearly a decade, has shown its high degree of sensitivity in detecting an abnormal RBC-df in diabetics. It can be able to detect differences between deformable and stiff cells in induced diabetic rabbits,[6] as well as in patients with renal disease.[7,15] Additionally, RBCs that had passed the 3μm pores were seen to maintain their binconcave discoid shape and, in general, showed no sign of crenation or hemolysis in the filtrate, as examined by light microscopy, indicating that movement of cells through the pores is not impaired by blocked pores.[4,6]

Blood was carefully drawn from an antecubital vein of subjects to avoid stasis into vacutainer tubes containing 20 USP U/ml sodium heparin. A pure suspension of washed erythrocytes was prepared for filtration studies by the following procedure: whole blood was filtered through Imugard IG 500 cotton

* This group comprised patients who were followed from 1990-91 before EPO treatment became the standard of care and before medicaid reimbursement. All of these patients refused EPO treatment.

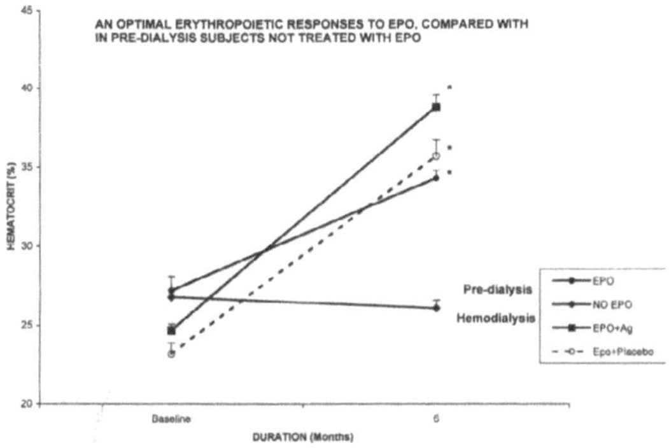

Figure 1. Six months after EPO treatment, an optimal erythropoietic responses, a consistently improve in their hematocrit were seen in both pre-dialysis and hemodialysis patients.
* Compared their own pre-EPO treatment values (P = 0.0005); But in pre-dialysis subjects not treated with EPO, the hematocrit was unchanged (p = 0.02).

layer were removed. Packed RBCs were washed three times in PBS solution (NaCl 8.3g, Kcl 0.2g, Na_2HPO_4wool. The effluent was centrifuged at 1000 x g for 10 minutes, and plasma, buffy coat, and uppermost RBC $0.7H_2O$ 0.94g, $NaH_2PO_4H_2O$ 0.2g, and 0.5g of bovine albumin, buffered to pH 7.4 with 0.1N Tris). The buffy coat was completely eliminated each time. Washed erythrocytes were aspirated from the middle of the packed erythrocyte column and resuspended in isotonic PBS to a final concentration of 4%. A qualitative measurement of RBC-df is expressed by the deformability index (DI) defined as: the time required for 5ml of red cell suspension to filter, divided by the time required for an equal volume of buffer to filter (a blank value). An increase in DI corresponds to a loss of filterability (reduction in deformability). Filtration results are reported as the average of two or three repeated tests and was normalized by a normal reference obtained from a group of age matched healthy adults (n =30). Normal DI =1.0. Sample preparation was performed at room temperature, and all filtration studies were maintained at $37C^0$ and performed within 3 hours of venopuncture.

Statistical Analyses

Results are presented as means ± SEM. Evaluation of the effects of Ag and EPO therapy on the RBC-df was performed by paired and unpaired tests. A p value < 0.05 were considered statistically significant. Correlation was performed using Pearson r. A p value less than 0.05 were considered significant.

Results

As shown in **Figure 1**, six months after EPO treatment, there was significant and optimal erythropoie-tic responses in dialysis and pre-dialysis patients treated with EPO, compared with their own pre-EPO treatment values (p = 0.0005). But in pre-dialysis subjects not treated with EPO, the hematocrit was unchanged (p = 0.02).

In the pre-dialysis group, nine azotemic patients treated with EPO showed significant improvement in RBC-df at 6 months (DI from 2.7 ± 0.1 to 1.6 ± 0.2, p = 0.005). This effect was sustained at 12 months (p = 0.005), In addition, a significant correlation existed between the absolute percent increase in hematocrit and the improvement in impaired RBC-df, as shown in **Figure 2** (p=0.04, r = 0.68). But in five pre-dialysis patients receiving usual care without EPO, there was no improvement in RBC-df (DI from 2.5 ± 0.1 to 2.6 ± 0.1, p = 0.2) (**Figure 3**).

As described above, all uremic patients on hemodialysis who received EPO during the 2 to 4 months prior to study had optimal erythropoietic responses. Mean hematocrit at the beginning study in uremic patients was remarkably improved (32.3 ± 0.9%) compared with pre- EPO treatment levels (23.9 ± 0.7% , P = 0.0005), as shown in **Table 1**. Simultaneously, DI shown at baseline was lower in hemodialysis group (2.1 ± 0.1) than in pre-dialysis group (2.6 ± 0.1) (meaning more deformable RBC in uremic patients than in azotemic patients, p = 0.005) (**Figure 3**). These results suggest that the better RBC-df observed in uremic patients group may be induced by the effect of EPO. In uremic patients, however, this effect seems to be limited. In a group treated with EPO and placebo there was no further significant improvement in RBC-

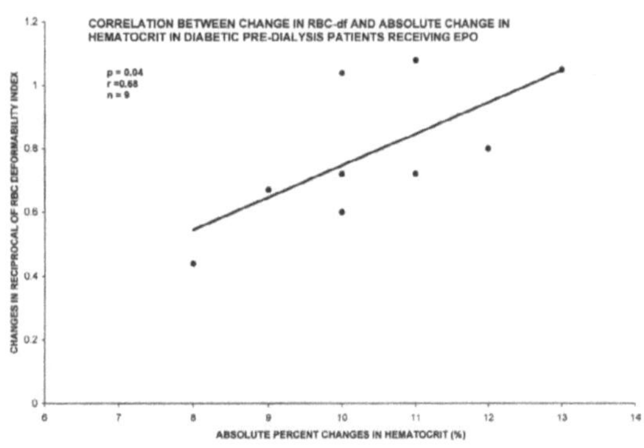

Figure 2. A significant (p = 0.04) correlation (r = 0.68) between absolute percent changes in hematocrit and changes (improvement) in RBC deformability impairment in nine pre-dialysis patients treated with EPO.

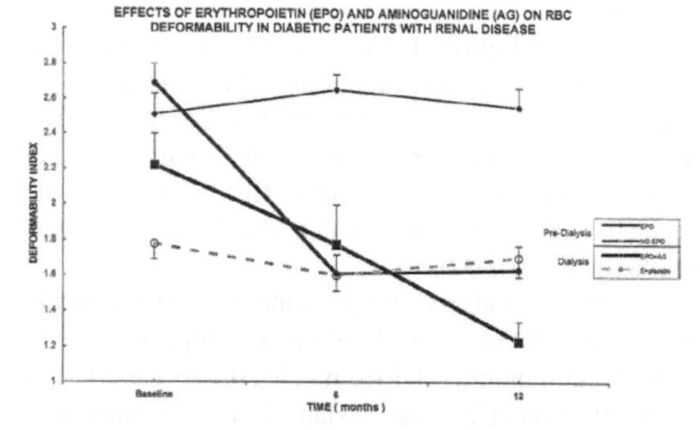

Figure 3. EPO improved RBC-df significantly at 12 months (p=0.005) in diabetic pre-dialysis patients(●), but no significant change in RBC-df seen in the same group patients without EPO treatment (◆). In diabetic patients with ESRD treated with EPO and placebo (O), there was no further improvement in RBC-df, although the early effect of EPO may exist. There was progressive improvement in RBC-df at 6 (p=0.01), 12 months (p=0.001) in diabetic patients with ESRD treated with EPO plus Ag (■). Normal RBC-df index = 1.0. Data are expressed as the mean ± SEM.

df (DI from 1.8 ± 0.1 to 1.7 ± 0.2, p = 0.3) despite continuing use of EPO.

In contrast, there was significant and progressive improvement in RBC-df at 6 months (DI from 2.2 ±0.2 to 1.8 ± 0.2, p = 0.01) and 12 months (1.2 ± 0.1, p = 0.001) in six uremic patients treated with EPO and Ag (**Figure 3**).

MCV levels in each of group, measured by centrifugation at 12,500g for 10 min., were shown in **Table 1**. There was no significant difference in MCV at baseline between pre-dialysis and hemodialysis groups. Furthermore, no appreciable changes in MCV was observed between before and after treatment in each group treated with EPO alone, EPO and placebo or the combination of EPO and Ag.

Discussion

In this study, we assessed and compared the effects of EPO alone and combined EPO plus AG treatment on RBC-df in both diabetic azotemic (pre-dialysis) and uremic patients (on maintenance hemodialysis). We found that treatment with EPO significantly improved RBC-df in diabetic azotemic patients; but in uremic patients, although EPO alone may have had an early effect on RBC-df shown at beginning study, there was no further improvement on RBC-df. However, the combination of EPO and AG restores RBC-df to near normal in diabetic patients with ESRD.

The mechanism underlying reduced RBC-df observed in diabetes remain unknown. However, Ag, an agent known to specifically block AGEs formation,[16,17] effectively corrects impaired RBC-df in diabetes.[6,7] This observation suggests that AGEs may contribute to the pathogenesis of RBC-df impairment observed in diabetes. This inference is unproved, since AGEs were not measured in this experiment. Supporting evidence does, however, implicate AGEs as an etiologic factor for RBC–df impairment include: 1) chronic hyperglycemia causes accelerated formation of AGEs;[18-20] 2) the relative long half-life of erythrocyte makes them a prime target for the formation of AGEs (in the membrane and hemoglobin);[21,22] and the evidence has been shown that alteration of rheological properties of human erythrocytes caused by crosslinking of membrane proteins.[23] The link between AGEs and RBC-df is further supported by the observations that tissue and serum AGEs levels rise as renal function declines in diabetic patients with nephropathy.[24] We have reported a highly significant direct correlation between severity of impairment in RBC-df and loss of renal function in diabetic patients.[15] Moreover, we have demonstrated that treatment with Ag both in diabetic rabbits and diabetic patients with ESRD corrects impaired RBC-df and that withdrawal of Ag resulted in the return of RBC-df to pre-treatment impairment.[6,7] Taken together, these observations prompt the hypothesis that excessive accumulation of AGEs (and/or AGE mediated action such as oxidative stress)[25] has a major adverse effect on RBC-df in diabetes.

A significant improvement in RBC-df was noted in pre-dialysis patients treated with EPO (p = 0.005) (**Figure 3**). It has been established that regulation of normal erythropoiesis is primarily under the control of erythropoietin.[26] As shown in **Figure 1**, a brisk improvement in hematocrit was noted in each group given EPO treatment (p = 0.0005). A link between erythropoiesis and RBC-df is supported by the finding that improvement in the absolute percent change in hematocrit correlated highly significant with improvement in mean RBC-df measured at baseline and at 6 months after treatment with EPO (Fig.2, p= 0.04, r = 0.68). The effect of EPO on RBC-df may presumably be mediated by enhancing the synthesis and influx of younger erythrocytes. The difference in rheologic properties between young and old RBCs have been demonstrated, and age-dependent decreases in RBC-df have been explained by various mechanisms.[27-29]

In diabetes, the decrease in RBC-df of aging RBC may be further altered by glycation. Schleicher et al.[30] noted that older RBCs, which are exposed for a longer time to glucose in the circulation, exhibit a higher (1.7 fold) amount of lysine-bound glucose of RBC membrane proteins and hemoglobin compared to young RBCs. The foregoing evidence led us to speculate that the significant improvement in RBC-df observed in

EPO treated azotemic patients may be related to increased synthesis and influx of young and relatively more deformable erythrocytes.

In uremic patients, the early (pre-baseline) effect of EPO (improvement in RBC-df) therapy may explain why mean RBC-df index shown at starting study was significantlly lower (2.1 ± 0.1) compared to in pre-dialysis groups (2.6 ± 0.1, p = 0.005) (**Figure 3**). But the rheologic effect of EPO appears to be limited, since there was no further improvement in RBC-df beyond 6 months of treatment (**Figure 3**). In contrast, in uremic patients treated with Ag and EPO, there was a significantly progressive improvement in RBC-df throughout 12 months of treatment (**Figure 3**).

There are two likely reasons that may explain the different effect on RBC-df in diabetic patients between treatment with EPO and Ag plus EPO. As mentioned above, the beneficial effect of EPO may be related to enhancing synthesis and influx of young erythrocytes, with no effect on glycation of RBCs. Because of the elevated ambient glucose concentration and glycation, RBCs remain susceptible to pathologic modification by AGEs, leading to deterioration in RBC-df. That may explain why the RBC-df response to EPO observed in pre-dialysis patients plateaus after 6 months of treatment. Another reason that EPO treatment failed to sustain and improve RBC-df in uremic patients may be the degree of renal insufficiency. The kidney plays a critical role in the catabolism of AGE.[31] Circulating AGE peptides, tissue-derived degradation pro-ducts of AGE-modified proteins, enter the circulation as low molecular weight species and are filtered by glomeruli, reabsorbed in the proximal tubule, degraded or modified, and finally excreted in the urine by the kidney.[31] Renal clearance of AGE peptides was not significantly different in diabetics with normal glomerular filtration (0.61 ± 0.2 ml/min) compared with normal subjects (0.72 ± 0.23 ml/min).[19] In renal failure, plasma AGE peptides increase directly with the severity of renal impairment. In diabetic patients with ESRD, serum AGEs can be increased by eightfold compared with normal subjects.[24] Furthermore, serum AGE pep-tides are not effectively removed by hemodialysis.[33] Intact renal function, therefore, plays an important role in the accumulation of AGEs in diabetic patients with ESRD.

On the other hand, a combination of EPO and Ag treatment restores impaired RBC-df to near normal in diabetic patients with ESRD (in **Figure 3**). Obviously, since treatment with EPO alone has a limited effect on RBC-df in uremic patients, this enhanced effect on RBC-df could be attributed to blockade of AGE by Ag.

Because multiple pharmacological action of Ag have been reported, in addition to blockade of AGEs formation, other actions of Ag may impact on RBC-df in diabetes, for example inhibition of aldose reduction,[33] diamine oxidase and NO production.[34] It is not known whether improvement in RBC-df impairment by Ag involves more than one mechanism.

References

1. Schmid-Schonbein H, Volger E: Red cell aggregation & red cell deformability in diabetes. Diabetes 25 (suppl. 2): 897-902, 1976
2. McMillan DE, Utterback NG, La puma J, Barbara,S: Reduced erythrocyte deformability in diabetes. Diabetes 27 (9): 895-901, 1978
3. Barnes AJ, Loeke P, Scudder PR, Dormandy JA, Slack J: Is hyperviscosity a treatable component of diabetic microcirculatory disease ? Lancet 2: 789-91, 1977
4. Brown CD, Zhao ZH, Berweek S, De Alvaro F, Chan S, Friedman EA: Effects of Alloxan-induced diabetes on hemorheology in rabbits. Horm Metabol Res 24 (6): 254-7,1992
5. Skalak R, Hanss M, Chien S: Indices of filterability of red blood cell suspensions. Biorheology 20: 311-16, 1983
6. Brown CD, Zhao ZH, De Alvaro F, Chan S, Friedman EA: Correation of erythrocyte deformability defect in ALX-induced diabetic rabbits after treatment with Aminoquanidine. Diabetes 16- 590-93,1993
7. Brown CD, Zhao ZH, Thomas LL, Wuerth JP, Friedman EA: Pimagedine improves RBC deformability in diabetic patients with ESRD. FASEB. J A6: 14 (4),2000
8. Reid HL, Barnes AJ, Lock PJ, Dormandy JA, Dormandy TL: A simple method for measuring erythrocyte deformability. J Clin Pathol 29: 855-58, 1976
9. Rainhart WH, Usami S, Schmalzer EA, Lee MML, Chien S: Evaluation of red blood cell filterability test: influences of pore size on hematocrit level, and flow rate. J Lab Clin med 104: 501-16,1984
10. Kenny MW, Meakin M, Stuart J: Methods for removal of leucocytes and platelets prior to study of erythrocyte deformability. Clinical Hemorheology. 3: 191-200, 1983
11. Stuart J, Stone PCW, Bareford D, Caldwell JE, Baar S: Evaluation of leucocyte remaval methods for studies of erythrocyte deformability. Clin Hemorheol. 5: 137- 47, 1985
12. Stuart J, Stone P.C,W., Bareford D, Bilto,YY: Effect of pore diameter and cell volume on erythrocyte filterability. Clinical hemorheology (5): 449-61,1985
13. Leblond PF, Coulombe L:The measurement of erythrocyte deformability using micropore membranes. A sensitive technique with clinical application. J Lab Clin Med 94: 133,1979
14. Gregersen MI, Bryant CA, Hammerle WE, Usami S, Chien S: Flow characteristics of human erythrocytes through polycarbonate sieves. Science 157: 825-27,1967
15. Brown CD, Zhao Z, Ghali H, Thomas L, Feiedman EA: Association of reduced RBC deformability and diabetic nephropathy (abstract) ASAIO 45 (2): 209,1999
16. Lewis BS, Harding JJ: The effects of aminoguanidine on the glycation (non- enzymic glycosylation) of lens proteins. Exp Eye Res 50: 463-67,1990
17. Edelstein D, Brownlee M: Mechanistic studies of advanced glycosylation end-product inhibition by aminoguanidine. Diabetes 41: 26-9,1992
18. Brownlee M, Cerami A, Vlassara H: Advanced glycosylation end products in tissue and the biochemical basis of diabetic complication. N Engl J Med 318: 1315-21,1988

19. Vlassara H: Serum advanced glycocylation end products: a new class of uremic toxin? Blood purif 12 (1): 54-9,1994
20. Cerami A, Vlassara H, Brownlee M: Role of advanced glycosylation products in complication of diabetes. Diabetes care 11 (suppl. 1): 73-9, 1988
21. Miller JA, Gravallese E, Bunn HF: Nonenzymatic glycosylation of erythrocyte membrane proteins: relevance to diabetes. J Clin Invest 65: 896-901,1980
22. Makita Z, Vlassara H, Bucala R: Hemoglobin AGE: A circulating marker of advanced glycosylation. Science 258: 651-53, 1992
23. Maeda N, Kon K, Imaizumi K. Sekiya M, Shiga T: Alteration of rheological properties of human erythrocytes by crosslinking of membrane proteins. Biochim Biophys Acta 735: 104-12, 1983
24. Makita Z, Radoff S, Rayfield E, Yang Z, Skolnik E, Delaney V, Friedman EA, Cerami A, Vlassara H: Advanced glycosylation end product in patients with diabetic nephropathy. N Engl J Med 325: 836-42, 1991
25. Baynes J: Role of oxidative stress in development of complications in diabetes. Diabetes 40-405-12, 1991
26. Lai PH, Everett R, Wang FF, Arakawa T, Goldwasser E: The primary structure of human erythropoietin. J Biol Chem 261: 3116-21, 1986
27. Tillmann W, Levin C, Prindull G, Schroter W: Rheological properties of young and Aged human erythrocytes. Klin Wochenschr 58: 569, 1980
28. Corry WD, Meiselman HJ: Centrifugal method of determining red cell deformability. Blood 51: 693-97, 1978
29. Shiga T, Maeda N, Suda T, Kon K, Sekiya M: The decreased membrane fluidity of in vivo aged, human erythrocytes. Biochim Biophys Acta 553: 84-7, 1979
30. Schleicher E, Scheller L, Wieland OH: Quantitation of lysine-bound glucose of normal and diabetic erythrocyte membranes by HPLC analysis of furosine. Biochem Biophys Res Commun 99(3): 1011-19,1981
31. Miyata T, Yasuhiko Ueda, Katsunori Horie, Masaomi Nangaku, Shuichi Tanaka,Charles Van Ypersele DE Strihou, Kiyoshi Kurokawa: Renal catabolism of advanced Glycation end products: The fate of pentosidine. Kidney Int 53: 416-22,1998
32. Papanastasiou P, GrassL, Rodela H, Patrikarea A, Oreopoulos D,Diamandis EP: Immunological quantification of advanced glycosylation end-products in the serum of patients on hemodialysis or CAPD. Kidney Int 46:216-22,1994
33. Kumari K, Umar S, Bansal V, Sahib MK: Inhibition of diabetes associated complication by nucliophilic compounds. Diabetes 40: 1079-84,1991
34. Corbett JA, Tilton RG, Chang K, Hasan KS, Ido J,Wang JC, Sweetland MA, Lancaster JR,Williamson JR, Mcdaniel ML: Aminoguanidine, a novel inhibitor of Nitric oxide formation, prevents diabetic vascular dysfunction. Diabetes 41:552-57, 1992

13 Characterization of the PKD1 Gene Product, Polycystin-1

ALESSANDRA BOLETTA, PHD, FENG QIAN, PHD, LUIZ F. ONUCHIC, MD, PHD, ALESSANDRA BRAGONZI, PH.D., MARINA CORTESE, M.SC., PIERRE J. COURTOY, MD, PHD, PETER M. DEEN, MD, PHD, MARCO R. SORIA, MD, PHD, OLIVIER DEVUYS, MD, PHDT, LUCIA MONACO, PHD, GREGORY G. GERMINO, MD

Summary

The most common form of autosomal dominant polycystic kidney disease results from mutation of the *PKD1* gene on chromosome 16p13.3. The gene encodes a 14kb mRNA that is predicted to result in a 462kDa membrane protein. The gene product, polycystin-1, has a large extracellular portion comprised of a novel combination of protein-protein interacting domains and is postulated to be a plasma membrane receptor involved in cell-cell/matrix interactions. Slow progress has been made in the characterization of polycystin-1 or the determination of its function, however. We attribute this delay to the lack of suitable reagents. In fact, the protein is expressed at very low levels in tissues and cell lines and previous efforts directed at expression of recombinant protein had been largely unsuccessful. We have recently developed constructs of full-length human *PKD1* cDNA that can be expressed in both a stable and transient fashion in mammalian cells. We used these systems to characterize our antibodies and to track the protein *in vivo*. We report here the first biochemical characterization of recombinant polycystin-1 and show that the protein is a 520kDa glycosylated polypeptide with an unglycosylated core of 460kDa. Subcellular fractionation as well as biotinylation studies confirmed that the protein is plasma-membrane associated. Furthermore, we show that the recombinant protein localizes to cell-cell junctions in polarized MDCK cells as revealed by indirect immunofluorescence. Our data represent the first characterization of polycystin-1 performed under highly controlled conditions.

Introduction

Autosomal Dominant Polycystic Kidney Disease (ADPKD) is one of the most common genetic diseases with an incidence of 1/1000. The main clinical manifestation is bilateral renal cyst formation; but ADPKD is a systemic disorder, since cysts can occur in other organs such as liver, pancreas and spleen and is associated with aortic and intracranial aneurysms.[1] Linkage studies have determined that the disease is genetically heterogeneous, with most cases resulting from mutations of either *PKD1* on chromosome 16 (~85%) or *PKD2* on chromosome 4 (~15%).

PKD1 encodes a 14kb mRNA that is predicted to yield a translation product of 4302 amino acids with an estimated molecular weight of at least 462kDa. The protein, polycystin-1, is predicted to have an extremely large extracellular amino terminus (~3000 residues) with numerous glycosylation sites, an odd number of transmembrane-spanning (TM) segments and a short intracellular carboxy-terminus.[2-4] The cytoplasmic carboxy terminus has a coiled-coil structure and a potential tyrosine phosphorylation site and appears to mediate the interaction of polycystin-1 with a number of other proteins including the *PKD2* gene product, polycystin-2.[5] The extracellular portion of polycystin-1 has a novel assortment of motifs[2-4,6] that suggest a role for the protein in mediating cell-cell and cell-matrix interactions but direct evidence supporting this model is lacking.

A major obstacle that has delayed characterization of polycystin-1 has been the lack of suitable, well-characterized reagents. Immunolocalization studies of polycystin-1 in tissues and cultured cells have reported contradictory results with respect to its pattern of expression at both the cellular and sub-cellular level. Similarly, a broad range of molecular weights (from 100 up to 600kDa) has been observed by Western blot analysis, with bands of ~400/450kDa most commonly described.[7-24] It is unclear whether these discrepancies are the result of non-specificity of the antisera that have been used or to the presence of several forms of the protein. One problem has been the absence of

M.M. Avram (ed.), Improving Prognosis for Kidney Disorders, 109-118.

proper negative and positive controls that could be used to verify the results.

Theoretically, over-expression of the full length cDNA for *PKD1* could be used to achieve this purpose. While a complete cDNA has been available for several years, previous attempts at expressing it in mammalian cells had been unsuccessful.[24-25] We have recently overcome this problem and established a series of Madin Darby Canine Kidney Cell (MDCK) lines with stable expression of full-length polycystin-1, which we used to define the first functional model for polycystin-1.[26] In the current study, we used these cell lines along with an epitope-tagged version of the full-length cDNA that can be transiently expressed in multiple cell types to characterize the protein. We provide the first biochemical characterization of *bona fide* polycystin-1 as well as its *in vitro* sub-cellular distribution. Furthermore, we employed our expression systems to characterize our antibodies and to track the protein presence *in vivo*.

Experimental Procedures

Expression Constructs

The β–globin intron and full length human *PKD1* cDNA was released from the pTRE-β-PKD1 vector[26] by digestion with *Spe*I and *Hind*III and cloned into the *Nhe*I/*Hind*III sites of pCI. The Flag epitope was inserted in-frame at the 3'end of the cDNA using a multi-step, PCR-based strategy. Primers 5'-TTTGATCAT CCTCCTTCCTGGCGGG-3' (Forward) and 5'- ACC TGATCACTTGTCATCGTCGTCCTTGTAGTCAGC TGCTGGGGTGGA-3' (Reverse) were used to amplify a 1000bp fragment using the *PKD1* cDNA KG8 as template.[3] The PCR product was digested with *Aat*II and then cloned into KG8 after an *Aat*II/*Hind*III fragment had been released and its *Hind*III site destroyed using Klenow. After verifying its sequence, we digested the modified KG8 with *Sal*I, treated with Klenow to create a blunt end, then digested again with *Sap*I to release a 1000bp fragment. The *Sap*I-blunt end fragment was cloned into pCI-β-PKD1 after a *Hind*III/*Sap*I fragment had been released and the *Hind*III site blunted as above. The correct sequence of the final construct was verified by sequencing.

RT-PCR

1μg of total RNA, isolated from cells using Trizol (Gibco) was reverse transcribed using MmLuV (New England Biolabs). PCR on cDNA was performed using the following primers and conditions: 5'-TCTTGA ATTCCACGCCTTGCGTGGAGAGFQ-3' (forward) and 5'-ATGGGCCACGGGAAGATC-3' (reverse) 30 cycles were performed at annealing temperature of 60°C. GAPDH primers (FQ-F33 5'-TCCTGCACCAC CAACTGCTTAG-3' and FQ-R35 5'-TGCTTCACCA CCTTCTTGATGTC-3') were used as controls.

Western Blot and Immunoprecipitation Studies

The C-T antiserum was generated using a fusion protein encoding the last 215 amino acids of human polycystin-1.[26] Affinity purification of the antibodies was performed by immobilizing the immunizing antigen to resin, followed by affinity chromatography according to the manufacturer's directions (AminoLink Plus kit, Pierce). Cell lysates were prepared by subjecting cells to three freeze/thaw cycles in lysis buffer (250 mM Sucrose, 20mM imidazole and 1mM EDTA, pH 7.4, 0.5% Triton-X 100). Total lysates were loaded on to 4%, 7.5% or 12% polyacrylamide gels for analysis of polycystin-1, Na+/K+ATPase, or aquaporin-2, respectively. Gels were blotted onto PVDF membranes, blocked in 5% milk in TBS-T. Antibodies were diluted in 2% BSA in TBS-T. The following dilutions were used for the various antisera: α-C-term (affinity purified) 1:100; α-C-term (affinity depleted) 1:1000; polyclonal α-Flag (Santa Cruz) 1:1000; anti-human AQP2, raised in rabbit (affinity-purified) 1:1,000 (reference); anti-Na/K-ATPase, α1 subunit, mouse monoclonal IgG, (Upstate Biotechnology) 1:2,000. The high molecular weight markers of Sigma were used with a urea-based buffer as recommended by the manufacturer.

For the immunoprecipitation studies, cells were resuspended in IP buffer (20mM NaH_2PO_4, 150mM NaCl, 10% glycerol, pH7.2, 0.5% Triton-X 100) and incubated on ice for 30 min. After the addition of α-C-term, the samples were rocked for 2 hrs at 4°C. G-Protein Sepharose beads (Amersham) were added, and the slurry was rocked for an additional 2h. The beads were pelleted, washed three times in lysis buffer, resuspended in 1X Laemli buffer, and loaded onto gels.

Biochemical Analyses

For the biotinylation assay, cells were grown to 50-60% confluence in P150 dishes, washed three times in borate buffer pH 9.00 and incubated for two 20 minute cycles at 4°C in the presence of 2.5 mg of NHS-SS-biotin (Pierce) diluted in borate buffer. The biotinylation reaction was arrested by using a quenching buffer containing TrisHcl (20 mM Tris, 120mM NaCl, pH 7.4) for 10 minutes, rinsed 3 times with PBS and lysed in IP buffer. Biotinylated proteins were immunoprecipitated using Streptavidin MagneSpheres (Promega), washed three times in lysis buffer, re-suspended in 1X Laemli buffer and processed for Western blot as above. PNGase (New England Biolabs) was used for the de-glycosylation studies according to the manufacturer's instructions. Identical samples treated in the absence of enzyme were included as negative controls.

Indirect Immunofluorescence

MDCK^{PKD1Zeo} and MDCK^{Zeo} cells were plated on 12mm transwells at a density of 2.5×10^5 cells/well and allowed to grow in 5% FCS for 4-6 days. Indirect immunofluorescence on polarized cells was performed as follows: cells were fixed in 4% paraformaldehyde, quenched in 75mM NH4Cl, 20mM glycine in PBS, washed with PBS and incubated for 15 min at 37°C in the presence of permeabilizing solution (0.7% gelatin, 0.016% saponin on PBS). Cells were then incubated in the presence of primary followed by secondary antibody in permeabilizing solution rocking at 37°C for 1hr or 30 min, respectively. Antibody dilutions were as follows: α-C-Term, 1:20. α-E-cadherin (clone C20820, Transduction Laboratories) 1:20; α-ZO-1 (Zymed) 1:50. TRITC-α-rabbit and FITC-α-mouse antibodies (Sigma) were used as secondary antibodies for α-C-Term/α-ZO-1 and α-E-cadherin, respectively. Samples were analysed using a Noran OZ confocal microscopy.

Tissue Sub-Cellular Fractionation

A sample from human kidney was obtained directly at surgery. The sample originated from the tumour-free pole of a kidney removed for polar hypernephroma. The use of such human sample has been approved by the University of Louvain Ethical Review Board. The sample was rinsed thoroughly with ice-cold PBS, the inner part of the medulla was dissected and collected into cold homogenization buffer.

Membrane and sub-cellular fractions were prepared as previously described.[27,29] Briefly, 0.5 g of medulla was homogenized in ice-cold 250mM sucrose, 3 mM imidazole, pH 7.4. The homogenate was centrifuged at 1000 *g* for 10 min. The pellet was re-suspended and centrifuged again at 1000 *g* for 10 min. The supernatants were pooled and defined as post-nuclear (E) extracts. The post-nuclear extract was centrifuged at 40,000 rpm for 30 min (3×10^6 g x min) in a fixed angle rotor to obtain a fraction combining all post-nuclear particles (fraction MLP) separated from the soluble components of the cells (fraction S). The post-nuclear particles were then re-suspended in buffer, layered on linear sucrose gradients (1.05 – 1.30 g/ml in density), and centrifuged at 49,000 rpm for 2 h (8×10^6 g x min) in a vertical rotor. After centrifugation, 14 fractions were collected, weighed and analyzed for density, and protein. Fraction #1 was collected at the bottom (high density) whereas fraction #14 was on the top (low density).

Results

1) Validation of α-PKD1 Antisera and Western Blot Analysis of Polycystin-1

As noted above we have recently developed a series of MDCK cell lines with stable expression of either human polycystin-1 (MDCK^{PKD1Zeo}) or empty vector (MDCK^{Zeo}). Each of the five independent MDCK^{PKD1Zeo} clones was shown by Western blot analysis to express a new protein >500kDa that is not present in 14 control cell lines. Three antisera generated using different portions of the protein detected the same band, confirming its identity as polycystin-1.[26]

One of the antiserum (α-C-Term), however, detected an additional >400 kDa band that was prominent in both the MDCK^{PKD1Zeo} and MDCK^{Zeo} lysates (**Figure 1A**, arrowhead). Given that MDCK cells express endogenous *PKD1* and that the size of this band is very close to what is predicted for polycystin-1 (462kDa), we queried whether the >400kDa band was in fact canine polycystin-1 or a non-specific signal. Our initial studies suggested that the signal was likely to be specific since neither the corresponding pre-immune serum nor α-C-term that had been depleted of its α-PKD1 activity by passage over a column containing the immunizing antigen yielded the same result. We speculated that differences in the length of the coding sequence in the two species could account for the size discrepancy. Alternatively, recombinant polycystin-1 could be subject to different post-translational modifications when expressed using a heterologous system.

The discovery that a band of identical size was recognized by the same antibody in multiple human and non-human cell lines (HeLa, Hek293, LLCPK, CHO, COS7, mIMCD) and tissues (human, mouse and rat brain and kidney) excluded both possibilities (data not shown). This result prompted us to consider alternative explanations for the phenomenon. One possibility was that endogenous *PKD1* was subject to splicing, yielding a slightly smaller mRNA and protein than that which results from forced over-expression of the full-length cDNA. Alternatively, recombinant polycystin-1 might be subject to different post-translational modifications than the endogenous form of the protein. Finally, it raised additional questions about the specificity of the antiserum.

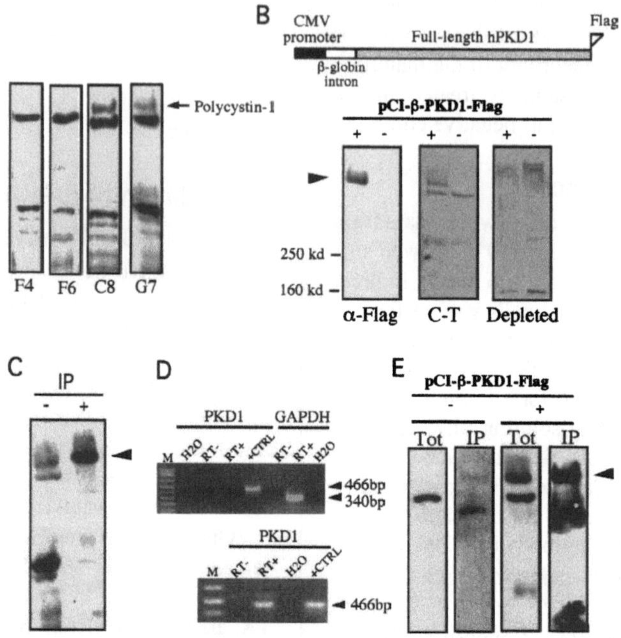

Figure 1. Western blot analysis of polycystin-1 and characterization of α-C-Term.
A. Immunoblot of 50µg of total cell lysates of two $MDCK^{PKD1Zeo}$ clones, C8 & G7, and two negative control lines ($MDCK^{Zeo}$), F4 & F6 that had been treated with 20mM sodium butyrate overnight. A new band was specifically observed in C8 & G7 (arrow), which is absent in F4 & F6.
B. Top: Schematic representation of the pCI-β-PKD1Flag insert. Bottom: Immunoblot of HeLa cells transiently transfected with the pCI-β-PKD1Flag construct. α-Flag detected a novel high molecular weight protein in cell lysates from transfected HeLa cells (+) which is absent in untransfected cells (-). A protein of identical size was detected by α-C-Term after re-probing the same membrane post-stripping. A second, slightly smaller protein of >400kDa was detected by α-C-Term in both the transfected and untransfected samples. The immunodepleted serum (far right) did not recognize either band and instead detected non-specific bands also recognized by the crude immune serum (data not shown).
C. Immunoblot of total cell lysate (-) and immunoprecipitation product (+) of the $MDCK^{PKD1Zeo}$ clone C8/68 probed with α-C-Term. α-C-Term was used to perform the immunoprecipitation (IP).
D. Top: HeLa cells are negative for *PKD1* mRNA expression as measured by RT-PCR. The pTRE-β-PKD1 vector (26) was used as a positive control for the *PKD1*-specific primers. In contrast, GAPDH primers yielded a specific product only in the RT+ lane, confirming the integrity of the HeLa mRNA used as template for both reactions. **Bottom:** Hek293 cells are positive for *PKD1* mRNA expression as measured by RT-PCR. The identical pair of primers and positive control used in Figure 1D was used for this experiment (35 cycles).
E. Polycystin-1 can be immunoprecipitated (IP) from Hek293 by α-C-Term. Lane 1, 50µg of total cell lysate of untransfected (-) Hek 293 cells. Lane 2, IP products of 1mg of total cell lysate of Hek293 cells. Lane 3, 50µg of total cell lysate of Hek293 cells transfected (+) with pCI-β-PKD1Flag. All samples were separated by PAGE on the same 4% polyacrylamide gel and immunoprobed using α-C-Term. An extremely faint band identical in size to the recombinant form of polycystin-1 was immunoprecipitated from Hek293 (lane 2).

In order to investigate the nature of such a band further, as well as to validate the specificity of our antibodies, we generated an epitope-tagged (Flag) form of polycystin-1that could be transiently expressed in a wide variety of different cell lines and easily detected using commercially available antibodies (**Figure 1B**, top). **Figure 1B** shows the results of transient expression of pCI-β–PKD1-Flag in the human cell line, HeLa. A >500kDa band was specifically recognized in the *PKD1*-transfected (+) and not in the untransfected (-) cells s by a polyclonal antibody specific for the Flag epitope (SantaCruz).

We next tested whether our α-C-term antiserum recognized the identical band. The same membrane was stripped, tested for residual signal and then re-probed using α-C-term. In parallel, we probed "sister" blots containing aliquots of the same samples with α-C-term and α-C-term antiserum depleted of its α-PKD1 activity. The affinity-purified antibody detected the same >500kDa band recognized by the α-Flag antiserum exclusively in the transfected samples (**Figure 1B**, bottom). It also detected the >400kDa band in both transfected and untransfected cells. In contrast, the affinity-depleted serum did not detect either band in any of the samples (**Figure 1B**, bottom). Using immunoprecipitation assays we found that we could immunoprecipitate the >500 kDa band with either the α-Flag or α-C-term antisera and then detect it with the other (data not shown). These data conclusively show that the C-term antiserum is capable of recognizing full-length polycystin-1 if present in sufficient quantities.

These studies raised additional questions about the identity of the >400kDa band, however. On the one hand, the affinity-enrichment/depletion strategy suggested some degree of specificity of α-C-term for the >400 kDa band. On the other hand, it could not be immunoprecipitated by α-C-term from any source tested (**Figure 1C** and data not shown). The latter result indicated that a splicing variant was unlikely to be the source of the smaller protein. The only way one could explain how the antiserum could recognize both *PKD1* gene products by Western blot but only one by immunoprecipitation is if the alternatively spliced product lacked the epitope responsible for the latter properties. While not strictly impossible, since α-C-term is polyclonal in nature, it is very unlikely, given that we and others have failed to find alternatively spliced products involving exons 45 and 46, the segment of *PKD1* used to generate the antiserum.

The results of the immunoprecipitation studies also suggested that different patterns of post-translational modification are unlikely to account for the size differences. If this were the cause, one would expect both forms of the protein to be immunoprecipitated by α-C-term. Moreover, the fact that α-Flag also failed to detect the smaller product on Western blot suggested that the latter was unlikely to be either an alternatively processed form of polycystin-1 or one that had been subject to proteolysis. Taken together, these findings suggested that the >400 kDa band was unlikely to be polycystin but rather a non-specifically recognized product.

Gene expression studies ultimately proved this to be the case. Previous studies had reported that HeLa cells do not express polycystin-1.[2] We confirmed these data by RNAse protection employing a probe spanning the whole KG8 region[3] (data not shown). Furthermore, employing primers specific for exon 46, we excluded the expression of even very low levels of *PKD1* in these cells (**Figure 1D**, top). We, therefore, conclude that α-C-Term is capable of detecting both full-length polycystin-1 and an abundant, widely expressed >400 kDa protein that is not a product of *PKD1*.

Finally, we sought to determine whether we could detect an endogenous protein in any cell line that had detectable levels of expression of *PKD1* mRNA. **Figure 1D** presents the results of our studies of Hek293 cells. RT-PCR was used to confirm the expression of *PKD1* in this cell line (**Figure 1D**, bottom). Under standard gel loading conditions (50 μg/lane), only the >400kDa band could be detected by α-C-term (**Figure 1E**, lane 1). We were, however, able to detect the >500 kDa band by immunoprecipitation using α-C-term when a sufficiently large amount of total cell lysate was used as starting material for the reaction (**Figure 1E**, lane 2). In contrast, a canine product of similar size could not be detected in MDCK cells even when a large quantity (>1mg) of total cell lysate was used for immunoprecipitation. These studies suggest that endogenous human polycystin-1 is identical in size to the recombinant form of the protein (**Figure 1E**, lane 3). We, therefore, conclude that ectopic expression of polycystin-1 generates a product identical in size to the native protein; and we proceeded further in its characterization.

2) Polycystin-1 is a 520kDa Glycosylated Protein

As already noted, the specific product generated by expression of the full-length cDNA for polycystin-1 was estimated to be >500 kDa. However, the standard high molecular weight markers (10 to 250 kDa) fall in a range far below the actual size of our band and cannot provide accurate information about the protein's molecular weight. Given the fact that this represents one of the debated issues in the literature, we determined more precisely its size using a panel of high molecular weight markers that range from 97 to

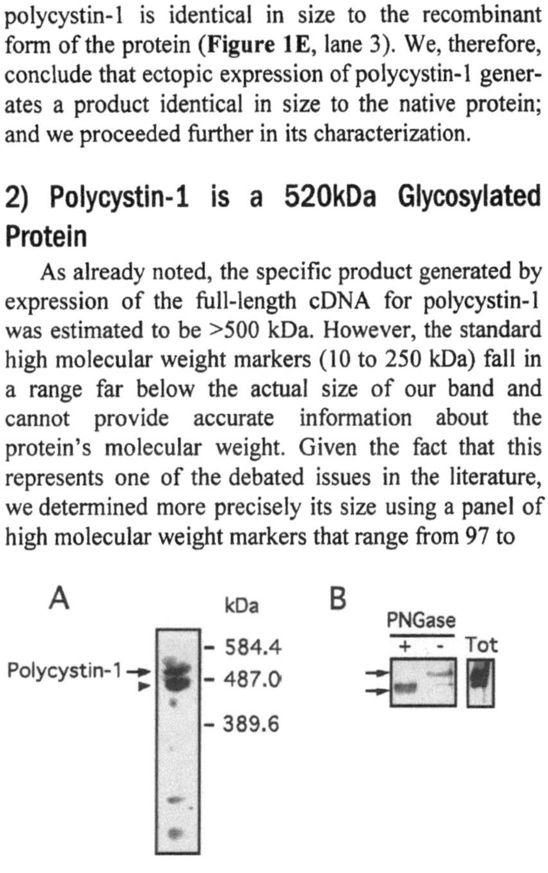

Figure 2. Polycystin-1 is a 520 kDa glycosylated protein
A. High molecular weight markers ranging from 97 to 584.4kDa (Sigma) were loaded on a 4% polyacrylamide gel beside an aliquot of cell extract of the MDCK[PKD1Zeo] clone, C8/68, electrophoresed using a urea-based buffer, immunoblotted and probed with α-C-Term. Using three markers that span a range which includes polycystin-1, we generated a standard curve and determined that polycystin-1 has a MW of 520kDa.
B. 50μg of total cell lysate of C8/68 treated with PNGase (+, left lane), subject to identical reaction conditions but in the absence of PNGase (-, middle lane), or freshly prepared without additional manipulation (+ CTRL, right lane) was immunoblotted and probed with α-C-Term.

584.4kDa (Sigma). In order to generate an accurate standard curve, we employed a 4% polyacrylamide gel and a urea-based buffer. Using this system we were able to determine that the size of our expressed product is, in fact, 520kDa (**Figure 2A**, arrow) while the ubiquitous non-specific band is 480kDa (**Figure 2A**, arrowhead).

The apparent size of polycystin-1 is considerably larger than predicted by its primary sequence (462 kDa molecular weight). Given that the sizeable extracellular amino terminal segment contains a number of potential glycosylation sites, we postulated that post-translational modifications of the protein were likely responsible for the discrepancy. We tested this hypothesis by treating cell lysates of the C8/68 clone with PNGase, an enzyme that removes N-linked glycosyl residues. We found that the product shifted down in size after treatment, with the core of the protein migrating at the expected size of ~460kDa (**Figure 2B**). Similar results were observed using the Flag-tagged version of the protein, while no such a shift was observed in the 480 kDa band (data not shown). These data strongly suggest that polycystin-1 is, indeed, heavily glycosylated.

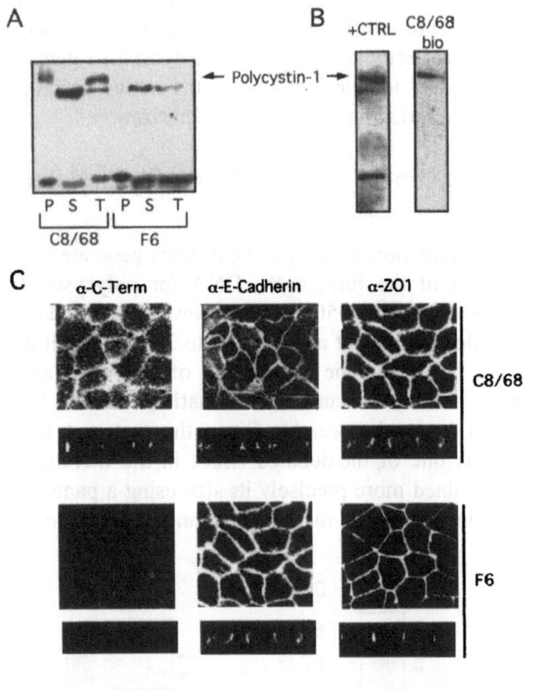

Figure 3. Polycystin-1 is a plasma-membrane protein and localizes to cell-cell junctions

A. Aliquots of total cell lysate (T), supernatant (S) and plasma membrane fraction (P) of C8/68 and F6 were loaded on a 4% polyacrylamide gel and analysed by Western blot using α-C-Term. Polycystin-1 sedimented exclusively with the plasma membrane fraction (P).

B. Immunoblot of total cell lysate (+ CTRL) and biotinylated cell surface proteins of the C8/68 cell line (bio), isolated using streptavidin-coated beads, probed with α-C-Term. This study shows that polycystin-1 is biotinylated under the conditions used whereas the non-specific 480kDa band is not.

C. Indirect immunofluorescence studies of C8/68 and F6 clones grown as monolayers on filters and stained with α-C-Term, α-E-cadherin or α-ZO1 antibodies. α-E-cadherin and α-ZO1 gave similar patterns of plasma membrane staining in both cell lines (top squares). In contrast, plasma membrane staining for Polycystin-1 was only observed in the C8/68 clone and absent in F6. XZ section analysis of the staining in these cells is shown in the bottom rectangles.

3) Polycystin-1 is a Plasma-Membrane Protein and Localizes to the Cell-Cell Junctions

Polycystin-1 is predicted to be a protein with multiple transmembrane spanning elements. A sucrose-gradient membrane preparation of cell lysates from C8/68 and F6 was prepared using serial centrifugation steps according to a previously published protocol.[27] Total lysates, as well as the supernatants (S) and sucrose-gradient purified pellets (P) of each sample, were analyzed by immunoblot using α-C-term. As shown in **Figure 3A**, the 520kDa polycystin-1-specific product was present exclusively in the pellet fraction; while the non-specific 480kDa band was isolated with the supernatant fraction. Interestingly, a 520kd band was not recognized by our antiserum in the pellet of F6 cells nor those of any other negative control cell line even when lanes were heavily loaded. This result suggests that endogenous canine polycystin-1 is not detectable by this antiserum under these conditions in MDCK cells.

To further verify whether polycystin-1 is plasma membrane bound, we performed a cell-surface biotinylation assay on intact cells of the C8/68 subclone and the F6 negative control followed by precipitation with streptavidin-coated beads. The products were analyzed by Western blot using α-C-term. The results show that polycystin-1 is biotinylated under these conditions (**Figure 3B**). As a negative control, we tested for biotinylation of TonEBP, a transcription factor known to be localized to the cytoplasm and nucleus (antiserum was a kind gift of Dr. M.Kwon).[28] We found that the protein was not biotinylated in the same lysate (data not shown).

We further investigated this point by indirect immunofluorescence (IF) using α–C-Term on sets of three independently-derived $MDCK^{PKD1Zeo}$ and $MDCK^{Zeo}$ clones grown as monolayers on filters. Endogenous E-cadherin and ZO-1 were employed as markers for plasma membrane distribution. As shown in **Figure 3C**, the pattern of staining observed using α-C-term on $MDCK^{PKD1Zeo}$ cells was typical for plasma membrane proteins and very similar to the one observed for E-cadherin and ZO-1 (C8/68 top squares). In contrast, no signal was observed for the $MDCK^{Zeo}$ clones using α-C-term though E-cadherin and ZO-1 had a normal staining pattern (F6, top squares). Control studies using the secondary antibody alone on $MDCK^{PKD1Zeo}$ cells yielded no signal (data not shown). Furthermore, analysis of XZ-sections revealed that polycystin-1 localized to the cell-cell junctions in all of the MDCK ^{PKD1Zeo} clones (C8/68 bottom rectangles and data not shown) in a pattern similar to that observed for E-cadherin and ZO-1 (bottom rectangles) and was absent in all of the $MDCK^{Zeo}$ clones (F6 bottom rectangles and data not shown) under these conditions.

4) Polycystin-1 is Expressed at Very Low Levels in Human Kidneys and Sediments with the Plasma Membrane Fractions

We next sought to identify polycystin-1 in human kidney, since it is the organ most frequently affected by mutations of *PKD1*. Whole tissue homogenates were subject to a sucrose gradient centrifugation protocol that yielded 15 different fractions, each of which had been characterized using biochemical and enzymatic assays.[29] The 520kDa band could not be detected in the initial nuclear (N) and postnuclear (S and MLP) fractions (**Figure 4**). However, when the MLP fraction was equilibrated in a linear sucrose gradient, the 520 kDa band corresponding to polycystin-1 was considerably enriched in fractions #7 and #8 (**Figure 4**). The gel was stripped and re-probed using a second α-polycystin antiserum and found that it recognized the same band (data not shown). Thus, polycystin-1 is associated with sub-cellular particles that can be sedimented in a pattern consistent with a membrane protein distribution. This distribution was similar although slightly different from that of the α1 subunit of Na+/K+ ATPase, which is enriched in fractions #8 and #9. In contrast, this pattern is identical to what is observed for the 29 kDa band corresponding to the water channel, aquaporin 2 (**Figure 4**). These results show that polycystin-1 has an enrichment pattern similar to that of two other known plasma membrane proteins and suggest a similar sub-cellular localization for polycystin-1.

Discussion

Little progress has been made in understanding the function of polycystin-1 since its original description in 1994. Inconsistent results have been reported for its localization in tissues and cells, and all functional

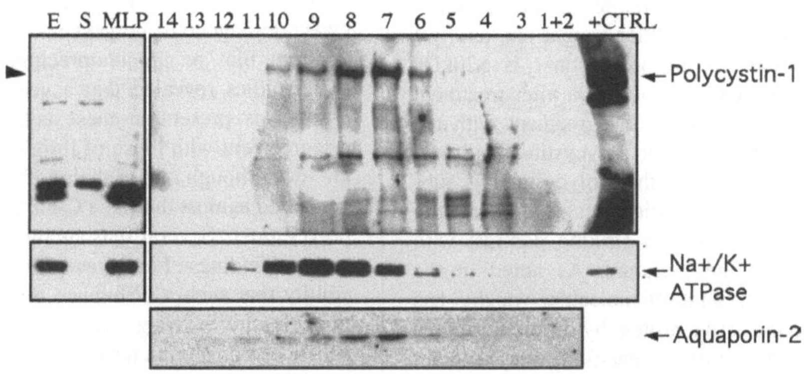

Figure 4. Polycystin-1 is a low-abundance 520kDa protein in human adult kidney.
Left Panel: Immunoblot analysis of the sub-cellular fractionation products of human kidney inner medulla probed with α-C-Term (top) or an antibody specific for the α1-subunit of the plasma membrane protein, Na+/K+ATPase (bottom). Lane E contains a sample of the entire extract after sedimentation of nuclei. Lane MLP contains an aliquot of all membrane particles that sediment from E after high-speed centrifugation (see methods) while S contains the soluble components that remained. A 520kDa band was not detected by α-C-Term in any fraction (arrowhead) whereas a protein of the correct size was identified by the α1 subunit antibody.
Right Panel: Immunoblot analysis of 14 sub-fractions of MLP separated by sucrose gradient fractionation (see methods). A specific band of 520kDa, identical in size to that detected in the C8/68 sample employed as a positive control (CTRL), was identified by α-C-Term in fractions 5-10. The α1 subunit of Na+K+ATPase and aquaporin2 (AQ2) had similar patterns of distribution.

studies have been limited to use of small segments of the complete protein.[7-24] A major limitation has been the lack of adequate tools that could be used for its study. Although a full-length cDNA has been available for several years, all prior attempts at expressing the complete protein in mammalian cells have been unsuccessful.[24-25] Not only has the lack of an expressible full-length construct prevented investigators from initiating functional studies, it has also precluded the complete characterization of α-polycystin-1 antisera.

We have recently reported the first successful stable expression of the full-length cDNA for polycystin-1 and shown that multiple independently-derived α-polycystin-1 antisera recognize the same product.[26] In the current study, we report a further validation of our system by demonstrating that the stable expression product in MDCK cells is identical to a newly developed, epitope-tagged version that has been transiently expressed in a variety of cell lines. We show that both the commercially available α-Flag antibodies as well as our α-polycystin-1 antisera detect the same protein. Moreover, both sets of antisera can be used to immunoprecipitate the identical 520kDa product. Finally, we have immunoprecipitated a product of the same size from Hek293 cells and shown that the 520kDa band is also present in low abundance in normal human kidney. These studies provide validation of our expression system and the ability of our antisera to recognize polycystin-1, when present.

Our expression system has now made it possible to define some of the basic properties of polycystin-1. Using a ladder of high molecular weight markers, we determined that the size of polycystin-1 is 520kDa under normal conditions and ~460kDa after treatment with PNGase. These data are in agreement with the predicted molecular weight for polycystin-1 and present the first direct evidence that polycystin-1 is subject to post-translational modifications. It is interesting to note that these data are in striking contrast with published results in the literature. As noted in the introduction, a broad range of molecular weights has been assigned to the native protein by different groups. While problems of antibody specificity may explain some of the observed differences (discussed below), a second reason is that most previous studies have not used a sufficiently high range of molecular weight markers or adequate PAGE conditions to allow accurate assessment of the protein's size. The size differences are unlikely to be due to differences between the processing of endogenous vs. transfected *PKD1* mRNA and polycystin-1, since we have identified the 520kDa product as an endogenous protein in Hek293 cells and normal human kidney.

Our studies suggest that polycystin-1 is present at very low levels in mammalian cell lines and tissues, and enrichment strategies must be employed in order to detect it. Other investigators have reported different results. One explanation that has been offered to account for the discrepant findings is that polycystin-1 is a highly labile molecule subject to rapid degradation.[17] Although this might be the case for the native protein in tissues, we did not observe this property for either recombinant or endogenous polycystin-1 isolated from Hek293 cells. Indeed, cell lysates could be stored in a freezer for prolonged periods of time and subject to multiple freeze-thaw cycles without affecting the protein's stability.

We have used three independent methods to show that polycystin-1 is indeed likely to be a membrane protein, as predicted on the basis of its primary sequence. Firstly, the sucrose-gradient protocol used to analyze the $MDCK^{PKD1Zeo}$ cell line and the more complete fractionation method used to analyze endogenous polycystin-1 in human kidney tissue yielded a pattern observed or other plasma membrane proteins. Secondly, the *in vivo* biotinylation studies provided direct evidence that polycystin-1 is localized to the plasma membrane. Finally, the immunofluorescence analyses have shown that polycystin-1 is localized to cell-cell junctions in MDCK cells grown as a monolayer on filters. These data support the hypothesis that polycystin-1 functions as a receptor involved in mediating cell-cell or cell-matrix interactions.

In both this and our previous study, we did not detect endogenous polycystin-1 in MDCK cells by Western blot or immunoprecipitation; although RT-PCR studies revealed that a very low level of Polycystin-1 is present in these cells.[26] Our data are in disagreement with those of Ibrighimov-Beskrovnaya et al.[25] even though one of their antibodies, like ours, was generated against the same C-terminal region of human polycystin-1. Several reasons might explain these discrepant findings. Firstly, we cannot exclude the possibility that such a difference reflects true differences in expression levels given the heterogeneity of MDCK cell lines and the number of passages they underwent in different laboratories since they were first cloned. Secondly, it is possible that their antisera are more sensitive for immunolocalization studies of canine polycystin-1. The fact that the localization pattern for polycystin-1 reported by them as well as by Peters et al.[10,30] is similar to what we have observed supports this conclusion. Thirdly, these authors' antisera may be recognizing protein(s) other than polycystin-1. The specificity of their antibodies was assessed using more limited criteria as defined below. Furthermore, Peters et al. do not comment on the pattern observed in Western blots of MDCK cell lysates. Further studies will be required to reconcile these findings.

We suspect that one of the factors that has most confounded the study of polycystin-1 is the uncertain specificity of the various antisera that have been used to trace its expression. Our data very clearly illustrate the point. We have presented compelling evidence that our affinity-purified α-C-term antiserum is capable of detecting polycystin-1 when the protein is present. We also found, however, that the antiserum can recognize a second, slightly smaller molecule of 480kDa that is much more abundant than the 520kDa band. Studies using the affinity-purified and immunodepleted sera suggest that this is a specific recognition; yet we have shown that, in at least one source where the 480kDa band is present, the mRNA for *PKD1* is not expressed. This was a fortuitous discovery, because *PKD1* mRNA is detectable in most cell lines and tissues. In the absence of suitable positive and negative controls, it is likely that the 480kDa band would have been mistaken for polycystin-1. It is clear that affinity-depleted or peptide-competed antibody cannot serve as an adequate negative control for its specificity.

It has been argued that the use of multiple antisera that recognize unique segments of one's target protein may help distinguish "specific" vs. non-specific binding. Our data, as well as those of Nauta et al,[7] show that this, too, is an inadequate measure of specificity. In our study, a second affinity-purified antiserum developed by us using the same immunogen that yielded our P4 antiserum[26] also detected the 480kDa protein by Western blot in HeLa cells (data not shown). Similarly, Nauta et al generated 14 different polyclonal antisera against fragments of polycystin-1 and found that many stained the epithelial cells of fetal, adult and cystic kidney sections in patterns similar to those reported by others. Further investigations, however, convinced them that the patterns they observed were not specific for polycystin-1. Both their data and ours suggest that results obtained using reagents that have not been validated using a panel of proven negative and positive controls should be interpreted cautiously.

In conclusion, we have established the first expression system for full-length polycystin-1 and used it to perform the initial characterizations of this low abundance protein. This system represents a very powerful tool to study polycystin-1 function *in vitro* and is an invaluable reagent for the characterization of α-polycystin-1 antisera.

Acknowledgments

A Boletta was supported by AHA and the NKF of Maryland. This work was supported by the PKRF, the NIH (DK48006, DK51042, NIH P50-DK57325), Italian Telethon (A.112), Fondation Alphonse and Jean Fonds de la Recherche Scientifique Medicale and Fonds National de la Richerche Scientifique. The authors are grateful to S. Akhter for help with the biotinylation studies, J. Lipschutz for protocols and helpful comments regarding the immunofluorescence studies of polarized MDCK cells, V. Chauvet and M. Leruth for helping in the characterization of the tissue sub-cellular fractions. GGG is the Blum Scholar of JHU School of Medicine. The investigators are members of the Johns Hopkins PKD Center of Excellence (NIH P50-DK57325).

References

1. Gabow, P.A: Autosomal Dominat Polycystic Kidney Disease. N Engl J Med 329: 332-42, 1993
2. The European Polycystic Kidney Disease Consortium: The polycystic kidney disease gene encodes a 14kb transcript and lies within a duplicated region on chromosome 16. Cell 77: 881-94, 1994.
3. The American PKD1 Consortium: Analysis of the genomic sequence for the autosomal dominant polycystic kidney disease (PKD1) gene predicts the presence of a leucine-rich repeat. Hum Mol Gen 4: 575-82, 1995.
4. The International Polycystic Kidney Disease Consortium: Polycystic kidney disease: the complete structure of the *PKD1* gene and its protein. Cell 81: 289-98, 1995.
5. Qian, F., Germino, F.J., Cai, Y., Zhang, X., Somlo, S., Germino, G.G: PKD1 interacts with PKD2 through a probable coiled-coil domain. Nat Genet 16, 179-83, 1997.
6. Moy GW, Mendoza LM, Schulz JR, Swanson WJ, Glabe CG, Vacquier VD: The sea urchin sperm receptor for egg jelly is a modular protein with extensive homology to the human polycystic kidney disease protein, PKD1. J Cell Biol 133: 809-17, 1996.
7. Nauta J, Goedbloed MA, van den Ouweland AM, Nellist M, Hoogeveen AT: Immunological detection of Polycystin-1 in human kidneys. Histochem Cell Biol 113: 303-11, 2000.
8. Ong AC, Harris PC, Davies DR, Pritchard L, Rossetti S, Biddolph S, Vaux DJ, Migone N, Ward CJ: Polycystin-1 expression in PKD, early onset PKD1, and TSC2/PKD1 cystic tissue. Kidney Int 56: 1324-33, 1999.
9. Griffin MD, Torres VE, Grande JP, Kumar R: Vascular expression of Polycystin. J Am Soc Nephrol 8: 616-26, 1997.
10. Peters DJ, van de Wal A, Spruit L, Saris JJ, Breuning MH, Bruijn JA, de Heer E: Cellular localization and tissue distribution of Polycystin-1. J Pathol 188: 439-46, 1999.

11. Ong AC, Ward CJ, Butler RJ, Biddolph S, Bowker C, Torra R, Pei Y, Harris PC: Coordinate expression of the autosomal dominant Polycystic kidney disease proteins, Polycystin-2 and Polycystin-1 in normal and cystic tissue. Am J Pathol 154: 1721-9, 1999.
12. Guillaume R, D'Agati V, Daoust M, Trudel M: Murine Pkd1 is a developmentally regulated gene from morula to adulthood: role in tissue condensation and patterning. Dev Dyn 14: 337-48, 1999.
13. Aguiari G, Piva R, Manzati E, Mazzoni E, Augello G, Chiari E, Moretti S, Neri LM, del Senno L: K562 erythroid and HL60 macrophage differentiation downregulates polycystin, a large membrane-associated protein. Exp Cell Res 244: 259-67, 1998.
14. Weston BS, Jeffery S, Jeffrey I, Sharaf SF, Carter N, Saggar-Malik A, Price RG: Polycystin expression during embryonic development of human kidney in adult tissues and ADPKD tissue. Histochem J 29: 847-56, 1997.
15. Aguiari GL, Bozza A, Piva R, Volinia S, Reali E, Maestri I, Magri E, Cavazzini L, del Senno L: Expression of protein fragments from the human PKD1 gene and production of rabbit polyclonal antibodies to the recombinant proteins. Contrib Nephrol 122: 49-52, 1997.
16. Griffin MD, O'Sullivan DA, Torres VE, Grande JP, Kanwar YS, Kumar R: expression of Polycystin in mouse metanephros and extra-metanephric tissues. Kidney Int 52: 1196-205, 1997.
17. Van Adelsberg J, Chamberlain S, D'Agati V: Polycystin expression is temporally and spatially regulated during renal development. Am J Physiol 272: F602-9, 1997.
18. Geng L, Segal Y, Pavlova A, Barros EJ, Lohning C, Lu W, Nigam SK, Frischauf AM, Reeders ST, Zhou J: distribution and developmentally regulated expression of murine polycystin. Am J Physiol 272: F451-9, 1997.
19. Geng L, Segal Y, Peissel B, Deng N, Pei Y, Carone F, Rennke HG, Glucksmann-Kuis AM, Schneider MC, Ericsson M, Reeders ST, Zhou J: Identification and localization of polycystin, the PKD1 gene product. J Clin Invest 98: 2674-82, 1996.
20. Palsson R, Sharma CP, Kim K, McLaughlin M, Brown D, Arnaout MA: Characterization and cell distribution of polycystin, the product of autosomal dominant polycystic kidney disease gene 1. Mol Med 2: 702-11, 1996.
21. Peters DJ, Spruit L, Klingel R, Prins F, Baelde HJ, Giordano PC, Bernini LF, de Heer E, Breuning MH, Bruijn JA: Adult, fetal, and polycystic kidney expression of polycystin, the polycystic kidney disease-1 gene product. Lab Invest 75: 221-30, 1996.
22. Griffin MD, Torres VE, Grande JP, Kumar R: Immunolocalization of polycystin in human tissues and cultured cells. Proc Assoc Am Physicians 108: 185-97, 1996.
23. Ward CJ, Turley H, Ong AC, Comley M, Biddolph S, Chetty R, Ratcliffe PJ, Gattner K, Harris PC: Polycystin, the polycystic kidney disease 1 protein, is expressed by epithelial cells in fetal, adult, and polycystic kidneys. Proc Natl Acad Sci U S A 93: 1524-8, 1996.
24. Ibraghimov-Beskrovnaya, O.,Dackowski, W.R., Foggensteiner, L., Coleman, N., Thiru, S., Petry, L.R., Burn, T.C., Connors, T.D., Van Raay, T., Bradley, J., Qian F, Onuchic LF, Watnick TJ, Piontek K, Hakim RM, Landes GM, Germino GG, Sandford R and Klinger KW: Polycystin: in vitro synthesis, in vivo tissue expression, and subcellular localization identifies a large membrane-associated protein. Proc. Natl.Acad. Sci. USA 94: 6397-402, 1997.
25. Ibraghimov-Beskrovnaya O, Bukanov NO, Donohue LC, Dackowski WR, Klinger KW, Landes GM: Strong homophilic interactions of the Ig-like domains of polycystin-1, the protein product of autosomal dominant polycystic kidney disease gene, PKD1. Hum Mol Genet 9:1641-9, 2000.
26. Boletta, A, Qian, F., Onuchic, L.F., Bhunia, A.K., Phakdeekitcharoen, B., Hanaoka, K., Guggino, B., Monaco, L.,Germino, G.G: Polycystin-1, the gene product of PKD1, induces resistance to apoptosis and spontaneous tubulogenesis in MDCK cells. Mol Cell 6: 1267-73, 2000.
27. Devuyst O, Christie PT, Courtoy PJ, Beauwens R, Thakker RV : intra-renal and subcellular distribution of the human chloride channel, CLC-5, reveals a pathophysiological basis for Dent's disease. Hum Mol Genet 8: 247-57, 1999.
28. Woo, S.K., Dahl, S.D., Handler, J.S., Kwon, H.M. Bidirectional regulation of tonicity-responsive enhancer binding protein in response to changes in tonicity. Am J Renal Physiol 278: 1006-12, 2000.
29. Kishore BK, Fuming Lu, Maldague P, Tulkens PM, Courtoy PJ. Mechanism of thesaurismosis and altered lysosomal dynamics induced by poly-D-glutamic acid in kidney proximal tubular cells Lab Invest 74: 1025-37, 1996.
30. Scheffers, M.S., Van Der Bent, P., Prins, F., Spruit, L., Breuning, M.H., Litvinov, S.V., de Heer, E., Peters, D.J. Polycystin-1, the product of the polycystic kidney disease 1 gene, co-localizes with desmosomes in MDCK cells. Hum Mol Genet 9: 2743-50, 2000.

14 Nutrition and Blood Pressure

JOEL D. KOPPLE, M.D.

Introduction

Nutrition may affect blood pressure in at least two ways: the body habitus of the patient and the intake of nutrients may each have major effects on blood pressure.

Obesity

Obesity may directly increase blood pressure. Blood pressure has been correlated with both fat cell size and/or number.[1] Also, obese individuals are more likely to have elevated blood pressure than non-obese subjects. The distribution of fat in an individual also influences the blood pressure. The ratio of the circumference of the waist to the hip correlates directly with both systolic and diastolic blood pressure (i.e., the male fat distribution is correlated with the blood pressure level).

A number of lines of evidence indicate that the renin-aldosterone system is also altered in obese individuals. Plasma renin activity (PRA), relative to the sodium chloride (NaCl) intake, may be disproportionately high in obese subjects. PRA and plasma aldosterone both decrease in obese individuals with weight reduction independent of the sodium intake. The sympatho-adrenal system may also be altered in obesity. Obese subjects have higher supine plasma norepinephrine, epinephrine and PRA levels and a greater norepinephrine response to upright posture and to isometric hand-grip exercise. Weight reduction in these individuals leads to more normal plasma hormone levels. Also, glucose ingestion is reported to increase plasma norepinephrine levels. Overeating may also increase triiodothyronine production from thyroxine. Triiodothyronine may also increase beta-adrenaline receptors.

Obese individuals often have increased dietary sodium intake, which may also promote hypertension. Moreover, hyperinsulinemia, which is often present in obesity, promotes renal sodium reabsorption. It is important to remember that very obese individuals may have a falsely elevated blood pressure when measured with a normal-sized blood pressure cuff. For accurate blood pressure measurements, the cuff size should be increased for individuals with large arm circumferences.

Nutrient Intake

Weight Reduction (Low Calorie) Diets

Fat reduction per se often lowers blood pressure in obese individuals. A low calorie diet appears to have an independent blood pressure lowering effect in these individuals. In one study, blood pressure was monitored in severely overweight individuals before and after they began a protein-sparing modified fast.[1] Blood pressure fell substantially after inauguration of the diet and in association with weight loss. After finishing dietary therapy and after commencing a more liberal diet, a number of these individuals regained most of their body weight. A comparison of the blood pressure at the same level of body weight showed that the blood pressure was significantly higher when the patients were ingesting a higher calorie diet and gaining weight than when they were at the same weight but ingesting the protein-sparing modified fast and losing weight.

The reduction in blood pressure that occurs with weight reduction is not exclusively due to a single factor. A reduction in sodium intake with lower calorie diets also may contribute to lowering of blood pressure. However, a study in which patients undergoing low-calorie weight reduction therapy were given each day an amount of sodium that was equal their sodium losses was still associated with a reduction in blood pressure levels.

Health Enhancing Diets

The recently completed DASH (Dietary Approaches to Stop Hypertension) Study provides much relevant information concerning appropriate dietary therapy to control blood pressure.[2] The DASH study was a multi-center study that compared a "control" typical American diet (low in fruits, vegetables, dairy products, essential

M.M. Avram.(ed.), Improving Prognosis for Kidney Disorders, 119-123.

minerals and fiber and high in saturated and total fat) to a diet rich in fruits and vegetables and also to a combination diet rich in fruits, vegetables and low-fat dairy products and with a reduced saturated and total fat content. The study was carried out in 459 adults, with a mean age of about 44 years. The control diet was fed for three weeks and individuals were then randomly assigned to remain on this diet or to receive the diet rich in fruits and vegetables or the combination diet. The maximum systolic and diastolic blood pressures were less than 160 mm Hg and 85 to 95 mm Hg, respectively, at the onset of study; and the mean blood pressures at baseline were 131 mm Hg systolic and 85 mm Hg diastolic. Hence many individuals had only high-normal blood pressure. About 65 percent of the study subjects were racial minorities, especially African-Americans. All meals were prepared for the participants, and five meals per week were ingested on the study site. The study used food rather than non-food sources of calcium. As can be seen from **Table 1**, the pre-study diet was very low in calcium.

The results indicated that there was a rapid, significant and sustained fall in systolic and diastolic blood pressure with both the fruits and vegetables diet and combination diet.[2] The fruits and vegetables diet reduced systolic and diastolic blood pressure by 2.8 mm Hg ($P<0.001$) and 1.1 mm Hg ($P=0.07$), respectively, more than the control diet. The combination diet decreased systolic and diastolic blood pressure by 5.5 and 3.0 mm Hg, respectively, more than the control diet ($P<0.001$ for each comparison). The combination diet also decreased systolic and diastolic blood pressure by 2.7 mm Hg ($P=0.001$) and 1.9 mm Hg ($P=0.002$) more than the fruits and vegetables diet. These declines in blood pressures with both experimental diets occurred within 2-3 weeks and essentially persisted throughout the rest of the 8-week period of study. Thus, this study indicated that a diet high in fruits and vegetables significantly reduces blood pressure. Moreover, addition of about 3 daily servings of dairy products, predominately low-fat milk, in association with a reduced saturated and total fat intake approximately doubled the degree of blood pressure reduction observed with the fruits and vegetables diet. It should be pointed out that these diets were provided for only 8 weeks; and therefore, the long-term effects of these two diets were not investigated.

Table 1. Composition of the DASH Diets (By Chemical Analyses)*

	Control Diet†	Fruits and Vegetables Diet†	Combination Diet†
Fat (% total kcal)	36	36	26
Saturated	14	13	7
Polyunsaturated	6	7	7
Carbohydrate (% total kcal)	50	49	56
Protein (% total kcal)	14	15	18
Cholesterol (mg/day)	233	184	151
Potassium (g/day)	1.75	4.10	4.42
Magnesium (mg/day)	176	423	480
Calcium (mg/day)	443	534	1265
Sodium (g/day)	3.03	2.82	2.86

*DASH: Dietary Approach to Stop Hypertension[2]

† Values are for diets designed to provide 2100 kcal/day

Calcium

It is possible that the greater blood pressure lowering effects observed with the DASH combination diet were due to the higher calcium intake. Indeed, there is a substantial controversy in the literature concerning whether high calcium intakes do lower blood pressure. McCarron and co-workers have conducted a series of studies suggesting that calcium supplementation does lower blood pressure.[3] Indeed, there is a correlation across populations and ethnic groups indicating that the mean dietary calcium intakes of these groups are inversely correlated with blood pressure.[3]

Bucher and associates performed a meta-analysis that described a significant reduction in systolic blood pressure of 4.3 mm Hg in hypertensive individuals and no decrease in diastolic blood pressure individuals.[4] There was no reduction in blood pressure in non-hypertensive subjects. Allender and co-workers carried out a meta-analysis of 22 randomized clinical trials in 1,231 individuals.[5] In this meta-analysis, calcium supplementation was observed to cause a significant but clinically unimportant reduction in systolic blood pressure (1.68 mm Hg) and no significant change in diastolic blood pressure in hypertensive individuals. Calcium supplements (that resulted in a median total daily calcium intake of about 1 g/day) did not effect systolic or diastolic blood pressure in normotensive individuals. It has been suggested that some of the confusion in the literature is related to the possibility that a low calcium diet predisposes to hypertension; whereas in individuals who are already eating an adequate calcium intake, higher intakes of calcium have little or no blood pressure lowering effect.[5,6] Further studies may be needed to resolve this latter question.

Fish Oil

It is also possible that the combination diet lowered blood pressure more because of the higher percentage of polyunsaturated fatty acids. Two meta-analyses of controlled clinical trials of the use of omega-3 fatty acids, often given as fish oil but sometimes provided as omega-3 polyunsaturated fatty acid enriched eggs or certain fishes, indicated that there was a significant reduction in blood pressure in hypertensive individuals but probably not in normotensive subjects.[7,8] The mean reduction in systolic and diastolic blood pressure in one study averaged 1.0 and 0.5 mm Hg in normotensive individuals and 5.5 ($P<0.001$) and 3.5 mm Hg ($P<0.001$) in untreated hypertensive individuals.[7] In the normotensive individuals the reduction in systolic blood pressure was of borderline significance ($P=0.05$), and the reduction in diastolic blood pressure was not statistically significant. The decrease in systolic and diastolic blood pressure in the untreated hypertensive individuals was statistically significant. In the second meta-analysis, there was a significant reduction in systolic (3.4 mm Hg) and diastolic (2.0 mm Hg) blood pressure in hypertensive individuals, whereas again there was no reduction in blood pressure in normotensive individuals.[8]

Thus, it may be concluded that fish oil significantly lowers blood pressure in hypertensive but not in normotensive individuals. The mechanism by which this occurs is not entirely clear. It may be related to enhanced elaboration of prostaglandins which, in turn, may increase sodium and water excretion, promote vasodilation, or inhibit the release of thromboxane (a vasoconstrictor). Also, it is possible that prostaglandins may regulate renin release or decrease responsiveness to vasopressor hormones. The preponderance of studies with fish oil were of short duration (less than 3 months), and longer term studies will be necessary to determine whether fish oil has a sustained anti-hypertensive effect in persons with hypertension. There were a number of side effects with the fish oil intake including, most commonly, eructation and a bad or fishy taste.[7]

Sodium Chloride

There is much evidence for an association between sodium chloride intake and elevated blood pressure.[9-12] NaCl intake correlates directly with blood pressure across population groups. The association of NaCl intake with blood pressure increases with age, blood pressure level, and among individuals with a family history of hypertension. The chloride salt of sodium appears to have a greater effect on hypertension than do other sodium salts. The blood pressure of some individuals tends to be sensitive to high NaCl intakes; whereas in other individuals, the blood pressure does not appear to be affected by the NaCl intake. NaCl sensitivity is determined by a reduction in blood pressure associated with NaCl depletion and/or an increase in blood pressure with NaCl loading.

The International Study of Salt and Blood Pressure (INTERSALT) indicated that in about 10,000 adults, aged 20-59 years old, at 52 centers in 32 countries around the world, 24-hour urine sodium excretion correlated significantly with the median systolic and diastolic blood pressure, the upward slope of systolic and diastolic blood pressure that occurs with age, and the prevalence of elevated blood pressure. Moreover, two recent meta-analyses indicate consistent reductions in blood pressure in individuals in response to a lower intake of NaCl.[11,12]

Potassium

Two meta-analyses of clinical trials concerning potassium supplementation support the thesis that potassium supplements (e.g., 60-120 mEq/day) lower blood pressure. In hypertensive individuals, systolic and diastolic blood pressures were lowered on average by 8.2 and 4.5 mm Hg in the meta-analysis of Cappuccio and MacGregor[13] and by 4.4 and 2.5 mm Hg in the meta-analysis by Whelton and co-workers.[14]

Magnesium

The anti-hypertensive effects of magnesium supplements in hypertensive individuals is controversial. Some studies show that magnesium reduces blood pressure levels, where other studies do not show such an effect.[15] The anti-hypertensive effects of magnesium supplements is small in those studies that suggest such an effect.

Fiber and Protein

There are a few randomized controlled clinical trials suggesting that dietary fiber intake may reduce blood pressure. Clinical trials do not confirm an effect of low-protein diets in reducing blood pressure.

Alcohol

Excessive alcohol intake often increases blood pressure. However, these effects are generally transient; and blood pressure falls rapidly when individuals stop drinking alcohol.[16]

The Trials of Hypertension Prevention (TOHB)

The TOHB evaluated the effects of non-pharmacological therapy on blood pressure in adults with high-normal blood pressure. The study was divided into two phases. In phase I, systolic and diastolic blood pressure were observed to decrease with either body weight loss or reduction of NaCl intake over an 18-month period but not by dietary supplementation with calcium, magnesium or potassium over an interval of 6 months. In phase II of

Table 2. A Suggested Dietary Approach to Prevent or Treat Hypertension*

1. Maintain desirable body weight.
2. Recommended calcium intake (about 1000 mg/day for persons aged 19-50 years and 1200 mg/day for persons older than 50 years).
3. Limit daily NaCl consumption to 6 g/day or lower.
4. Maintain adequate potassium and magnesium intake.
5. For individuals who drink alcohol, no more than two rinks (3 to 4 units) per day.
6. Consider the DASH combination diet (a diet high in fruits, vegetales and low-fat dairy products and low in saturated and total fat).
7. For individuals with hypertension, consider a high omega-3 fatty acid diet (i.e., about 3-6 of fish oil per day).

*These recommendations can be considered to be part of a health-enhancing lifestyle. This nutritional lmanagement should not be substituted for pharmacological therapy for individuals with established hypertension. Rather, in hypertensive patients, unless and until the nutritional therapy has been demonstrated to lower the blood pressure adequately without medicinal therapy.
Regular exercise training shoud also be considered.

the study, overweight adults with high-normal blood pressure were treated with dietary-induced weight loss or decreased NaCl intake alone or in combination for 3-4 years. The results indicated that weight loss was associated with a decrease in systolic (-6.0 mm Hg) and diastolic (-5.5 mm Hg) at 6 months. A reduction in NaCl intake was also associated with a decrease in both systolic (-5.1 mm Hg) and diastolic (-4.4 mm Hg) at 6 months. The effects of weight loss and decreased NaCl intake combined were not additive. After 6 months of treatment, the two interventions were less effective at maintaining both weight loss and NaCl intake; and, possibly for this reason, the reduction in blood pressure was also attenuated.

Exercise

Some studies have suggested that regular exercise training may reduce blood pressure. Exercise, particularly when combined with a low fat intake, may have a serum cholesterol lowering effect. Exercise may also accelerate weight reduction in obese individuals who are ingesting a low calorie diet. It is important to remember that in hypertensive individuals, the increase in blood pressure that normally occurs when individuals are actually exercising may be greatly exaggerated. Thus, blood pressure should be monitored carefully in hypertensive individuals who are embarking on exercise training until it has been ascertained that dangerous levels of hypertension do not occur.

Conclusions and Recommendations

A dietary approach to either prevent or to treat hypertension is indicated in **Table 2**. It should be emphasized that for patients who have major elevations in blood pressure, it is very uncommon for the hypertension to respond adequately to dietary management alone. These individuals will almost certainly require pharmacological management as well. However, appropriate dietary management may prevent the onset of hypertension, may correct mild hypertension, and can be a useful adjunct to pharmacological therapy for the treatment of established hypertension. Individuals who are obese or have other dietary habits that may predispose to hypertension (e.g., high NaCl intake) should be encouraged to inaugurate appropriate dietary therapy. However, if the blood pressure is substantially elevated, a reasonable approach would be to start pharmacological anti-hypertensive therapy concomitantly with dietary management. If the dietary management is effective at maintaining an appropriately lowered blood pressure, attempts may be made to gradually withdraw the anti-hypertensive medicines. This approach will be of particular value for those individuals who are unable or unwilling to maintain an appropriate dietary regimen or in whom blood pressure reduction does not respond sufficiently to dietary therapy. Exercise training should be encouraged but only after a careful medical evaluation.

References

1. Dornfield LP, Maxwell MH, Waks A, Tuck M: Mechanisms of hypertension in obesity. Kidney Int 32(Suppl 32):S254-8, 1987.
2. Appel LJ, Moore TJ, Obarzanek E, Vollmer WM, Svetkey LP, Sacks FM et al: A clinical trial of the effects of dietary patterns on blood pressure. N Eng J Med 336:1117-24, 1997.
3. McCarron DA: Epidemiological evidence & clinical trials of dietary calcium's effect on blood pressure. Contrib Nephrol 90:2-10, 1991.
4. Bucher HC, Cook RJ, Guyatt GH, Lang JD, Cook DJ, Hatala R, Hunt DL: Effects of dietary calcium supplementation on blood pressure: A meta-analysis of randomized controlled trials. JAMA 275:1016-22, 1996.
5. Allender PS, Cutler JA, Follmann D, Cappuccio FP, Pryer J, Elliott P: Dietary calcium and blood pressure: A meta-analysis of randomized clinical trials. Ann Intern Med 124:825-31, 1996.
6. Dwyer JH, Dwyer KM, Scribner RA, Sun P, Li L, Nicholson LM, Davis IJ, Hohn AR: Dietary calcium, calcium supplementation, and blood pressure in African American adolescents. Am J Clin Nutr 68:648-55. 1998.
7. Appel LJ, Miller ER III, Seidler AJ, Whelton PK: Does supplementation of diet with 'fish oil' reduce blood pressure? A meta-analysis of controlled clinical trials. Arch Intern Med 153:1429-38, 1993.

8. Morris MC, Sacks F, Rosner B: Does fish oil lower blood pressure? A meta-analysis of controlled trials. Circulation 88:523-33, 1993.
9. Dyer A, Elliott P, Chee D, Stamler J: Urinary biochemical markers of dietary intake in the INTERSALT Study. Am J Clin Nutr 65(suppl):1246S-53S, 1997.
10. Kotchen TA and McCarron DA: Dietary electrolytes and blood pressure: A statement for healthcare professionals from the American Heart Association Nutrition Committee. Circulation 98:613-7, 1998.
11. Midgley JP, Matthew AG, Greenwood CM, Logan AG: Effect of reduced dietary sodium on blood pressure: A meta-analysis of randomized controlled trials. JAMA 275:1590-7 , 1996.
12. Cutler JA, Follmann D, Allender PS: Randomized trials of sodium reduction: An overview. Am J Clin Nutr 65:643S-651S, 1997.
13. Cappuccio FP and MacGregor GA: Does potassium supplementation lower blood pressure? A meta-analysis of published trials. J Hypertens 9:465-73, 1991.
14. Whelton PK, Jiang H, Cutler JA, Brancati FL, Appel LJ, Follmann D, Klag MJ: Effects of oral potassium on blood pressure: Meta-analysis of randomized controlled clinical trials. JAMA 277:1624-32, 1997.
15. Cappuccio FP, Markandu ND, Beynon GW, Shore AC, Sampson B, MacGregor GA: Lack of effect of oral magnesium on high blood pressure: a double blind study. Br Med J 291:235-8, 1985.
16. MacGregor GA: Nutrition and blood pressure. Nutr Metab Cardiovasc Dis(Suppl 9):6-15, 1999.
17. The Trials of Hypertension Prevention Collaborative Research Group: The effects of non-pharmacological interventions on blood pressure of persons with high normal levels: Results of the Trials of Hypertension Prevention, Phase I. JAMA 267:1213-20, 1992.
18. The Trials of Hypertension Prevention Collaborative Research Group: Effects of weight loss and sodium reduction intervention on blood pressure and hypertension incidence in overweight people with high normal blood pressure: The Trials of Hypertension Prevention, Phase II. Arch Intern Med 157:657-67, 1997.

15 How to Minimize Bone Disease in Renal Failure

KEVIN J. MARTIN, M.B., B.CH., F.A.C.P., AND ESTHER A. GONZÁLEZ

Introduction

Bone disease is common in patients with renal insufficiency and can result in substantial morbidity. The renal bone diseases are a heterogenous group of disorders that can be divided into three groups: those with high bone turnover, or osteitis fibrosa, due to secondary hyperparathyroidism; those with low bone turnover, or adynamic bone; and patients who show features of both of these abnormalities, which are termed mixed renal osteodystrophy.[1,2] Strategies to minimize skeletal complications in the setting of renal disease are based on the elucidation of the pathogenesis of these complex disorders from studies by many investigators over the past 30 years. The major factors involved in the pathogenesis of secondary hyperparathyroidism are the consequences of phosphate retention as GFR falls and decreases in the levels of calcitriol as renal mass is reduced, with the consequent effect on the levels of serum calcium. These three factors, calcium, phosphorus and calcitriol are closely interrelated; and all directly or indirectly result in the increase of PTH secretion with the attendant effects upon the skeleton. Thus, the skeletal effects of hyperparathyroidism can lead to osteitis fibrosa, demineralization of the skeleton, loss of structural stability of bone, and easy fracturability. The control of hyperparathyroidism is indicated not only for its effects on the skeleton but also because of the many extrarenal effects of parathyroid hormone in multiple organ systems. The treatment strategy to minimize the complications of hyperparathyroidism on bone is listed in **Table 1**.

Role of Phosphorus Retention

From the extensive studies of Slatopolsky and Bricker, the role of phosphorus in the pathogenesis of secondary hyperparathyroidism has been well defined.[3,4] These studies were initially interpreted to indicate that phosphorus retention led to a decrease in the levels of ionized calcium which, in turn, stimulated parathyroid hormone secretion. Validation of this concept was achieved by dietary restriction of phosphate in proportion to the

Table 1. The Principles of the Management of Renal Bone Disease. For full description, see text.

Management of Renal Bone Disease
Control serum phosphorus
Maintain serum calcium within normal limits and minimize the calcium burden
Prevent the development of parathyroid hyperplasia
Suppress secondary hyperparathyroidism
Prevent or reverse complications of treatment

reduction of GFR and showed, with this maneuver, that secondary hyperparathyroidism can be substantially ameliorated.[5] Further work has extended the understanding of the mechanisms by which phosphate retention contributes to secondary hyperparathyroidism. Thus, phosphorus has been shown to directly stimulate the secretion of PTH from the parathyroid gland,[6-8] and further study has indicated that phosphorus levels also appear to affect parathyroid cell growth.[9,10] The effects of phosphorus on parathyroid growth are extremely important and appear to occur very early in the course of renal insufficiency, within days in experimental animals, and progress thereafter.[10] The consequences of this early increase in parathyroid growth must be addressed in our treatment strategies. Thus, as illustrated in **Figure 1**, it is now clear that phosphate retention and hyperphosphatemia can directly affect PTH secretion and parathyroid growth and can also affect these two fundamental processes by a variety of indirect means, by changes in the levels of serum calcium, by altering levels of calcitriol, and by inducing resistance to parathyroid hormone at the level of the skeleton. Accordingly, in order to control parathyroid hormone secretion and parathyroid growth, it is imperative that phosphorus levels be controlled. In addition, there is now substantial evidence that phosphate retention can also contribute to metastatic calcification and has been shown to be an independent risk factor for death.[11,12] Therefore, the initial strategy for the management of the hyperparathyroidism component of renal osteodystrophy, is to control serum phosphorus. This is usually accomplished by modest dietary restriction. However, efforts

M.M. Avram (ed.), Improving Prognosis for Kidney Disorders, 125-131.

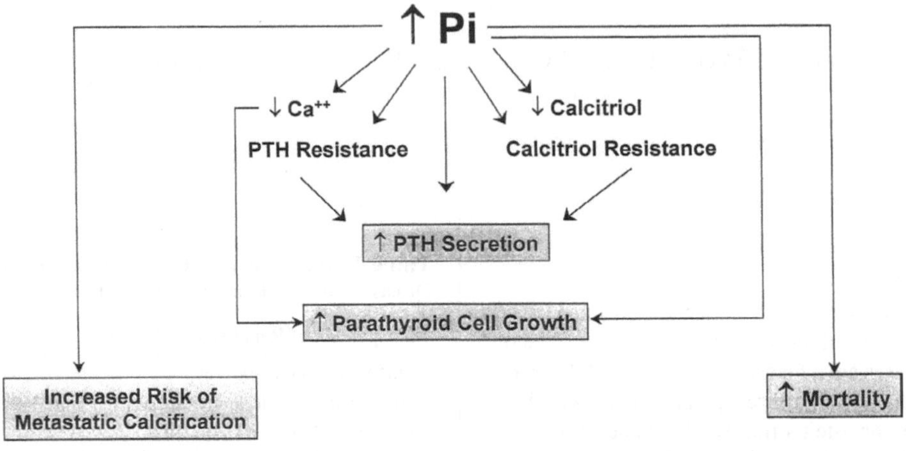

Figure 1. Diagramatic representation of the consequences of phosphate retention. Hyperphosphatemia may result in decreases in ionized calcium, resistance to PTH, decreases in calcitriol, and calcitriol resistance, which can all contribute in stimulating the secretion of parathyroid hormone. Phosphate also directly increases PTH secretion and directly and indirectly increases parathyroid cell growth. Hyperphosphatemia is also a risk factor for metastatic calcification and for mortality.

to restrict dietary phosphorus have decreased in recent years as emphasis has been placed on maintaining the protein intake in patients with renal insufficiency and it is difficult to separate phosphate from protein in the diet. Accordingly, it is necessary to use phosphate binders to prevent the absorption of phosphorus from the intestine. For the last number of years, this has been accomplished with calcium-containing salts, usually calcium carbonate and calcium acetate; and if these salts are taken with meals, satisfactory control of serum phosphorus can be achieved.[13-17] However, it is now well recognized that rather large amounts of calcium salts are necessary to achieve satisfactory control of serum phosphate if protein intake is maintained in the 1-1.2 g/kg per day which is recommended for nutritional purposes.[16] It has been emphasized in recent years that this may impose a substantial calcium burden upon the patient in that the ingestion of large amounts of calcium, some of which is absorbed in the intestine, cannot be excreted in the absence of renal function and, therefore, must accumulate in the body.[11,12] While it was initially hoped that this accumulation would be in bone, substantial concern exists now that this accumulation of calcium is in extra-skeletal sites, particularly in the blood vessels. Accordingly, in the management strategy of renal osteodystrophy, it is important to emphasize that, as efforts are undertaken to control serum phosphorus, this must be done in the context of keeping serum calcium within the normal range and with efforts to minimize the calcium burden.

Prevention of Parathyroid Hyperplasia

In order to prevent the development of hyperparathyroidism and parathyroid hyperplasia, it is obviously necessary to initiate the interventions when this process begins in the course of renal failure. There is substantial evidence in experimental animals that the process of parathyroid hyperplasia begins early in the course of chronic kidney disease,[9,10] and hyperparathyroidism is evident in patients with modest reductions in renal function (GFR < 60 ml/min);[18] and accordingly, it would be appropriate to begin interventions at this stage of renal insufficiency if the opportunity is presented. Unfortunately, however, many patients are initially seen by nephrologists with already marked decreases in renal function; and hyperparathyroidism has already been established by the time they are seen. Accordingly, at this stage of renal insufficiency, it is also necessary to undertake maneuvers to suppress existing secondary hyperparathyroidism.

Suppression of Established Hyperparathyroidism

In addition to controlling serum phosphorus, an additional treatment strategy is to replace the deficiency in calcitriol that occurs in chronic kidney disease. This maneuver has been shown to be extremely effective in the past 15 years resulting in effective suppression of the levels of parathyroid hormone.[19-21] Detailed study on the role of vitamin D in the control of parathyroid hormone secretion has revealed multiple mechanisms by which this can occur. There are a number of direct actions of calcitriol on the parathyroid glands, which include direct effects on the transcription of the PTH gene[22] and the regulation of vitamin D receptor expression in the parathyroid gland.[23] There are also direct effects of calcitriol on parathyroid cell proliferation,[9] and it has also been shown that vitamin D may regulate the expression of the calcium-sensing receptor in the parathyroid gland.[24] In some circumstances, vitamin D can alter the setpoint for calcium. All of these maneuvers can result in the direct inhibition of PTH secretion by calcitriol. In addition to these direct effects, calcitriol also affects parathyroid hormone by indirect means. Thus, it increases the intestinal absorption of serum calcium, resulting in elevations of serum calcium, which can control parathyroid hormone secretion. It has also been suggested that calcitriol can improve skeletal resistance to the calcemic action of PTH.[25] Both of these effects would tend to increase serum calcium and lead to control of hyperparathyroidism.

It is often less well recognized, however, that calcitriol, in addition to increasing the intestinal absorption of serum calcium, also increases intestinal phosphorus absorption.[26] This can counteract efforts to control hyperphosphatemia, which is a significant problem with the use of calcitriol in this context. As concern builds over extraskeletal calcifications, not only of soft tissues but in blood vessels, it becomes necessary, as we use this treatment strategy, to try to minimize the consequences of calcitriol therapy on the levels of calcium and phosphorus in the serum in order to minimize these calcification problems.

This consideration has led to the development of calcitriol analogs, which have demonstrated that it was possible to modify the calcitriol molecule, retaining the effects of calcitriol on parathyroid hormone gene expression, while at the same time, having lesser effects on elevating serum calcium and phosphorus. This strategy has been applied not only to patients with chronic renal failure but to a wide variety of disorders throughout human disease, including disorders of the skin, cancer treatment, immunosuppressive treatments, and also for osteoporosis.[27]

There are five vitamin D analogs listed in **Table 2** that are currently approved or under evaluation for the control of secondary hyperparathyroidism. Two of these are approved in the USA and include paricalcitol (19-nor-1,25-dihydroxyvitamin D_2), which is available in intravenous form, and doxercalciferol (1-α-hydroxy-vitaminD_2), which is available in both oral and parenteral form. This latter compound requires hydroxylation in the 25 position in order to become biologically active. Both of these vitamin D analogs have been applied to the treatment of patients with end stage renal disease.[28,29] 22-oxa-calcitriol and falecalcitriol[30,31] are approved and under evaluation in Asia respectively and 1-α-hydroxy-vitamin D_3 is widely used outside the United States.[32,33]

Paricalcitol was evaluated extensively in experimental renal failure and was demonstrated to be an effective inhibitor of PTH secretion with about one-third the potency of calcitriol. However, this compound was found to have one-tenth the ability of calcitriol to raise serum calcium and, importantly, one-tenth the ability of calcitriol to raise serum phosphorus.[34-36] Taken together, these data indicate that 19-nor-1,25-dihydroxyvitamin D_2 had a three-fold increase in selectivity for PTH suppression and, accordingly, was evaluated in clinical trials for patients with hyperparathyroidism in end stage renal disease. These studies revealed that 19-nor-1,25-dihydroxyvitamin D_2 could effectively decrease PTH levels in patients on hemodialysis with minimal effects on serum calcium and suggest that this analog may offer a wider therapeutic window for the use of vitamin D metabolites to control hyperparathyroidism.[28,37] The few episodes of hypercalcemia that occurred with this compound all appear to occur when PTH levels were brought to values close to 100 pg/ml of the intact PTH assay.[37] Therefore, it appears that hypercalcemia occurs as a result of overtreatment; and as experience has grown with the use of this compound, hypercalcemic episodes appear to have diminished. Longer term studies with paricalcitol have been conducted and shown that parathyroid levels can be effectively controlled in patients on hemodialysis with calcium and phosphorus levels remaining within the normal range (unpublished results). Additional clinical studies have been conducted to try to validate the selectivity suggested by the results obtained from experimental animals. Studies in patients on dialysis have shown that a dose ratio of 1:4, calcitriol to paricalcitol, appears to be equivalent in terms of controlling PTH levels in human subjects, close to the 1:3 ratio found in experimental animals.[37] Similarly, with

Table 2. The vitamin D analogs that are in use or under evaluation for the control of secondary hyperparathyroidism. 19-Nor-1,25-$(OH)_2D_3$ and 1-α-$(OH)D_2$ are both approved in the United States. 1-α-$(OH)D_3$ is widely used **outside** of the United States and 22-oxacalcitriol and 1,25-$(OH)_2$-26,27-F_6D_3 is under evaluation in Asia.

19-Nor-1,25$(OH)_2D_2$
1α-$(OH)D_2$
1α-$(OH)D_3$
22-oxa-calcitriol
1,25$(OH)_2$-26,27-F_2-D_3

regard to mobilization of calcium from bone, paricalcitol has been found in patients to have one-eighth the ability to raise serum calcium compared to calcitriol.[38] Again, these observations are similar to what had been found in experimental animals. In terms of the ability of paricalcitol to elevate serum phosphorus, studies have been presented to suggest that paricalcitol appears to be less phosphatemic than calcitriol,[39] again, confirming that the apparent selectivity observations from experimental animals can be extrapolated to human subjects.

The other vitamin D analog approved for use for the therapy of secondary hyperparathyroidism in the USA is 1-α-hydroxyvitamin D_2. As noted above, this has to undergo hydroxylation in the 25 position for biological activity and perhaps then can enter other metabolic pathways as well. The use of 1-α-hydroxyvitamin D_2 has stemmed from observations that appear to indicate that vitamin D_2 compounds appear to be somewhat less toxic than vitamin D_3 compounds in LD-50 studies in animals.[40] This decrease in toxicity appears to correlate with kidney calcium content, although it could not be demonstrated that there was a difference in intestinal calcium transport or in the ability to elevate serum calcium between 1-α-hydroxyvitamin D_2 or 1-α-hydroxyvitamin D_3.[40] While initial studies appeared to confirm the suggestion that 1-α-hydroxyvitamin D_2[41] might be less calcemic, more recent studies by the same group of investigators have shown that in terms of the ability to elevate serum calcium, to elevate serum phosphorus, and to lower levels of intact PTH in an ovariectomized rat model, 1-α-hydroxyvitamin D_2 and 1-α-hydroxyvitamin D_3 were identical.[42] Thus, at the present time, there appears to be no evidence for selectivity of 1-α-hydroxyvitamin D_2 of parathyroid hormone suppression.

Clinical trials, however, with 1-α-hydroxyvitamin D_2 in patients on hemodialysis have shown that, like other vitamin D compounds, both the oral and intravenous forms effectively suppress the levels of PTH; and under the study conditions, effects on the serum levels of calcium and phosphorus were minimal.[29] There appears to be an advantage by giving the compound intravenously in terms of lesser increases in serum calcium, lesser increases in serum phosphorus, while achieving equivalent suppression of PTH.[43] Hypercalcemic episodes, defined as greater than 10.5 mg/dL, occurred between 8 and 15 percent of determinations, with the patients on IV or oral 1-α-hydroxy-vitamin D_2, respectively. Similarly, hyperphosphatemic episodes occurred between 14 and 17 percent of measurements of IV and oral treatments, respectively.[43] Further studies will be required to compare 19-nor-1-α-dihydroxyvitamin D_2 with 1-α-hydroxyvitamin D_2 in patients to confirm the results in animals that there is an intrinsic advantage with the 19-nor conformation.

Prevention of Complications of Therapy

As these measures are undertaken to control hyperparathyroidism, it is important to prevent or reverse further complications as a result of these treatment measures. In this context, it is important not to suppress parathyroid hormone to the degree that bone turnover would be made abnormally low and contribute to adynamic renal bone disease. The pathogenesis of adynamic bone is extremely complex, as illustrated in **Figure 2**; but central to its

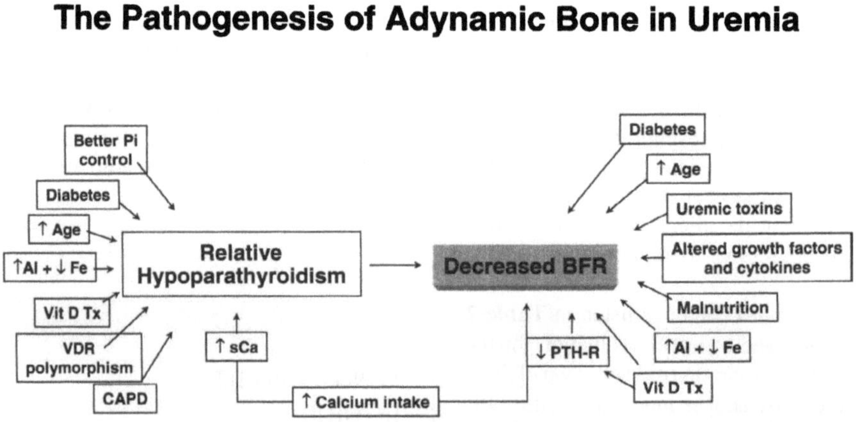

Figure 2. Diagramatic representation of the pathogenesis of adynamic bone in uremia. Many factors contribute to a relative degree of hypoparathyroidism. Similarly, there are a variety of factors in uremia that contribute to decrease bone formation rate. Thus, bone formation rate may be decreased directly by a number of factors in uremia, as well as by relative degree of hypoparathyroidism.

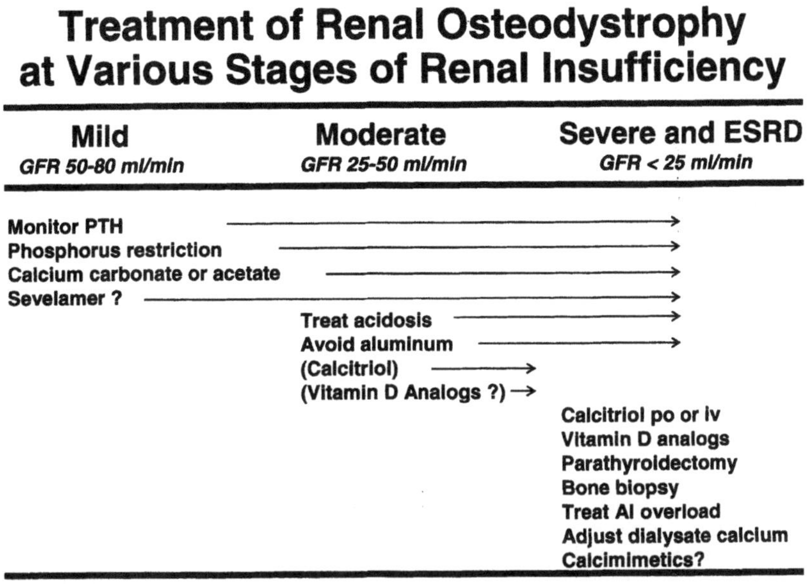

Figure 3. The treatment of renal osteodystrophy, according to the stage of renal insufficiency. For full description, see text.

pathogenesis appears to be a relative degree of hypoparathyroidism, perhaps as a result of high calcium intake or vitamin D treatment or numerous other factors.[44] At any rate, low levels of PTH undoubtedly contribute to decreased bone formation rate; and this observations raises the important issue as to what are the appropriate targets for parathyroid hormone as treatment is undertaken. Both Wang *et al.* and Quarles *et al.* have suggested that PTH levels in the 150 to 300 pg/ml range in the intact PTH assay appear to be appropriate targets to achieve and would be expected to result in normal bone formation in this patient group.[45,46] However, further studies in the current era with bone biopsy are needed to verify the appropriate target levels for PTH at the present time.

Integration of Therapeutic Strategies

In **Figure 3** are summarized the treatment strategies for renal bone disease at various stages of renal insufficiency. Based upon the evidence discussed above, it would be appropriate to begin monitoring PTH when GFR is reduced to the 50 to 80 ml/min range and if elevated, measures should be undertaken with dietary phosphorus restriction or perhaps to use calcium-containing phosphate binders at this point in time. As renal failure becomes more advanced, these measures need to be continued and intensified. If acidosis is present, it should be treated; since it is deleterious to the skeleton in terms of demineralization and in amplifying the effects of parathyroid hormone. Whether use of calcitriol or vitamin D analogs should be considered at this stage of renal function will require further study before definitive recommendations can be made. Most of the studies have been conducted in patients on dialysis with end stage renal disease, and the principles of management here include frequent monitoring of PTH, and phosphorus restriction and phosphate binders with attention to minimizing the calcium burden. There are now non-calcium-containing phosphate binders available, such as sevelamer hydrochloride, which may be a useful agent to achieve phosphate control while minimizing the calcium burden.[47] Calcitriol or vitamin D analogs may be administered to these patients for the control of hyperparathyroidism; and evidence is accumulating that these analogs can achieve the desired effects of calcitriol on the parathyroid with lesser effects on calcium and phosphorus and, therefore, appear to be poised to supplant calcitriol for this purpose.[37,43] Parathyroidectomy continues to be a satisfactory option for treatment, particularly if hyperparathyroidism is severe or if phosphate control cannot be achieved, which precludes the use of vitamin D therapy. Additional therapeutic agents, such as calcimimetic agents, which act directly on the parathyroid gland and may become a useful addition to the armamentarium to try to control hyperparathyroidism.[48]

Therefore, following decades of extensive work, we now have a clear understanding of the pathogenesis of renal bone diseases; and with an understanding of these pathogenetic factors with appropriate therapies targeted at these issues, a satisfactory control of hyperparathyroidism can be achieved. Further progress is likely to reveal new therapeutic agents that will improve our ability to deal with this problem with minimal complications.

References

1. Malluche H, Faugere MC: Renal bone disease 1990: an unmet challenge for the nephrologist. Kidney International 38:193-211, 1990
2. Sherrard DJ, Hercz G, Pei Y, Maloney NA, Greenwood C, Manuel A, Saiphoo C, Fenton SS, Segre GV: The spectrum of bone disease in end-stage renal failure--an evolving disorder. Kidney International 43:436-42, 1993
3. Slatopolsky E, Caglar S, Pennell JP, Taggart DD, Canterbury JM, Reiss E, Bricker NS: On the pathogenesis of hyperparathyroidism in chronic experimental renal insufficiency in the dog. Journal of Clinical Investigation 50:492-9, 1971
4. Slatopolsky E, Bricker NS: The role of phosphorus restriction in the prevention of secondary hyperparathyroidism in chronic renal disease. Kidney International 4:141-5, 1973
5. Rutherford WE, Bordier P, Marie P, Hruska K, Harter H, Greenwalt A, Blondin J, Haddad J, Bricker N, Slatopolsky E: Phosphate control and 25-hydroxycholecalciferol administration in preventing experimental renal osteodystrophy in the dog. Journal Of Clinical Investigation 60:332-41, 1977
6. Slatopolsky E, Finch J, Denda M, Ritter C, Zhong M, Dusso A, MacDonald PN, Brown AJ: Phosphorus restriction prevents parathyroid gland growth. High phosphorus directly stimulates PTH secretion in vitro. J Clin Invest 97:2534-40, 1996
7. Almaden Y, Canalejo A, Hernandez A, Ballesteros E, Garcia-Navarro S, Torres A, Rodriguez M: Direct effect of phosphorus on PTH secretion from whole rat parathyroid glands in vitro. Journal of Bone & Mineral Research 11:970-6, 1996
8. Almaden Y, Hernandez A, Torregrosa V, Canalejo A, Sabate L, Fernandez Cruz L, Campistol JM, Torres A, Rodriguez M: High phosphate level directly stimulates parathyroid hormone secretion and synthesis by human parathyroid tissue in vitro. Journal Of The American Society Of Nephrology 9:1845-52, 1998
9. Naveh-Many T, Rahamimov R, Livni N, Silver J: Parathyroid cell proliferation in normal and chronic renal failure rats. The effects of calcium, phosphate, and vitamin D. Journal Of Clinical Investigation 96:1786-93, 1995
10. Denda M, Finch J, Slatopolsky E: Phosphorus accelerates the development of parathyroid hyperplasia and secondary hyperparathyroidism in rats with renal failure. Am J Kidney Dis 28:596-602, 1996
11. Block GA, Port FK: Re-evaluation of risks associated with hyperphosphatemia and hyperparathyroidism in dialysis patients: recommendations for a change in management. Am J Kidney Dis 35:1226-37., 2000
12. Block GA, Hulbert-Shearon TE, Levin NW, Port FK: Association of serum phosphorus and calcium x phosphate product with mortality risk in chronic hemodialysis patients: a national study. Am J Kidney Dis 31:607-17., 1998
13. Pflanz S, Henderson IS, McElduff N, Jones MC: Calcium acetate versus calcium carbonate as phosphate-binding agents in chronic haemodialysis. Nephrol Dial Transplant 9:1121-4, 1994
14. Almirall J, Veciana L, Llibre J: Calcium acetate versus calcium carbonate for the control of serum phosphorus in hemodialysis patients. Am J Nephrol 14:192-6, 1994
15. Delmez JA, Tindira CA, Windus DW, Norwood KY, Giles KS, Nighswander TL, Slatopolsky E: Calcium acetate as a phosphorus binder in hemodialysis patients. J Am Soc Nephrol 3:96-102., 1992
16. Slatopolsky E, Weerts C, Lopez-Hilker S, Norwood K, Zink M, Windus D, Delmez J: Calcium carbonate as a phosphate binder in patients with chronic renal failure undergoing dialysis. N Engl J Med 315:157-61, 1986
17. Hercz G, Kraut JA, Andress DA, Howard N, Roberts C, Shinaberger JH, Sherrard DJ, Coburn JW: Use of calcium carbonate as a phosphate binder in dialysis patients. Mineral & Electrolyte Metabolism 12:314-9, 1986
18. Malluche H, Ritz E, Lange H: Bone histology in incipient and advanced renal failure. Kidney International 9:355-62, 1976
19. Andress DL, Norris KC, Coburn JW, Slatopolsky EA, Sherrard DJ: Intravenous calcitriol in the treatment of refractory osteitis fibrosa of chronic renal failure [see comments]. N Engl J Med 321:274-9, 1989
20. Cannella G, Bonucci E, Rolla D, Ballanti P, Moriero E, De Grandi R, Augeri C, Claudiani F, Di Maio G: Evidence of healing of secondary hyperparathyroidism in chronically hemodialyzed uremic patients treated with long-term intravenous calcitriol. Kidney International 46:1124-32, 1994
21. Slatopolsky E, Lopez-Hilker S, Delmez J, Dusso A, Brown A, Martin KJ: The parathyroid-calcitriol axis in health and chronic renal failure. Kidney Int Suppl 29:S41-7, 1990
22. Silver J, Naveh-Many T, Mayer H, Schmelzer HJ, Popovtzer MM: Regulation by vitamin D metabolites of parathyroid hormone gene transcription in vivo in the rat. Journal Of Clinical Investigation 78:1296-301, 1986
23. Naveh-Many T, Marx R, Keshet E, Pike JW, Silver J: Regulation of 1,25-dihydroxyvitamin D3 receptor gene expression by 1,25-dihydroxyvitamin D3 in the parathyroid in vivo. Journal Of Clinical Investigation 86:1968-75, 1990
24. Brown AJ, Zhong M, Finch J, Ritter C, McCracken R, Morrissey J, Slatopolsky E: Rat calcium-sensing receptor is regulated by vitamin D but not by calcium. Am J Physiol 270:F454-60, 1996
25. Massry SG, Stein R, Garty J, Arieff AI, Coburn JW, Norman AW, Friedler RM: Skeletal resistance to the calcemic action of parathyroid hormone in uremia: role of 1,25 (OH)2 D3. Kidney International 9:467-74, 1976
26. Ramirez JA, Emmett M, White MG, Fathi N, Santa Ana CA, Morawski SG, Fordtran JS: The absorption of dietary phosphorus and calcium in hemodialysis patients. Kidney Int 30:753-9., 1986
27. Brown AJ, Dusso A, Slatopolsky E: Selective vitamin D analogs and their therapeutic applications. Semin Nephrol 14:156-74, 1994
28. Martin KJ, González EA, Gellens M, Hamm LL, Abboud H, Lindberg J: 19-Nor-1-α-25-Dihydroxyvitamin D_2 (Paricalcitol) Safely and Effectively Reduces the Levels of Intact PTH in Patients on Hemodialysis. Journal of the American Society of Nephrology 10:1427-32, 1998
29. Frazao JM, Elangovan L, Maung HM, Chesney RW, Acchiardo SR, Bower JD, Kelley BJ, Rodriguez HJ, Norris KC, Robertson JA, Levine BS, Goodman WG, Gentile D, Mazess RB, Kyllo DM, Douglass LL, Bishop CW, Coburn JW: Intermittent doxercalciferol

(1alpha-hydroxyvitamin D(2)) therapy for secondary hyperparathyroidism. Am J Kidney Dis 36:550-61., 2000

30. Akiba T, Marumo F, Owada A, Kurihara S, Inoue A, Chida Y, Ando R, Shinoda T, Ishida Y, Ohashi Y: Controlled trial of falecalcitriol versus alfacalcidol in suppression of parathyroid hormone in hemodialysis patients with secondary hyperparathyroidism. American Journal of Kidney Diseases 32:238-46, 1998
31. Kurokawa K, Akizawa T, Suzuki M, Akiba T, Ogata E, Slatopolsky E: Effect of 22-oxacalcitriol on hyperparathyroidism of dialysis patients: results of a preliminary study. Nephrol Dial Transplant 11:121-4, 1996
32. Lind L, Wengle B, Wide L, Wrege U, Ljunghall S: Suppression of serum parathyroid hormone levels by intravenous alphacalcidol in uremic patients on maintenance hemodialysis. A pilot study. Nephron 48:296-9, 1988
33. Brandi L, Nielsen PK, Bro S, Daugaard H, Olgaard K: Long-term effects of intermittent oral alphacalcidol, calcium carbonate and low-calcium dialysis (1.25 mmol L-1) on secondary hyperparathyroidism in patients on continuous ambulatory peritoneal dialysis. J Intern Med 244:121-31., 1998
34. Finch JL, Brown AJ, Slatopolsky E: Differential effects of 19-nor-1,25-$(OH)_2 D_2$ on calcium and phosphate resorption in bone. J Am Soc Nephrol 8:573A, 1997
35. Slatopolsky E, Finch J, Ritter C, Denda M, Morrissey J, Brown A, DeLuca H: A new analog of calcitriol, 19-nor-1,25-$(OH)_2D_2$, suppresses parathyroid hormone secretion in uremic rats in the absence of hypercalcemia. Am J Kidney Dis 26:852-60, 1995
36. Takahashi F, Finch JL, Denda M, Dusso AS, Brown AJ, Slatopolsky E: A new analog of 1,25-(OH)2D3, 19-NOR-1,25-(OH)2D2, suppresses serum PTH and parathyroid gland growth in uremic rats without elevation of intestinal vitamin D receptor content. Am J Kidney Dis 30:105-12, 1997
37. Martin KJ, Gonzalez EA, Gellens ME, Hamm LL, Abboud H, Lindberg J: Therapy of secondary hyperparathyroidism with 19-nor-1alpha,25-dihydroxyvitamin D2. Am J Kidney Dis 32:S61-6., 1998
38. Coyne DW, Grieff M, Ahya S, Giles K, Norwood K, Slatopolsky E: Differential Potencies of 1,25$(OH)_2D_3$ and 19-Nor-1,25$(OH)_2D_2$ on Bone resorption in Hemodialysis Patients. Journal Of The American Society Of Nephrology 11:574A, 2000
39. Lerma EV, D.P. M, Ghanekar HP, Abraham M, Sprague SM, Batlle D: A Comparative Study between 19-Nor-1-alpha--25-dihydroxyvitamin D_2 and Intravenous calcitriol on PTH Suppression in Hemodialysis patients. Journal Of The American Society Of Nephrology 11:578A, 2000
40. Sjoden G, Smith C, Lindgren U, DeLuca HF: 1 alpha-Hydroxyvitamin D2 is less toxic than 1 alpha-hydroxyvitamin D3 in the rat. Proc Soc Exp Biol Med 178:432-6., 1985
41. Erben RG, Bante U, Birner H, Stangassinger M: 1alpha-hydroxyvitamin D2 partially dissociates between preservation of cancellous bone mass and effects on calcium homeostasis in ovariectomized rats. Calcif Tissue Int 60:449-56., 1997
42. Weber K, Goldberg M, Stangassinger M, Erben RG: 1alpha-hydroxyvitamin D2 is less toxic but not bone selective relative to 1alpha-hydroxyvitamin D3 in ovariectomized rats. J Bone Miner Res 16:639-51., 2001
43. Maung HM, Elangovan L, Frazao JM, Bower JD, Kelley BJ, Acchiardo SR, Rodriguez HJ, Norris KC, Sigala JF, Rutkowski M, Robertson JA, Goodman WG, Levine BS, Chesney RW, Mazess RB, Kyllo DM, Douglass LL, Bishop CW, Coburn JW: Efficacy and side effects of intermittent intravenous and oral doxercalciferol (1alpha-hydroxyvitamin D(2)) in dialysis patients with secondary hyperparathyroidism: a sequential comparison. Am J Kidney Dis 37:532-43., 2001
44. Couttenye MM, D'Haese PC, Verschoren WJ, Behets GJ, Schrooten I, De Broe ME: Low bone turnover in patients with renal failure. Kidney Int Suppl 73:S70-6., 1999
45. Wang M, Hercz G, Sherrard DJ, Maloney NA, Segre GV, Pei Y: Relationship between intact 1-84 parathyroid hormone and bone histomorphometric parameters in dialysis patients without aluminum toxicity. American Journal of Kidney Diseases 26:836-44, 1995
46. Quarles LD, Lobaugh B, Murphy G: Intact parathyroid hormone overestimates the presence and severity of parathyroid-mediated osseous abnormalities in uremia. Journal of Clinical Endocrinology & Metabolism 75:145-50, 1992
47. Chertow GM, Burke SK, Dillon MA, Slatopolsky E: Long-term effects of sevelamer hydrochloride on the calcium x phosphate product and lipid profile of haemodialysis patients [In Process Citation]. Nephrol Dial Transplant 15:559, 2000
48. Goodman WG, Frazao JM, Goodkin DA, Turner SA, Liu W, Coburn JW: A calcimimetic agent lowers plasma parathyroid hormone levels in patients with secondary hyperparathyroidism. Kidney Int 58:436-45., 2000

Index

O

P

R

T

U

V

MIX
Papier aus verantwortungsvollen Quellen
Paper from responsible sources
FSC® C105338

If you have any concerns about our products,
you can contact us on
ProductSafety@springernature.com

In case Publisher is established outside the EU,
the EU authorized representative is:
Springer Nature Customer Service Center GmbH
Europaplatz 3, 69115 Heidelberg, Germany

Printed by Libri Plureos GmbH
in Hamburg, Germany